ADVANCES IN
Pediatrics

Editor-in-Chief
Carol D. Berkowitz, MD, FAAP, FACEP

Division of General Pediatrics,
Department of Pediatrics,
Harbor-UCLA Medical Center,
Distinguished Professor of Pediatrics,
David Geffen School of Medicine at UCLA,
Torrance, California, USA

ELSEVIER

PHILADELPHIA   LONDON   TORONTO   MONTREAL   SYDNEY   TOKYO

ADVANCES IN
Pediatrics

VOLUMES 1 THROUGH 70 (OUT OF PRINT)

VOLUME 71

Editor: Kerry Holland
Developmental Editor: Malvika Shah

Reprints: For copies of 100 or more of articles in this publication, please contact the Commercial Reprints Department, Elsevier Inc., 1600 John F. Kennedy Boulevard, Suite 1600, Philadelphia, PA 1910, United States E-mail: reprints@elsevier.com.

Printed by Sheridan at 450 Fame Avenue, Hanover, PA 17331.

Publishing Office:
Elsevier Inc.
1600 John F. Kennedy Boulevard,
Suite 1600
Philadelphia, PA 19103
United States

International Standard Serial Number: 0065-3101
International Standard Book Number: 13: 978-0-443-34455-8

ADVANCES IN
Pediatrics

Editor-in-Chief

CAROL D. BERKOWITZ, MD, FAAP, FACEP, Chief, Division of General Pediatrics, Department of Pediatrics, Harbor-UCLA Medical Center, Distinguished Professor of Pediatrics, David Geffen School of Medicine at UCLA, Torrance, California

Associate Editors

JANE D. CARVER, PhD, MS, Professor Emeritus, Adjunct Professor, Department of Pediatrics, University of South Florida Morsani College of Medicine, Tampa, Florida

RONALD BRUCE HIRSCHL, MD, Arnold G. Coran Collegiate Professor of Pediatric Surgery, University of Michigan School of Medicine, Ann Arbor, Michigan

CHARLOTTE W. LEWIS MD, MPH, Professor, Department of Pediatrics, Division of General Pediatrics, University of Washington School of Medicine, Seattle, Washington

SURENDRA VARMA, MD, DSc (Hon), FAAP, FACE, FRCP(London), Grover E. Murray Professor, Ted Hartman Endowed Chair in Medical Education, Executive Associate Dean for GME & Resident Affairs, University Distinguished Professor & Vice-Chair, Pediatrics, Texas Tech University Health Sciences Center, School of Medicine, Lubbock, Texas

CONTRIBUTORS

WALID ABUHAMMOUR, MD, MBA, FAAP, FIDSA, Clinical Professor, Mohammad Bin Rashid University, Dubai, United Arab Emirates; Honorary Professor, The Jordan University- School of Medicine, Amman, Jordan; Department of Pediatric Infectious Diseases, Al Jalila Children's Hospital (AJCH), Dubai, United Arab Emirates

AMBIKA P. ASHRAF, MD, FNLA, Professor, Department of Pediatrics, The University of Alabama at Birmingham, Birmingham, Alabama, USA

NIDHI BANSAL, MD, MPH, Associate Professor, Division of Diabetes and Endocrinology, Department of Pediatrics, Baylor College of Medicine, Texas Children's Hospital, Houston, Texas, USA

JAVIER BENITO-FERNÁNDEZ, MD, PhD, Pediatric Emergency Department, Cruces University Hospital, Barakaldo, Bizkaia, Spain

JENNIFER BLASE, MD, PhD, Clinical Assistant Professor of Pediatrics and Pediatric Hematology-Oncology, C.S. Mott Children's Hospital, University of Michigan, Ann Arbor, Michigan, USA

IVANA BRAJKOVIC, MD, MPH, Clinical Assistant Professor, Division of Neonatology, Department of Pediatrics, Seattle Children's Hospital, University of Washington, Seattle, Washington, USA

DANIELLE CAMERON, MD, MPH, Assistant Professor of Surgery, Harvard Medical School Division of Pediatric Surgery, Mass General for Children, Department of Surgery, Mass General Brigham, Boston, Massachusetts, USA

ENITAN D. CARROL, MD, Professor of Paediatric Infection, Department of Clinical Infection, Microbiology and Immunology, University of Liverpool Institute of Infection, Veterinary and Ecological Sciences, Liverpool, United Kingdom

ISMAEL CORRAL, MD, MBA, Pediatric Cardiologist, Department of Pediatrics, Los Angeles County Department of Health Services, Harbor-UCLA Medical Center, Torrance, California, USA; Pediatric Cardiologist, Department of Pediatrics, Los Angeles County Department of Health Services, Olive View-UCLA Medical Center, Sylmar, California, USA

MEGHAN CRAVEN, MD, Assistant Professor, Division of Diabetes and Endocrinology, Department of Pediatrics, Baylor College of Medicine, Texas Children's Hospital, Houston, Texas, USA

KAYA CZYZ, BS, BA, Research Assistant, Institute on Inequalities in Global Health, University of Southern California, Los Angeles, Los Angeles, California, USA

BIREN J. DESAI, DO, FAAP, Fellow, Department of Pediatrics, University of Washington, Division of Gastroenterology, Hepatology, and Nutrition, Seattle Children's Hospital, Seattle, Washington, USA

PETER F. EHRLICH, MD, MSc, Pediatric Surgeon, Section of Pediatric Surgery, CS Mott Children's Hospital, University of Michigan, Ann Arbor, Michigan, USA

KAREN FUGATE, MSN RNC-NIC, CPHQ, LSSBB-C, Performance Improvement Supervisor, Department of Performance Improvement, Tampa General Hospital, Tampa, Florida, USA

KARYN GERSTLE, MD, MPH, IBCLC, Assistant Professor, Department of Pediatrics, University of South Florida, Tampa, Florida, USA

ALAIN GERVAIX, MD, Professor, Departments of Gynecology and Obstetric, Director, Department of Pediatrics, Geneva University Hospitals, University of Geneva, Children's Hospital, HUG, Geneva, Switzerland

CHERYL GODCHARLES, MD, NABBLM-C, IBCLC, Assistant Professor, Department of Obstetrics and Gynecology, University of South Florida, Tampa, Florida, USA

CHRISTÈLE GRAS-LE GUEN, MD, PhD, Professor of Medicine, Pediatric Emergency Department, Hôpital Mère – Enfant, CHU Nantes, Nantes, France

SOFIA GRUSKIN, JD, MIA, Distinguished Professor and Director, Institute on Inequalities in Global Health, University of California, Los Angeles, Los Angeles, California, USA

ROHAN K. HENRY, MD, MS, Associate Professor, Section of Endocrinology and Diabetes, Department of Pediatrics, Nationwide Children's Hospital, The Ohio State University College of Medicine, Columbus, Ohio, USA

BENJAMIN HOLLAND, BS, Student, Department of Pediatrics, Indiana University School of Medicine, Indianapolis, Indiana, USA

GRACE K. KIM, MD, Assistant Professor, Division of Diabetes and Endocrinology, Department of Pediatrics, Baylor College of Medicine, Texas Children's Hospital, Houston, Texas, USA

SERGEY KUNKOV, MD, MS, MBA, Professor and Chair, Department of Pediatrics, Texas Tech University Health Sciences Center, Lubbock, Texas, USA

JENNIFER M. LADD, MD, MSc, Assistant Professor, Section of Endocrinology and Diabetes, Department of Pediatrics, Nationwide Children's Hospital, The Ohio State University College of Medicine, Columbus, Ohio, USA

MEGAN LANGILLE, MD, Associate Clinical Professor of Pediatrics, David Geffen School of Medicine at UCLA, Torrance, California, USA

BEATRIZ FABIOLA MARIN RUIZ, MD, Assistant Professor, Division of Pediatric Nephrology, Department of Pediatrics, University of South Florida, Tampa, Florida, USA

JENNIFER MARKWOOD, DO, MPH, Resident Physician, Department of Pediatrics, University of South Florida, Tampa, Florida, USA

KELLY McGEE, MD, Resident Physician, Department of Pediatrics, University of South Florida, Tampa, Florida, USA

DEVIN McKISSIC, MD, Clinical Assistant Professor, Division of Neonatology, Department of Pediatrics, Seattle Children's Hospital, University of Washington, Seattle, Washington, USA

ROBERT H. PANTELL, MD, Professor, Department of Pediatrics, University of California San Francisco School of Medicine, San Francisco, California, USA

NICCOLÒ PARRI, MD, Pediatric Emergency Physician, Meyer Children's Hospital IRCCS, Florence, Italy

CHERLYN ANGELA PEREZ-CORRAL, MD, MPP, Hospitalist, Department of Medicine, Los Angeles County Department of Health Services, Harbor-UCLA Medical Center, Torrance, California, USA

ASHLEY PERRY, MD, Quality Improvement and Patient Safety Fellow, Department of Graduate Medical Education, University of South Florida, Tampa, Florida, USA

HANNIBAL PERSON, MD, FAAP, Assistant Professor, Department of Pediatrics, University of Washington, Division of Gastroenterology, Hepatology, and Nutrition, Seattle Children's Hospital, Seattle, Washington, USA

SABITHA SASIDHARAN PILLAI, MD, Clinical Assistant Professor, Department of Pediatrics, Keck School of Medicine, University of Southern California, Los Angeles, Center for Endocrinology, Diabetes and Metabolism, Children's Hospital Los Angeles, Los Angeles, California, USA

ANDREW C. SAYCE, MD, DPhil, Resident, Department of Surgery, University of Pittsburgh Medical Center, Pittsburgh, Pennsylvania, USA

STEFAN SCHOLZ, MD, PhD, FACS, Assistant Professor, Division of Pediatric General and Thoracic Surgery, UPMC Children's Hospital, University of Pittsburgh, Pittsburgh, Pennsylvania, USA

ALEJANDRO F. SILLER, MD, MSCI, Assistant Professor, Division of Diabetes and Endocrinology, Department of Pediatrics, Baylor College of Medicine, Texas Children's Hospital, Houston, Texas, USA

SHAILA SIRAJ, MD, Assistant Professor, Department of Pediatrics, Johns Hopkins All Children's Hospital, St Petersburg, Florida, USA

CARA L. SLAGLE, MD, Associate Professor, Division of Neonatology, Department of Pediatrics, Indiana University School of Medicine, Indianapolis, Indiana, USA

MICHELLE C. STARR, MD, MPH, Assistant Professor, Division of Nephrology, Department of Pediatrics, Division of Child Health Service Research, Department of Pediatrics, Indiana University School of Medicine, Indianapolis, Indiana, USA

DOROTHY STEARNS, MD, MPH, Postdoctoral Fellow, Institute for Firearm Injury Prevention, University of Michigan, Ann Arbor, Michigan, USA

ALYSSA STETSON, MD, MPH, Research Fellow, Division of Pediatric Surgery, Mass General for Children, Department of Surgery, Mass General Brigham, Boston, Massachusetts, USA; General Surgery Resident, University of Cincinnati, Cincinnati, Ohio, USA

CHRISTINE TABULOV, PharmD, Assistant Professor, Department of Pharmacotherapeutics and Clinical Research, University of South Florida Taneja College of Pharmacy, Tampa, Florida, USA

CHRISTOPHER B. WELDON, MD, PhD, Associate Professor of Surgery, Harvard Medical School, Senior Surgeons' Chair and Associate in Surgery and Anesthesia (Critical Care), Boston Children's Hospital, Affiliate Member, Dana-Farber Cancer Institute, Boston, Massachusetts, USA

ALYSSA WOODARD, MD, CLC, Assistant Professor, Department of Pediatrics, University of South Florida, Tampa, Florida, USA

ADVANCES IN
Pediatrics

CONTENTS VOLUME 72 • 2025

Attention to the interdependence of health and human rights has increasingly been recognized as vaualble to efforts to improve child health. Through application of a health and human rights analysis to two case examples, we hope to shed light on a valuable framework for use by health professionals with relevance to myriad health topics. This review briefly assesses relevant literature, defines key concepts, provides two examples of real-world application to children's sexual and reproductive health and rights, and concludes with a discussion on how a rights-based approach can be used in practice by child health professionals to support the rights and health of the children they work with.

Progress in Pediatric Firearm Research in the Last 5 years

Dorothy Stearns and Peter F. Ehrlich

Firearm injury has overtaken motor vehicle collision as the leading cause of death in children and young adults. To address this public health crisis, a comprehensive understanding of the problem is required. The purpose of this article is to highlight concepts that can help prevent and treat children affected by firearm violence.

Procalcitonin in Pediatric Emergency Medicine

Niccolò Parri, Robert H. Pantell, Enitan D. Carrol, Walid Abuhammour, Javier Benito-Fernández, Christèle Gras-Le Guen, and Alain Gervaix

Procalcitonin (PCT) has been increasingly evaluated as a biomarker in clinical situations where it is important to distinguish bacterial infection from viral and other inflammatory conditions. When added to other clinical and laboratory markers, PCT has comparably high sensitivity but markedly better specificity for detecting invasive bacterial infections in febrile young infants than decision algorithms not including PCT. For febrile infants, evidence shows PCT reduces unnecesary lumbar punctures (LPs), hospitalizations, and antibiotic use. PCT has also been documented to accurately distinguish between acute pyelonephritis and cystitis. Implementation strategies have succeeded in incorporating PCT into clinical care.

Seizures and Shaking in Newborns and Babies 41
Megan Langille

Babies and small children can make movements that look like seizures but are nonpileptic and call only for reassurance. Features more suggestive of seizure are vital sign changes, stereotyped, occur across different setting/situations, involve head/eye movement, cannot be stopped with repositioning, and are not stimulus induced/trigger. If a child's medical history is positive for risk factors for seizures, then further work up may be necessary. Risk factors include birth history concerning perinatal hypoxic-ischemic encephalopathy/prematurity/neonatal intensive care unit stay, genetic condition/diagnosis, developmental delay, and prior seizures. Electroencephalography and imaging may be necessary when seizure disorder is suspected and can clarify diagnosis.

The Ouchless Pediatric Emergency Department 57
Sergey Kunkov

The article "The Ouchless Pediatric Emergency Department" describes a comprehensive approach to reducing pain and anxiety in pediatric emergency care. By combining nonpharmacologic methods (eg, distraction and cognitive-behavioral techniques), pharmacologic interventions (eg, topical anesthetics and sedation), and environmental changes (eg, sensory-friendly spaces), this model can turn a pediatric emergency department into a compassionate care setting. Parental involvement and child life specialists can further support children through emotional reassurance, reducing the need for sedation and improving cooperation. This "ouchless" model aims to enhance patient and family satisfaction, promote positive health care experiences, and establish a new standard in pediatric emergency medicine.

Vascular and Gastrointestinal Access in Children 69
Andrew C. Sayce and Stefan Scholz

The concept of vascular and enteral access is a core component of modern pediatric care. Administration of appropriate fluid, nutrition, and medication depends upon reliable delivery. As such, an understanding of techniques for obtaining reliable vascular and enteral access is essential for delivery of patient care. Pediatric patients present unique challenges due to their smaller anatomy and the need for long-term nutritional strategies in certain conditions. This review details considerations for decision-making regarding means of access and the technical considerations required for establishing and maintaining vascular and enteral access. We focus on practical application to the pediatric patient.

Pediatric Lymphadenopathy 93
Danielle Cameron, Alyssa Stetson, Jennifer Blase, and Christopher B. Weldon

Lymphadenopathy (LAD) is common in children, and often nonpathologic, but requires a thorough evaluation with a detailed history and physical before being designated as "benign idiopathic." Cervical LAD is the most common location in children. History should focus on patient and lymph node characteristics and patient exposures, while physical should include characteristics of the lesion, evaluation of the region, and systemic findings. Based on these findings, a differential can be generated, which includes infectious, malignant, immunologic, or iatrogenic etiologies. Options for further testing include imaging (most often with ultrasound and/or chest radiograph), laboratory markers, and biopsy in rare instances.

Quality Improvement in Pediatrics 103
Ashley Perry and Shaila Siraj

Quality improvement has been successful in improving patient safety and the value of care that is provided to patients. Continued provider involvement in quality improvement activities is necessary to continue to advance patient care. This article provides clinicians with basic tools to start to build a foundation in quality improvement methodologies. Overall, a quality improvement initiative should outline the problem, aim, scope, change ideas, and measures. Further work remains to address barriers to implementation of quality improvement, improve education on quality improvement during training, and use quality improvement to promote health equity.

Helping Support Our Families Reach Their Breastfeeding Goals: Innovative Skill-Based Breastfeeding Education for Pediatric Residents 115
Jennifer Markwood, Karen Fugate, Alyssa Woodard, Cheryl Godcharles, and Karyn Gerstle

General pediatricians have a unique role in supporting breastfeeding goals of families due to the frequency of well visits and weight checks during the first few weeks of life. Many interventions to improve breastfeeding longevity such as the "baby friendly" initiatives have focused primarily on hospital policies, with special attention given to the immediate postpartum period. While this is a crucial time to support the mother/infant dyad, most dyads do not encounter many common challenges to breastfeeding until after hospital discharge. This article outlines the current state of pediatric resident competency in supporting a family's breastfeeding goals.

Neonatal Resuscitation Program: Then and Now   131
Devin McKissic and Ivana Brajkovic

This article begins by reviewing the history of the Neonatal Resuscitation Program (NRP), including the rationale for its inception, and how NRP has evolved over time. It reviews the basic tenets of NRP and then summarizes the important changes and revisions to the program over time. It concludes with a review of how select technologies are currently being studied and utilized in NRP education and practice.

Renal Physiology: From Fetus to Newborn and Beyond   143
Benjamin Holland, Cara L. Slagle, and Michelle C. Starr

Developmental renal physiology concepts can best be divided into prenatal, perinatal, and postnatal periods. Structural kidney development and a maximum number of nephron formations predominate the prenatal period with kidney function playing a primary role in amniotic fluid production. Kidney function reaches near-adult maturation around 2 y of age, with variation depending on gestational age at birth and neonatal complications. Neonatal kidneys are particularly sensitive to injury, which impacts both short- and long-term health outcomes. A greater understanding of developmental renal physiology facilitates increased awareness of kidney health, thus improving overall care.

Neonatal Endocrine Emergencies   157
Grace K. Kim, Alejandro F. Siller, Meghan Craven, and Nidhi Bansal

Neonatal endocrine emergencies may be associated with high morbidity and mortality. Recognizing subtle clinical features of neonatal endocrine emergencies is important for early diagnosis and acute stabilization and treatment. This article reviews the presentation, evaluation, and initial management of common neonatal endocrine emergencies.

Ethical Issues in Pediatric Endocrinology: A Primer for the Practitioner   171

Jennifer M. Ladd and Rohan K. Henry

With technologic advancements and the use of existing therapeutic modalities to treat new patient populations, practitioners of pediatric endocrinology may face ethical dilemmas in providing care. The 4 ethical pillars of clinical practice are outlined in this review and serve as the basis for discourse surrounding 5 broad categories of clinical care, which pediatric endocrinology practitioners may encounter.

Artificial Intelligence in Pediatric Endocrinology   185

Sabitha Sasidharan Pillai and Ambika P. Ashraf

The rapid technological progress over the last couple of decades has paved the way for innovative methods capable of solving scientific questions at a rate far exceeding human capabilities. One prime example is the field of artificial intelligence (AI). AI comprises several technologies, such as machine learning, deep learning, natural language processing, robotics, speech processing, and other automation technologies. A human-in-the-loop approach makes sure that the AI systems are guided, communicated, and supervised by human expertise while the AI technology complements and enhances the skills of clinicians resulting in improved safety and quality of health care services and patient outcomes.

Pharmacology in Pediatric Renal Solid Organ Transplantation 197

Christine Tabulov, Kelly McGee, and
Beatriz Fabiola Marin Ruiz

In pediatric renal transplantation, managing immunosuppression is critical to prevent graft rejection while also reducing the risks of infection, cancer, and medication side effects. This review covers both induction and maintenance immunosuppression agents. Pediatric patients face unique challenges due to their continuous growth and development, requiring careful dosing adjustments and comprehensive education for both patients and caregivers. Collaboration among multidisciplinary professionals is essential to enhance patient outcomes and ensure long-term graft survival in this particularly at-risk population.

A Practical Approach to Functional Abdominal Pain and Irritable Bowel Syndrome in Children and Adolescents   219

Biren J. Desai and Hannibal Person

Disorders of gut-brain interaction (DGBI) are conditions contributing to chronic gastrointestinal symptoms related to alterations in normal gut physiology and sensation. They are encountered frequently in pediatric health care settings and require thoughtful conversation between providers and patients as the diagnosis is confidently made and treatments are initiated. Diagnostic testing should be limited to those patients who are experiencing what is known as alarm symptoms, which suggest an alternate etiology. When choosing treatment options, there should be an emphasis on preventing iatrogenic harm from overmedicalization as well as adverse drug side effects. Patients can often be successfully managed by general practitioners; however, select patients may benefit from referral to specialty services, including gastroenterology (GI), GI psychology, and pain medicine.

A Review of Wolff-Parkinson-White for the General Practitioner 235

Ismael Corral and Cherlyn Angela Perez-Corral

Wolff-Parkinson-White (WPW) syndrome was first described nearly a century ago and has been found to have a relatively high prevalence within the general population. The risk of sudden cardiac death due to a high-risk accessory pathway in pediatrics is substantially higher than in adults necessitating further risk stratification to identify and treat these high-risk patients. It is of upmost importance for the general practitioner to be able to identify patients with WPW, which is often diagnosed incidentally, and refer to a cardiologist for further evaluation.

ADVANCES IN PEDIATRICS

PREFACE

Two Steps Forward—One Step Back: Keeping Pace with Advances

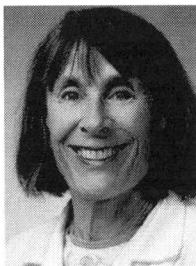

Carol D. Berkowitz, MD, FAAP, FACEP
Editor

T he medical community continues to confront challenges that raise concerns about what setbacks we may experience and about what advances we can sustain as we navigate an unpredictable health care environment. In many areas of medicine, there continue to be improvements in the management of diseases and new methods to better treat patients and to educate physicians and the public alike about this progress. None of us can become an expert in all domains of medicine yet we have an obligation to be knowledgeable about new ideas and advances as we care for our patients.

Foremost in many current discussions is to explore how to address the gaps in health care. Czyz and Gruskin introduce the intersection between health and human rights, focusing on the issue of sexual and reproductive rights, a topic not without controversy. Equally controversial is addressing the role of firearms as a leading cause of pediatric mortality. In 2020, firearms injury surpassed motor vehicle collisions as the number one cause of traumatic death in children. While there has been a lack of funded research in this area, more information has become available over the past 5 years, and there is value to using real-time data from emergency departments to craft more comprehensive interventions, as described by Stearns and Ehrlich.

Emergency departments are the sight of preliminary assessments of numerous serious illnesses, and the challenge is to define a valid and efficient

https://doi.org/10.1016/j.yapd.2025.04.001
0065-3101/25/© 2025 Published by Elsevier Inc.

way to make such an assessment. Pantell and his team focus on the value of procalcitonin, especially in helping to recognize bacterial infections, especially UTIs, and in reducing the unnecessary use of antibiotics. It is harder to diagnose and determine the cause of various motor movements in newborns and young infants. Langille describes the risk factors and features that help distinguish seizures from other movements and details the appropriate workup.

Kunkov advocate for an emergency department that is *ouchless*–"no pain, children gain," a notion introduced in 1997 by Dr Neil Schecter and colleagues. There are multiple modalities to consider, both pharmacologic and nonpharmacologic, including cognitive behavioral therapy.

Gaining either vascular or gastrointestinal access is described in detail by Sayce and Scholz. Many medical providers may only consider the issues of intravenous access for acute and limited conditions, but there are many circumstances in which more permanent vascular lines, or long-term direct gastrointestinal access, are needed to minimize the need for repeated intervention. Surgeons are helpful in securing such access. Surgeons often are also involved in the evaluation of lymphadenopathy. As Cameron and colleagues note, while lymphadenopathy is frequently infectious, and responds to antibiotics, there are features and location of the node or nodes that suggest the need for a biopsy and/or other treatments, including surgical excisions.

An overarching principle in all these updates is the emphasis on study, measurement, and improvement. Perry and Siraj describe how quality-improvement efforts can inform the safety and well-being of patients and promote health equity. Markwood and colleagues illustrate quality improvement with their innovative approach to augment breast-feeding skills for residents and pediatricians, thus assisting mothers to breast-feed their infants. McKissic and Brajkovic detail the evolution of neonatal resuscitation in "Neonatal Resuscitation Program Then and Now" and document how this life-saving course has saved thousands of infants around the world–"Helping Babies Breathe."

Neonatology continues to be in the forefront of advances in knowledge and interventions. Holland and team provide a better understanding of neonatal physiology and thereby help promote ways to reduce kidney injury. Kim and colleagues address neonatal endocrine emergencies, with a measurable reduction in endocrine-associated morbidity and mortality. New medications and treatments create new dilemmas and new ethical issues, especially in endocrinology. These issues are well detailed and articulated by Ladd and Henry, who include discussions of neurologically devastated youth, transgender individuals, diabetes, and obesity.

Use of artificial intelligence (AI), a term coined by John McCarthy, a computer and cognitive scientist in 1955, has permeated the medical scene at many levels, including endocrinology, as detailed by Pillai and Ashraf. AI has been helpful in improving determination of bone age and facial recognition of Turner syndrome.

Last, there are new methodologies and treatments in a number of other chronic conditions, including therapies to ensure the success of renal transplants, as discussed by Tabulov, McGee, and Ruiz. More common conditions, functional abdominal pain and irritable bowel syndrome, are seen frequently by primary care pediatricians. These disorders are now termed DGBI, Disorders of Gut-Brain Interaction, and Desai and Person clarify the biopsychosocial model to approach these disorders. Accuracy in recognizing and diagnosing WPW (Wolf-Parkinson-White) syndromes can prevent sudden cardiac deaths in children and teens. Corral and Perez-Corral present new information on risk stratification and treatment modalities.

Once again, we face challenges, controversies, and distractions. Our *North Star* remains our patients and what is in their best interest, be it injury preventions, dealing with emergencies, or early recognition and treatment of chronic disorders—a lot going and a lot to digest.

Disclosures

The author has no conflicts of interest to disclose.

Carol D. Berkowitz, MD, FAAP, FACEP
Division of General Pediatrics
Department of Pediatrics
Harbor–UCLA Medical Center
David Geffen School of Medicine at UCLA
1000 West Carson Street
Torrance, CA 90509, USA

E-mail address: Cberkowitz52@gmail.com

Advances in Pediatrics 72 (2025) 1–13

ADVANCES IN PEDIATRICS

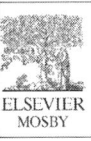

Bridging the Gap
Engaging the Health and Human Rights Paradigm to Support Children's Health in the United States

Kaya Czyz, BS, BA, Sofia Gruskin, JD, MIA*

Institute on Inequalities in Global Health, University of Southern California, Los Angeles, CA 90032, USA

Keywords
- Adolescents • Health care professionals • Health disparities • Human rights
- Sexual and reproductive health

Key points

- Attention to the rights of children is well correlated to result in benefits to their health.
- Despite interest in application of the health and human rights paradigm to child health, definitions, tools, and approaches to implementation are not yet well-known.
- Violations of children's human rights are on the rise, most dramatically in relation to their sexual and reproductive health and rights.
- Human rights methods and standards can be used concretely by health professionals to support the rights and health of the children they work with.

INTRODUCTION
Prioritizing the health and human rights of children

The right to the highest attainable standard of health is critical to both the underlying determinants of child health and to how services can optimally be delivered. Additionally, the health of children requires attention to a range of other rights, including nondiscrimination, participation, education, and

*Corresponding author. 1845 N. Soto Street, SSB 318J MC, Los Angeles, CA. *E-mail address:* gruskin@usc.edu

https://doi.org/10.1016/j.yapd.2024.12.004
0065-3101/25/

Abbreviations

3AQ	available, accessible, acceptable and quality
CRC	Convention on the Rights of the Child
CSE	comprehensive sexuality education
ECPCP	European Confederation of Primary Care Pediatricians
NSES	National Sex Education Standard
RBA	rights-based approach
SRH	sexual and reproductive health
SRHR	sexual and reproductive health and rights
STI	sexually transmitted infection
UNEPSA	Union of National European Pediatric Societies and Associations
WHO	World Health Organization

information [1]. Health care professionals working with children, defined by the Convention on the Rights of the Child (CRC) as all individuals under the age of 18, should rightly be concerned with children's access to, preference for, and motivation to use critical services as well as their representation within relevant health care settings [2]. Children benefit most when health professionals recognize them as rights holders on their own behalf. In drawing on the CRC, health professionals have the opportunity not only to use legal and normative standards to address the health of children, but also to explicitly consider rights in the approach taken to delivery of care, as well as the larger economic, social, cultural, and political environment that impact children's representation and health and well-being [1–4].

While prior human rights treaties placed no emphasis on age, the 1989 CRC provides a common ethical and legal framework for the realization of children's rights, formally recognizing the rights of children, prioritizing nondiscrimination, participation, health and well-being, and the child's best interests [2]. Legally binding now in all countries except for the United States, it has been effectively used by the child health community in multiple ways to assess and address relevant child health concerns with a particular focus on child survival and development, including within the larger economic and social environment with the implications for advocacy, policy, and programming [5].

Emphasizing human rights as beneficial to health

Public health professionals have only in the last few decades recognized the genuine value of the health and human rights paradigm to improve health outcomes for children [6]. Much of this recognition is due to empirical work which has shown that health and well-being are greatly impacted by the extent to which individuals and populations, including children, live in an enabling legal and policy environment, have the ability to participate in decisions that affect their health, have access to needed health and social services, and do not face stigma and discrimination.

With the increase in flagrant human rights violations in recent years that impact health and well-being, the need for providers to ensure attention to human rights has never been greater—in particular, the ways in which attention to the links between health and human rights can be important not only for analysis, but also for actions to positively impact health outcomes [6].

Integrating human rights standards in health

Health is often described as a state of complete physical, mental, and social well-being; while human rights as what governments and institutions of power can do to us, cannot do to us, and should do for us. The concepts of health and of human rights continue evolving independently and synergistically, as they are interconnected by their capacities to define, shape, and advance human well-being [7]. The relationship between health and human rights is bi-directional, with health policies and programs having the potential to both positively or negatively impact human rights—where, for example, the bans on any and all aspects of gender-affirming care which now exist in 25 US states can be seen to varying degrees to violate both the rights and health of children in need of these services, as compared with those states which recognize the right to access these services for those who experience gender dysphoria [8,9]. Second, and conversely, the promotions or violations of human rights have deep impacts on health. Access to comprehensive sexuality education (CSE) is a globally recognized right with huge impacts on health throughout the life course, including associations with higher contraceptive use, lower risk sexual activities, fewer unintended pregnancies, and healthy sexuality throughout the life course [10,11]. Within the United States, however, this right is not recognized at the federal level, and while sex education exists to varying degrees in a number of states, 45 states are silent on the matter, with documented egregious examples of misinformation and disinformation rampant. Only 5 states have laws requiring CSE, and of these only 3 require CSE to be taught in all schools, all with impacts on the health of children more broadly [12].

Our focus in this review is on sexual and reproductive health and rights (SRHR), even as myriad areas of child health could be used to illustrate the value of the health and human rights nexus. We do this because of the urgency driven by the increased assaults on SRHR, particularly for those who are under 18, increasingly happening in our country, all with significant impacts on health and well-being [13]. We envision this review bridging the application of human rights concepts and methods to children's health, particularly their sexual and reproductive health [14].

Below, Table 1 (Key Concepts and Definitions) offers definitions and key concepts to orient the reader, the text that follows offers concrete examples of these concepts as applicable to 2 case examples, and the discussion concludes with application of rights to health in practice.

APPLICATION TO CONCRETE EXAMPLES

The 2 examples later, access to sexual and reproductive health services and CSE, are used as the illustrations of issues where considering both health and rights can raise key and complementary issues to be considered in

Table 1
Key concepts and definitions

Key concepts	Definitions
Children	As per the United Nations Convention on the Rights of the Child, a child is every human being below the age of 18 years unless under the law applicable to the child, majority is attained earlier [2].
Human rights	Human rights define the relationship between the rights holder and the duty bearer, understood to include the state, institutions, health systems, and health professionals.
International human rights law	The obligations and duties by which States are bound to respect, protect, and fulfill human rights as well as provide accountability for curtailments of human rights. States undertake the responsibility to abide by such law through ratification of international human rights documents [15].
Equality and nondiscrimination	Human rights law proscribes any discrimination in access to health care and the underlying determinants of health, as well as to the means and entitlements for their procurement, on well-recognized grounds [16].
Participation	The right of individuals and groups to participate in decision-making processes, which may affect their health and development [17].
Legal and policy context	The legal and policy context can support or threaten the health and well-being of individuals and populations. This goes beyond those policies strictly recognized as within the health sector, such as criminal law, age of consent laws, and privacy protections [18].
RBA to health	An RBA to health requires the adoption of an approach explicitly shaped by human rights principles, including attention to the key elements of the right to health, participation, equality and nondiscrimination, the legal and policy context, and accountability [17].
Key elements of the right to health	As stated in General Comment 14 of the UN Committee on Economic, Social and Cultural Rights, key elements of the right to health include availability, accessibility, acceptability, and quality (3AQ) [19]. *Availability*—Functioning public health and health care facilities, goods and services, as well as programs, available in sufficient quantity. This includes the underlying determinants of health, such as safe and potable drinking water and adequate sanitation facilities, hospitals, clinics and other health-related buildings, trained medical and professional personnel receiving domestically competitive salaries, and essential drugs [20]. *Accessibility*—Health facilities, goods, and services have to be accessible without discrimination and must be physically and economically accessible, including for the most marginalized. *Acceptability*—All health facilities, goods, and services must be acceptable to the populations for whom they are intended, respectful of medical ethics and culturally appropriate, sensitive to gender and lifecycle requirements, as well as designed to respect confidentiality. *Quality*—Health facilities, goods, and services must be scientifically and medically appropriate and of good quality [21].
Sexual and reproductive health and rights	Sexual and reproductive health and rights ensure individuals can make decisions about their body, access the sexual and reproductive health services they need including accurate information, and be free from all forms of sexual violence, including forced abortion and forced sterilization, allowing for positive expressions of sexuality and well-being in relation to health and sexuality including sexual pleasure [22]

optimizing the health and rights of children. In each example, we begin by noting relevant global level health standards and human rights principles, then the current context is briefly described, followed with attention to alignment and synergies that can best support the health and human rights of children in the United States in the current moment.

Sexual and reproductive health services

According to the World Health Organization (WHO), comprehensive access to sexual and reproductive health (SRH) services "should cover access to contraception, fertility and infertility care, maternal and perinatal health, prevention and treatment of sexually transmitted infections (STIs), protection from sexual and gender-based discrimination and education on safe and healthy relationships" [23]. SRH services are recognized to be vital to ensuring access to the highest attainable standard of health including sexual and reproductive rights more generally. This access is particularly crucial for young people, and also includes counseling, provision of medical care and CSE. An SRHR focus on services is concerned with ensuring these services are available, accessible, acceptable, and of quality (3AQ), and importantly that as organized they are not simply disease-oriented but help individuals attain, support, and maintain a positive attitude toward their sexuality, including their sexual health.

While it is well recognized that the larger legal and policy environment can impact childrens' access and use of services, in addition to the 3AQ derived from right the health, operationalizing the human rights principles of equality and nondiscrimination, participation and accountability can all provide a critical check in determining if the SRH services available to young people truly meet the needs of their intended beneficiaries. Children's active engagement with rights-based SRH services is essential to affirm their SRHR, including but not limited to access to contraception, abortion, and gender affirming care as needed, and importantly for all young people to understand consent and the longer-term ability to establish positive sexual communication and build healthy relationships [24].

Within the United States, children consistently and increasingly are less likely to receive or be provided access to health services, including SRH services [25]. These discrepancies are further exacerbated when faced with already existing systemic inequities that children may face, for example, on the basis of race, class, gender, and other intersecting forms of discrimination. These systematic barriers to health and well-being in turn have long-lasting effects, far beyond simply whether or not the services are accessed and used, with important implications throughout the life-cycle [26,27]. Such inequities are further complicated by the growing lack of legal protections ensuring access to SRH services; the normative presence of or lack thereof of state-based policies to access SRH services is resulting in children's rights and health being increasingly dependent on the location where they live. This runs contrary to the international human rights principles of equality and nondiscrimination, prevents equality of opportunity in access to SRH services as well as to participate in relevant decision-making and accessing needed SRH information, all with lasting impacts on their ability as children and as they grow to achieve their highest attainable standard of health [24].

Differing state-by-state, location-based hierarchizations of health services and, therefore, health for children based on nothing more than a child's physical location, can have significant impacts on health and well-being over the life-course—particularly when interrelated with community-based histories of trauma and exclusion. Without continuous and universal access to comprehensive and confidential SRH services, children cannot autonomously make decisions regarding their SRHR nor can they be assured that their SRHR will be respected, protected, and fulfilled. Access to SRHR services is a key marker to support individual health, life and development; a health and human rights analysis clarifies that the current legal and political environment in the United States threatens the health and well-being of this and future generations.

Comprehensive sexuality education

Comprehensive sexuality education (CSE) as the term implies depicts age-appropriate, evidence-informed sexuality education with changes to curricula depending on whether children are in primary and secondary school. CSE is well recognized to be important for children as it provides (age-appropriate) accurate information and resources to understand sexuality, sexual and reproductive health, and sexual pleasure, which data have shown helps children over time form healthy relationships, prevent sexual abuse and violence, improve contraceptive use, as well as reduce unintended pregnancies, and the transmission of STIs and HIV [11,28,29].

Human rights principles, as outlined in international human rights documents, further ground the importance of CSE by depicting how children have a right to participation, equality and nondiscrimination but also a right to education, information, health, and bodily autonomy, all of which are central to CSE [2]. Secondarily, the restriction of these rights is only permissible in exceptional circumstances, noting the importance of CSE for health and well-being over time suggests that in the case of CSE such restrictions are nonjustifiable [30]. Within the United States, the National Sex Education Standards (NSES), a civil society partnership, seeks to promote institutionalization of quality sex education in schools, and in so doing protect human rights by addressing inconsistent implementation and content of CSE. The NSES note a desire for K-12 sexuality education to be evidence-based, age-appropriate, and planned within health education curricula and guidance programs, outlining and emphasizing diversity, equity, and inclusion in learnings for and with students, educators, and faculty engaging in CSE [31]. These national standards thus support the promotion of the rights to education, equality, health, nondiscrimination, and participation in the context of CSE.

Despite evidence of the value of CSE and the existence of these standards, according to a 2024 report by SIECUS, only 30 states and the District of

Columbia in the United States require some form of sexuality education by law or state standard, only 5 of those states require sexuality education to be CSE [12,32]. Of relevance, the Guttmacher Institute finds in 2022 that about half of young people in the United States are not receiving the sexuality education necessary to meet the Healthy People 2030 initiative goals [33]. Such differences on a state-by-state level are inconsistent with evidence-based public health and human rights standards. The United States thus largely and increasingly fails to uphold the rights of the child to learn about information and education related to their SRHR, while also failing these children as they grow into adulthood. In recent years, such faults have worsened as rollbacks against CSE curriculum have grown, allowing abstinence-only education and misinformation to persist [34,35]. Such rollbacks are known to create far-reaching consequences, as when this occurred in Europe, trends revealed declines in condom use, inclines in unprotected sex, and increases in population-based health inequities and disparities within SRHR for children [36]. Given what is known about CSE in the United States, a similar trend can be expected.

DISCUSSION

Health professionals who engage with children are well aware of the implications of restrictions on access to services and to CSE on the populations they work with and can address these gaps in a number of ways. In addition to a health and human rights analysis of the issues affecting children's health and well-being, it is also possible to draw on human rights principles in practice [37]. Often called a rights-based approach (RBA) to health, this includes centering analysis and action on addressing preexisting inequalities in the delivery, uptake and use of health services, including attention to the ever-changing legal and policy environment under which we now live as it impacts child health, as well as emphasizing the approach taken to the processes by which services are delivered, including ensuring attention on how best to serve the most marginalized populations, working toward equitable service delivery, and extending and deepening the participation of children in all services made available to them.

Health practitioners may consider this to make sense in theory but retain questions as to how to apply these principles to their work. In practice, an RBA to health requires actively engaging with the impacts of the legal and policy context and other structural determinants of health on the patient population, actively engaging with the availability, accessibility, acceptability, and quality of how services are delivered, including explicit attention to ensuring no discrimination occurs, ensuring mechanisms to support participation, and putting into place the mechanisms of accountability. A further explanation of each of these areas is articulated later. Table 2 (Questions to Consider when Integrating an RBA to Child Health) is intended to introduce a few questions that can guide such practice.

Legal and policy context

When integrating an RBA to child health, directly considering the legal and policy context can help health professionals understand not only the landscape

Table 2
Questions to consider when integrating an rights-based approach to child health

Key concepts	Questions to consider
Legal and policy context	What is the current legal environment in your city, county, and state that may impact the health and well-being of the children you serve? Which laws or policies will help and which will hinder your efforts? For those that are in conflict, what will it take to sustain and implement those that are helpful and to get rid of those that are harmful?
Availability, acceptability, accessibility, and quality (3AQ)	How can you do a better job of ensuring the availability, acceptability, accessibility, and quality of the services you provide? Considering each component of the 3AQ, what are the barriers to your patients having what you consider to be optimal care? Which specific efforts can you take to overcome the barriers in each of these domains?
Equality and nondiscrimination	What steps can be taken to identify the ways in which discrimination is impacting your patients' ability to be or remain healthy? How can you identify ways in which this discrimination can be addressed in how you deliver services?
Participation	Which efforts are being made to ensure children are helping shape the approach taken to the delivery of services? How are you ensuring the voice of the child is heard and considered in all decisions affecting their health?
Accountability	How are you ensuring transparency and accountability for the ways you do your work? How can you measure success and progress in ways that optimize both the rights and health of children?

they exist and practice within, but how this environment may be affecting their patients. The complex interplay of law and policy at the city, county, state, and federal levels has significant impacts on the health of children, offering at times contradictory emphases. In understanding where the legal and policy context is helpful, where its harmful, and where it varies based on topic or geography, child health professionals will better be able to support the health and questions of the communities they work with. This information is easily found through review of city, county, and state legal and policy databases, and can readily be integrated into practice.

The ubiquitous 3AQ

The 3AQ is at its root about how services are delivered. This framework provides 4 descriptors for health professionals to use in evaluating how services are provided [38]. With respect to *availability*, this includes ensuring the physical infrastructure of course, but also that services are available not only in highly dense areas but also through telemedicine or some other means to all children who need them. *Accessibility* requires services not only to be within safe reach but that, whether privately or publicly provided, they are affordable, and that the information children need to make informed decisions about their health is provided. *Acceptability* is about messaging, and how services are delivered, ensuring that services are culturally tailored, sensitive to gender and other underlying determinants of health, as well as designed to respect confidentiality. While *quality* is intended to ensure not only that information and services are scientifically and medically appropriate but also that they are of good quality.

Equality and nondiscrimination

Both attention to the legal and policy environment and to the 3AQ point to the need to actively consider how differences in a child's identity, culture, and intersecting markers of identity can impact their health, as well as their uptake and use of services on offer. In thinking about individuals in this way, including the levels of stigma and discrimination they may face on a daily basis, it becomes possible to tailor services to ensure they promote the rights to equality and nondiscrimination not only conceptually but also operationally. This awareness means that interactions can be tailored to reduce barriers and address experiences of discrimination as relevant to child health [39].

Participation

Aligned with a commitment to the 3AQ and equality and nondiscrimination, promoting participation entails ensuring the means to actively listen and engage with the children for whom services are provided, not simply informing them what to do. Enacting participation in this way goes beyond simply, for example, putting a comment box in the lobby but engaging children in their own health care including fostering understanding of how the individual's surrounding environment, including parents and homelife, can influence health [40]. Integrating participation in this way recognizes the child as an agent, not simply as a beneficiary, by engaging a holistic view of health and centering the child and their perception of their environment in discussions of health [41].

Accountability

A commitment to integrating a rights perspective into health practice requires also transparency in how decisions are made, including in determining what is working and what is not, and a metric to ensure that rights and health are actually being addressed in how services are delivered and the difference this can make over the long-term. Some examples of enacted accountability can be seen through commitments to creating an annual report on progress, opportunities, and constraints in implementation, an operational plan for enactment of a patients' bill of rights and/or the opportunity for monitoring of service delivery with explicit attention to the rights-based commitments made [42].

Prioritizing accountability as a part of how one envisions service delivery makes an RBA to health increasingly sustainable over time and ensures responsiveness to the community being served.

SUMMARY

In May 2019, the European Pediatric Association, which is the Union of National European Pediatric Societies and Associations (EPA/UNEPSA), and the European Confederation of Primary Care Pediatricians (ECPCP), together representing more than 200,000 European pediatricians, signed a memorandum of understanding to speak with one voice to advocate for the rights and health of children [43]. We hope this review can help to spark a similar trend among US child health professionals. Human rights are vital to understanding health and well-being, and if taken seriously can actually improve patient care [6]. The utility depends on the application of rights in concrete ways to practice and not simply rhetorical acknowledgment [44]. Through consideration of these rights principles in one's health practice, it becomes easier to frame who needs what sorts of services, who is being left behind and what actions are needed to support child health and well-being more generally. Of critical import here is for work in service delivery not to be done in isolation but for pediatricians to have the opportunity to join forces with others concerned with child health and well-being including those in public health as well as lawyers, social workers, teachers, and others from a variety of sectors all working together to ensure that the range of services on offer to children are rights-based, and that not only health care but systems more generally are seeking not to undermine but to optimize the health and well-being of children [8,45]. In so far as the United States is not likely to ratify the Convention on the Rights of the Child any time soon, attention to these principles can serve as a moral, ethical, and practical compass from which pediatricians and their allies can build toward ensuring the rights and health of all children in the United States no matter their material circumstances nor where they live [46].

Disclosure

The authors have nothing to disclose.

References

[1] Institute of Medicine (US). Child Health and Human Rights. Washington (DC): National Academies Press (US); 1994. Introduction. Available at: https://www.ncbi.nlm.nih.gov/books/NBK231322/

[2] United Nations. Convention on the rights of the child. United Nations general assembly document A/RES/44/25. 1989. Available at: https://www.un.org/en/development/desa/population/migration/generalassembly/docs/globalcompact/A_RES_44_25.pdf. Accessed November 1, 2024.

[3] Chapman AR, Brunelli L, Forman L, et al. Promoting children's rights to health and well-being in the United States. Lancet Reg Health Am 2023;25:100577.

[4] Centers for Disease Control and Prevention. A child's health is the public's health. CDC; 2019. Available at: https://www.cdc.gov/childrenindisasters/features/children-public-health.html. Accessed November 1, 2024.

[5] Frequently asked questions on the convention on the rights of the child. In: UNICEF. Available at: https://www.unicef.org/child-rights-convention/frequently-asked-questions. Accessed November 1, 2024.

[6] Gruskin S, Mills EJ, Tarantola D. History, principles, and practice of health and human rights. Lancet 2007;370:449–55.

[7] Mann JM, Gostin L, Gruskin S, et al. Health and human rights. Health Hum Rights 1994;1(6):7–23.

[8] Gruskin S. and Tarantola D., Health and human rights overview: the nexus of health and human rights in times of peace and crisis, In: Quah S., International Encyclopedia of public health, 3rd edition, 2023, Reference Modules in Biomedical Sciences, 1–11. Available at: https://www.sciencedirect.com/referencework/9780323972802/international-encyclopedia-of-public-health#book-description.

[9] Impact of gender affirming care bans on LGBTQ+ adults. In: Human Rights Campaign Foundation. 2023. Available at: https://hrc-prod-requests.s3-us-west-2.amazonaws.com/GAC-Ban-Memo-Final.pdf. Accessed November 1, 2024.

[10] The importance of access to comprehensive sex education. In: American Academy of Pediatrics. Available at: https://www.aap.org/en/patient-care/adolescent-sexual-health/equitable-access-to-sexual-and-reproductive-health-care-for-all-youth/the-importance-of-access-to-comprehensive-sex-education/?srsltid=AfmBOoqDXcnuNoTKntsd-f4U2ufSi5HeFQfCpSGD3omfVmV1QLrsktv4G. Accessed November 1, 2024.

[11] Goldfarb ES, Lieberman LD. Three decades of research: the case for comprehensive sex education. J Adolesc Health 2021;68(1):13–27.

[12] Sex Ed for Social Change. State profiles. In: SIECUS. Available at: https://siecus.org/siecus-state-profiles/. Accessed November 1, 2024.

[13] Gruskin S, Zacharias K, Jardell W, et al. Inclusion of human rights in sexual and reproductive health programming: facilitators and barriers to implementation. Glob Pub Health 2021;16(10):1559–75.

[14] Tobin J. Beyond the supermarket shelf: using a rights based approach to address children's health needs. Int J Child Rts 2006;14:275–306.

[15] United Nations Human Rights Office of the High Commissioner. International human rights law. In: United Nations. Available at: https://www.ohchr.org/en/instruments-and-mechanisms/international-human-rights-law. Accessed November 1, 2024.

[16] United Nations Human Rights Office of the High Commissioner. International covenant on economic, social and cultural rights, general assembly resolution 2200 (XXI). United Nations Document A/6316. 1966. Available at: https://www.ohchr.org/en/instruments-mechanisms/instruments/international-covenant-economic-social-and-cultural-rights. Accessed November 1, 2024.

[17] Gruskin S, Bogecho D, Ferguson L. Rights-based approaches to health policies and programs: articulations, ambiguities and assessment. J Pub Health Pol 2010;31(2):129–45.

[18] Gruskin S, Ferguson L. Government regulation of sex and sexuality: in their own words. RHM 2009;17(34):108–18.

[19] United Nations Committee on Economic, Social and Cultural Rights. Substantive issues arising in the implementation of the international covenant on economic, social and cultural rights, general comment No. 14. In: United Nations. 2000. Available at: https://docstore.ohchr.org/SelfServices/FilesHandler.ashx?enc=4slQ6QSmlBEDzFEovLCuW1AVC1NkPsgUedPlF1vfPMJ2c7ey6PAz2qaojTzDJmC0y%2B9t%2BsAtGDNzdEqA6SuP2r0w%2F6sVBGTpvTSCbiOr4XVFTqhQY65auTFbQRPWNDxL#:~:text=Health%20is%20a%20fundamental%20human,living%20a%. Accessed November 1, 2024.

[20] World Health Organization. WHO model list of essential medicines: 23rd list. In: World Health Organization. 2023. Available at: https://iris.who.int/bitstream/handle/10665/371090/WHO-MHP-HPS-EML-2023.02-eng.pdf?sequence=1. Accessed November 1, 2024.

[21] United Nations Committee on Economic, Social and Cultural Rights. Report on the twentieth and twenty-first sessions. In: United Nations. 2000. Available at: https://www.un.org/esa/documents/ecosoc/docs/2000/e2000-22.PDF. Accessed November 1, 2024.

[22] United Nations Human Rights Office of the High Commissioner. Sexual and reproductive health and rights. In: United Nations. Available at: https://www.ohchr.org/en/women/sexual-and-reproductive-health-and-rights. Accessed November 1, 2024.

[23] World Health Organization. Sexual and reproductive health and rights. In: World Health Organization. Available at: https://www.who.int/health-topics/sexual-and-reproductive-health-and-rights#tab=tab_1. Accessed November 1, 2024.

[24] Guttmacher Institute. An overview of consent to reproductive health services by young people. In: Guttmacher Institute. 2023. Available at: https://www.guttmacher.org/state-policy/explore/overview-minors-consent-law. Accessed November 1, 2024.

[25] Centers for Disease Control and Prevention. Sexual health services. In: Centers for Disease Control and Prevention. 2017. Available at: https://www.cdc.gov/healthyyouth/factsheets/sexual_health_services-detailed.htm. Accessed November 1, 2024.

[26] Why youth need equitable access to sexual and reproductive health services. In: American Academy of Pediatrics. 2024. Available at: https://www.aap.org/en/patient-care/adolescent-sexual-health/equitable-access-to-sexual-and-reproductive-health-care-for-all-youth/the-importance-of-equitable-access-to-sexual-and-reproductive-health-services/?srsltid=AfmBOop9hXnOvfujm8eBerXj85l2eKD6LE_t. Accessed November 1, 2024.

[27] Whitfield B, Lantos H, Manlove J. Offering sexual and reproductive health services to adolescents in school settings can create more equitable access. In: Child Trends. 2022. Available at: https://www.childtrends.org/publications/offering-sexual-and-reproductive-health-services-to-adolescents-in-school-settings-can-create-more-equitable-access. Accessed November 1, 2024.

[28] World Health Organization. Comprehensive sexuality education. In: World Health Organization. 2023. Available at: https://www.who.int/news-room/questions-and-answers/item/comprehensive-sexuality-education. Accessed November 1, 2024.

[29] Breuner CC, Mattson G. Sexuality education for children and adolescents. Clin Rep 2016;138(2):e1–11.

[30] An international human right: sexuality education for adolescents in schools. 2008. Available at: https://www.reproductiverights.org/sites/default/files/documents/SexualityEducationforAdolescents.pdf. Accessed November 1, 2024.

[31] Advocates for Youth. National sex education standards: core content and skills, K-12. Future Sex Ed; 2020. Available at: https://advocatesforyouth.org/wp-content/uploads/2020/03/NSES-2020-web.pdf.

[32] United Nations Educational, Scientific and Cultural Organization. International technical guidance on sexuality education: an evidence-informed approach. In: UNESCO. 2018. Available at: https://cdn.who.int/media/docs/default-source/reproductive-health/sexual-health/international-technical-guidance-on-sexuality-education.pdf?sfvrsn=10113efc_29&download=true. Accessed November 1, 2024.

[33] Guttmacher Institute. US adolescents' receipt of formal sex education. In: Guttmacher. 2022. Available at: https://www.guttmacher.org/fact-sheet/adolescents-teens-receipt-sex-education-united-states#. Accessed November 1, 2024.

[34] Forouzan K. Midyear 2024 state policy trends: many US states attack reproductive health care, as other states fight back. In: Guttmacher Institute. 2024. Available at: https://www.guttmacher.org/2024/06/midyear-2024-state-policy-trends-many-us-states-attack-reproductive-health-care-other. Accessed November 1, 2024.

[35] Hawkins SS. Expansion of comprehensive sexuality education. J Obstet Gynecol Neonatal Nurs 2024;53(1):14–25.

[36] World Health Organization. Alarming decline in adolescent condom use, increased risk of sexually transmitted infections and unintended pregnancies, reveals new WHO report. In: World Health Organization. 2024. Available at: https://www.who.int/europe/news/

item/29-08-2024-alarming-decline-in-adolescent-condom-use–increased-risk-of-sexually-transmitted-infections-and-unintended-pregnancies–reveals-new-who-report. Accessed November 1, 2024.

[37] World Health Organization. WHO recommendations on adolescent sexual and reproductive health and rights. In: World Health Organization. Available at: https://iris.who.int/bitstream/handle/10665/275374/9789241514606-eng.pdf. Accessed November 1, 2024.

[38] United Nations. Elevating rights and choices for all: guidance note for applying a human rights-based approach to programming. In: United Nations. 2020. Available at: https://www.unfpa.org/sites/default/files/pub-pdf/2020_HRBA_guidance.pdf. Accessed November 1, 2024.

[39] Gender, Human Rights and Culture Branch of the UNFPA, Harvard School of Public Health Program on International Health and Human Rights. A human rights-based approach to programming: practical implementation manual and training materials. New York: UNFPA; 2010.

[40] Koller D. Right of children to be heard. BMJ Paediatrics Open 2021;5(1).

[41] Ford K, Dickinson A, Water T, et al. Child centered care: challenging assumptions and repositioning children and young people. Family-Centered Care 2018;43:39–43.

[42] Phumaphi J, Mason E, Alipui NK, et al. A crisis of accountability for women's, children's, and adolescents' health. Lancet 2020;396(10246):222–4.

[43] EPA-UNEPSA 2019 Activities report at the annual 2020 meeting of the international pediatric association (IPA). In: European Paediatric Association. 2019. Available at: https://www.pediatr-russia.ru/news/2019%20EPA_UNEPSA%20activities.%20Annual%20Report%20for%20IPA.pdf. Accessed November 1, 2024.

[44] Gruskin S, Ferguson L. Using indicators to determine the contribution of human rights to public health efforts: why? What? And how? Bull WHO 2009;87:714–9.

[45] Yamin AE. Health systems as "core social institutions." In: Yamin AE, editor. Power, suffering, and the struggle for dignity: human rights frameworks for health and why they matter. Pennsylvania: University of Pennsylvania Press; 2015. p. 99–127.

[46] Lichtsinn H, Goldhagen J. Why the USA should ratify the UN convention on the rights of the child. BMJ Paediatr Open 2023;7(1):e001355.

Advances in Pediatrics 72 (2025) 15–23

ADVANCES IN PEDIATRICS

ELSEVIER
MOSBY

Progress in Pediatric Firearm Research in the Last 5 years

Dorothy Stearns, MD, MPH[a],*, Peter F. Ehrlich, MD, MSc[b]

[a]Institute for Firearm Injury Prevention, University of Michigan, 1109 Geddes Avenue, Suite 1000, Ann Arbor, MI 48109, USA; [b]Section of Pediatric Surgery, CS Mott Children's Hospital, University of Michigan, 1540 E Hospital Drive, Ann Arbor, MI 48109, USA

Keywords

• Pediatric • Firearm • Prevention • Injury • Screening • Clinician

Key points

• Firearm-related injuries are the leading cause of death among children, underscoring the need for effective screenings to assess firearm accessibility in the home.

• Clinicians can serve a vital role in the treatment and prevention of firearm-related injuries through screenings, risk assessments, and educating families on storage practices.

• Ongoing research areas include collecting real-time data on firearm violence for more comprehensive interventions and developing robust surveillance systems.

INTRODUCTION

In 2020 firearm injury surpassed motor vehicle collision (MVC) as the number one cause of traumatic death in children [1] (Fig. 1). In 2021 there were 4752 pediatric firearm-related fatalities (vs 4397 deaths from MVC). Even greater numbers of youth are injured by firearms each year, with estimates suggesting that 15,000 nonfatal pediatric firearm injuries occurred in 2022 alone. In 2023 the United States has had more than 20 school shootings involving youth and more than 300 mass shooting [2]. Over the past decade (2009–2019), pediatric firearm fatality rates have increased by 31.2%, and firearms were responsible for more than 15,000 fatalities and 70,000 visits from the pediatric population [1,3]. Furthermore, firearm mortality rates (8.27 per 100,000) for all older adolescents (age 14–17 years) are now 27.6% higher than for motor vehicle crashes (6.48 per 100,000) [1]. As a result, US high-school–age youth (age

*Corresponding author. E-mail address: dstearns@umich.edu

https://doi.org/10.1016/j.yapd.2025.03.001

Abbreviations

CAP	child access prevention
CDC	Centers for Disease Control and Prevention
ED	emergency department
HBVIPs	hospital-based violence intervention programs
MVC	motor vehicle collision

14–17 years) are now more likely to die from firearm injuries than any other cause of pediatric death.

Pediatric firearm injuries remain a substantial economic burden, Economic costs are substantial, approaching $630 million annually for the treatment of acute firearm assault injuries alone, before including long-term costs such as lost wages and productivity, long-term medical and disability care, and costs for legal and criminal justice proceedings [4]. Based on the Healthcare Costs and Utilization Project (HCUP), Kid's Inpatient Database (KIDS) median initial hospitalization cost for a pediatric firearm injury was $12,984 [5]. Compared with MVC, firearm injury hospital costs per child were nearly 5 times higher. Pediatric firearm morbidity and mortality is now recognized as a critical public health epidemic [6].

Firearm injury prevention has been challenging due to the diverse purposes of firearms, such as recreational hunting and self-defense, as well as sociocultural factors that complicate efforts to regulate firearm possession and storage practices. In addition, firearm injury outcomes often are associated with existing public health disparities. Firearm ownership has become an intrinsic part of American society as evidenced by the number of guns owned by US citizens: there are approximately 120.5 firearms per 100 persons living in the United States, which makes it a global outlier with regard to firearm ownership compared with other developed nations [7]. Increased firearm availability is associated with higher rates of firearm-related deaths and injuries, so effective firearm safety measures and an associated effort to combat this public health crisis are necessary [1,8]. Firearm injuries fall within the scope of practice of all medical professionals who interact and care for children and young adults, so a clear understanding of best practices for prevention, acute treatment, and long-term outcomes is important for our children.

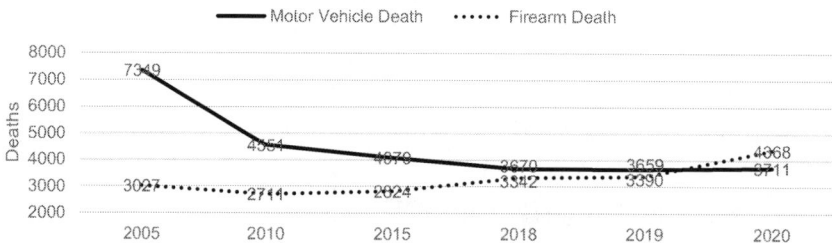

Fig. 1. Firearm versus motor vehicle death in children younger than 19 years.

SURVEILLANCE AND EPIDEMIOLOGY

One of the reasons why firearms have overtaken MVC as the number one cause of death in the pediatric/young adult population is that our understanding of the epidemiology of firearm injuries lags behinds what we know about MVC. There are national surveillance systems for firearm injuries, but these are mainly focused on firearm deaths and quite limited in terms of the data collected. They do not provide data on nonfatal firearm injury in children and offer little information about the social factors, context, or shooting types. This limits health professionals who are trying to impact locally because local data are hard to find [9].

Pediatric firearm injuries can differ by region due to various factors. In rural regions, there is a higher incidence of unintentional shootings and firearm suicides [10], and these areas face unique challenges because of limited mental health resources and emergency services. Racial disparities are evident in firearm injury outcomes, with most literature indicating that being black and male are significant risk factors for firearm injuries [9,11–13]. For example, Black youth are disproportionately affected by firearms, representing 46% of pediatric fatalities but only 14% of the population. [14–16]. Firearm violence against black women and girls is a growing concern because there has been an increase of 51% in firearm-related homicides from 2018 to 2022 according to the Giffords Law Center [17]. Proposed causes include structural racism, intergenerational trauma, exposure to violence at various developmental stages, and victimization, all of which have only recently begun to be examined in the context of firearm violence.

Neighborhood socioeconomic status significantly affects a child's risk of firearm-related injury [18]. One study in an urban area found that children from neighborhoods in the highest deprivation index quintile experienced 25% of all injuries but 57% of all firearm-related injuries. Furthermore, children from the neighborhoods in the highest quintile of deprivation had 30 times the risk of presenting for a firearm-related injury compared with children from the neighborhoods in the lowest deprivation index quintile [19]. Those who witness or experience gun violence are more likely to carry firearms for self-defense or to engage in high-risk behaviors, potentially fueling a cycle of violence [20].

High Brady state gun law strictness scores were associated with less firearm-related ED visits, as observed in the Northeast United States. [10]. In contrast, children in the South and West experience disproportionately high rates of firearm injuries and fatalities, possibly because of permissive gun laws and higher rates of gun ownership [11,21]. All of these factors underscore the need to explore pediatric firearm violence in the context of a health disparities and regional framework to discuss the psychological, sociocultural, and ecological circumstances of affected adolescents and children [22].

PRIMARY PREVENTION

Most primary prevention efforts have focused on safe storage. Parental firearm storage practices in the United States are vital in reducing the risk of accidental injuries and suicides among children and adolescents. Safe storage practices, such as keeping firearms locked and unloaded, significantly reduce the risk of access by children [23]. In contrast, households with firearms that are not securely stored have a greater risk for unintentional shootings and youth suicides [24,25]. At the time of the child's firearm death, 52.4% of firearms were reported unlocked and 38.5% loaded. Firearm deaths occurred primarily at the child's home (69.0%) or a friend or relative's home (15.9%), with most involving a handgun (80.6%), emphasizing the importance of primary prevention through secure firearm storage to prevent child firearm deaths. This is also an important consideration in examining school shootings. Using data from The American School Shooting Study (TASSS) on 262 adolescents who were school shooters, Klein and colleagues reported that approximately 82% of firearms were stolen from relatives [26].

Physicians have the potential for a major preventive impact if they do 3 things: (1) ask patients about access to firearms, (2) counsel patients about the safe use of those firearms, and (3) if necessary, intervene to thwart harm. However, lack of training is a significant barrier to conversations about gun access and safety in the clinical setting, especially among trainees. Even among postgraduate medical training programs with an emphasis on preventive medicine, the vast majority (75%) of programs provided no training related to firearm injury prevention [27]. The use of screening tools may help to identify situations where children are at risk for gun violence: the SaFEty Score [28] (Serious fighting, Friend weapon-carrying, community Environment, and firearm Threats) and FiGHTS (Fighting, Gender, Hurt while fighting, Threatened, Smoker) score are clinical screening tools designed to evaluate firearm risk in households, helping health care providers assess the likelihood of unsafe gun practices by focusing on factors such as access to firearms, the presence of children, and mental health conditions [29]. Providers can thus offer tailored advice on gun safety and storage practices and the accessibility of firearms to individuals at risk for suicide, thereby minimizing firearm-related injuries, particularly among vulnerable populations like children and individuals with mental health risks [30]. Furthermore, it is important to understand each firearm owner's preference for storage practices because ease of access is a major factor in storing firearms consistently [31]. Firearm owners may feel hesitant to remove firearms from the home, which is the most effective strategy to reduce firearm-related injuries in children [8]. Many studies have reported that gun safes and lock boxes are the preferred storage practice among firearm owners [32]. Guns that use biometric systems, such as fingerprint scanners or radio frequency identification, provide a new opportunity to enhance safety by preventing accidents, theft, or misuse by unauthorized users. However, concerns about reliability in high-stress situations, public acceptance, recalls, and regulatory gaps have challenged their widespread adoption [31,33].

Firearm primary prevention has been shown to be feasible in health care settings. Campbell and colleagues conducted a study in pediatric surgery clinics through the United States. Parents were shown a firearm safety video and then asked a series of questions related to firearm safety [34]. The study was completed by 543 parents from 15 states. Most parents (81%, n = 438) thought it was appropriate for physicians to provide firearm safety counseling. Two-thirds (63%) of gun owning parents who do not keep their guns locked said that the information provided in the module would change the way they stored firearms at home. Other studies have also demonstrated that most parents were receptive to receiving anticipatory guidance on firearm safety.

SECONDARY PREVENTION

Secondary prevention focuses on mitigating the consequences of a disease or disease process. Significant mental health issues can occur after a firearm injury in a child or young adult. Ehrlich and colleagues, found that children with firearm injuries were 50% more likely to have a new mental health diagnosis postinjury compared with after MVC [35]. Hospital admission/severity of injury increased the odds of a new mental health diagnosis compared with discharge from the ED. The increased risk of new mental health diagnoses was driven by increases in substance-related and addictive disorders and trauma- and stressor-related disorders. Preexisting mental health diagnosis were also noted in up to one-third of firearm injuries, which was significantly more than those in motor vehicle accidents. Despite this, 3 in 5 children do not receive mental health services after firearm injury [16]. These results suggest the hospital is an important setting for early intervention and secondary prevention for children and adolescents with firearm injuries.

Some hospitals and trauma centers have developed programs to address the secondary consequences of firearm injuries. These hospital-based violence intervention programs (HBVIPs) have arisen across the country in the past decade and show promise in mitigating the secondary impact of firearm injuries [36]. This program has mostly been used for the young adult population (16–24 years) and funded either by donors or the hospitals themselves. There is also some evidence that HBVIPs can be effective in providing psychological interventions for patients during their hospital admission. Nofi and colleagues, reported that HBVIPs helped reduce violent behaviors and risk of future reinjury and criminal involvement [36]. Community-based violence intervention programs involve reaching out to at-risk youth and connecting them with mentors who can serve as role models. Schools can use counselors and connect with community-based mental health services for individuals identified as high-risk for violence or firearm-related injury [37]. But taken together, there is a lot of work still needed to sort out the best role for HBVIPs.

THE IMPACT OF POLICY

A major positive step forward has been the change in rules for federal funding for firearm research, which was significantly restricted due to the Dickey Amendment in the 1990s, which prohibited the Centers for Disease Control and Prevention (CDC) from using funds to advocate for gun control [38]. With recent legislative changes in 2020, the CDC and the National Institutes of Health have begun funding research on gun violence [38]. The most prominent grant has been the Firearm Safety Among Children and Teens (FACTS) Consortium funded by the National Institute for Child Health and Human Development (NCIHD).The major aim of FACTS consortium [10] was to develop research resources for the field, including a pediatric-specific research agenda for firearm injury prevention that was published in 2019 [39].

The 3 most common pediatric firearm policy strategies have been legislative measures such as safe storage laws, child access prevention (CAP) laws, and extreme risk protection orders. All of these are associated with reduced firearm-related injuries and deaths [40–44]. ERPOs work by identifying individuals who may be at risk for firearm violence to themselves or others to prevent them from possessing or purchasing firearms. These measures vary across states, but they have been associated with decreased suicide rates [4]. CAP laws have variable standards and penalties, which has made assessing changes in firearm injury rates postimplementation historically difficult. Studies examining changes in pediatric firearm-related injuries following the implementation of CAP laws reported a decrease in injuries, with the severity of the laws affecting the degree of their impact.

NATIONAL INITIATIVES

National collaboratives derived from health care systems, national bodies, and new research societies have evolved to tackle the growing problem of firearm violence. For example, the Northwell Gun Violence Prevention Learning Collaborative consists of 600 hospitals from 38 states [45]. Its mission is to learn best practices from each other. As a result of the first phase of the collaborative, many hospitals reported either implementing their first firearm injury prevention program or expanding an existing one. By sharing their innovations in a collaborative group, health systems can improve the implementation and evaluation of new programs and use insights to inform best practices for the industry at large.

The American College of Surgeons has several working groups addressing firearm violence and has held 2 summits with more than 40 other medical organizations to address the challenges in a collaborative and multi-disciplinary manner [46,47].

Finally, the first national research meeting on firearm violence was held in Washington DC in 2022. Topics included criminal justice, public health, medicine, surgery, and community-based organizations dedicated to reducing the incidence and impact of firearm violence. The meeting also marked the establishment of the Research Society for Prevention of Firearm-Related Harms. This new group intends to promote and facilitate research on firearms- and gun-related topics to bridge the gap between researchers, practitioners, and policy makers.

Table 1
PubMed search limited to Jan 2020 to present (Oct 2024, English, human and age categories (all ages, 19–65 y, 0–18 y)

Research Area	All Ages	19–65	0–18
All	2499	1328	858
Epidemiology and surveillance	1274	782	545
Risk and protective factors	141	80	52
Primary preventive	135	101	70
Secondary preventive	40	27	20
Policy	600	303	204
Data enhancement	31	19	8

Numbers are from PubMed search, and there may be overlap. (Oct 2024).

SUMMARY

Fatal and nonfatal firearm violence has become a major pediatric public health problem. It is preventable, and strategies do exist to reduce risk. Although some progress has been made in advancing firearm injury prevention efforts for children, considerable work needs to be done. A comprehensive local, regional, and national approach is required to enhance understanding of the epidemiologic risk and protective factors. Finally targets for effective primary and second prevention interventions across different settings (school, hospital, community) are necessary (Table 1).

CLINICS CARE POINTS

- Routine screening for household firearms and counseling on safe storage practices (unloaded and locked) reduce pediatric firearm-related injury and mortality.
- Clinicians can help support community-based interventions and collaborate with schools, hospitals, and local organizations to raise awareness about firearm safety and prevention strategies.

Disclosure

The authors have nothing to disclose.

References

[1] Centers for Disease Control and Prevention. Web-Based injury statistics query and reporting system (WISQARS). Available at: https://www.cdc.gov/injury/wisqars/index.html. Accessed January 30, 2023.
[2] Gun Violence Archive. Mass shootings in 2022. Available at: https://www.gunviolencearchive.org/reports/mass-shooting. Accessed September 23, 2022.
[3] Carter PM, Cook LJ, Macy ML, et al. Individual and neighborhood characteristics of children seeking emergency department care for firearm injuries within the PECARN network. Acad Emerg Med 2017;24(7):803–13.
[4] Howell E, Abraham P, Hospital costs of firearm assaults. Urban Institute. 2013, 1-10. Available at: https://www.ojp.gov/ncjrs/virtual-library/abstracts/hospital-costs-firearm-assaults.

[5] Taylor JS, Madhavan S, Han RW, et al. Financial burden of pediatric firearm-related injury admissions in the United States. PLoS One 2021;16(6):e0252821.

[6] Christoffel KK. Firearm injuries: epidemic then, endemic now. Am J Publ Health 2007;97(4): 626–9.

[7] Karp A, Estimating global civilian-held firearms numbers. Small Arms Survey. 2018, 1-12. Available at: http://www.jstor.com/stable/resrep20049.

[8] Lee LK, Fleegler EW, Goyal MK, et al. Firearm-related injuries and deaths in children and youth. Pediatrics 2022; https://doi.org/10.1542/peds.2022-060071.

[9] Naik-Mathuria BJ, Cain CM, Alore EA, et al. Defining the full spectrum of pediatric firearm injury and death in the United States: it is even worse than we think. Ann Surg 2023;278(1): 10–6.

[10] Herrin BR, Gaither JR, Leventhal JM, et al. Rural versus urban hospitalizations for firearm injuries in children and adolescents. Pediatrics 2018;142(2); https://doi.org/10.1542/peds.2017-3318.

[11] Roberts BK, Nofi CP, Cornell E, et al. Trends and disparities in firearm deaths among children. Pediatrics 2023;152(3); https://doi.org/10.1542/peds.2023-061296.

[12] Kaufman EJ, Wiebe DJ, Xiong RA, et al. Epidemiologic trends in fatal and nonfatal firearm injuries in the US, 2009-2017. JAMA Intern Med 2021;181(2):237–44.

[13] Mulugeta MG, Bailey G, Parsons K, et al. Trends in pediatric firearm-related injuries and disparities in acute outcomes. Front Public Health 2024;12:1339394.

[14] Gramlich J, Gun deaths among US children and teens rose 50% in two years, 2023, Pew Research Center. Available at: https://coilink.org/20.500.12592/wjjkjr.

[15] Planey AM, Smith SM, Moore S, et al. Barriers and facilitators to mental health help-seeking among African American youth and their families: a systematic review study. Child Youth Serv Rev 2019;101:190–200.

[16] Hoffmann JA, Pulcini CD, Hall M, et al. Timing of mental health service use after a pediatric firearm injury. Pediatrics 2023;(1):152.

[17] GIFFORDS. Gun violence in black communities. Available at: https://giffords.org/lawcenter/report/gun-violence-in-black-communities/. Accessed October 15, 2021.

[18] Trinidad S, Kotagal M. Socioeconomic factors and pediatric injury. Curr Trauma Rep 2023;9(2):47–55.

[19] Sarnthiyakul S, Ross EE, Ourshalimian S, et al. Neighborhood deprivation and childhood opportunity indices are associated with violent injury among children in Los Angeles County. J Trauma Acute Care Surg 2023;95(3):397–402.

[20] Comer BP, Connolly EJ. Exposure to gun violence and handgun carrying from adolescence to adulthood. Soc Sci Med 2023;328:115984.

[21] Patel SJ, Badolato GM, Parikh K, et al. Regional differences in pediatric firearm-related emergency department visits and the association with firearm legislation. Pediatr Emerg Care 2021;37(11):e692–5.

[22] Bottiani JH, Camacho DA, Lindstrom Johnson S, et al. Annual Research Review: youth firearm violence disparities in the United States and implications for prevention. JCPP (J Child Psychol Psychiatry) 2021;62(5):563–79.

[23] Doh KF, Morris CR, Akbar T, et al. The relationship between parents' reported storage of firearms and their children's perceived access to firearms: a safety disconnect. Clin Pediatr (Phila) 2021;60(1):42–9.

[24] Aitken ME, Minster SD, Mullins SH, et al. Parents' perspectives on safe storage of firearms. J Community Health 2020;45(3):469–77.

[25] Hartman HA, Seewald LA, Weigend Vargas E, et al. Contextual factors influencing firearm deaths occurring among children. Pediatrics 2024;154(Suppl 3).

[26] Klein BR, Trowbridge J, Schnell C, et al. Characteristics and obtainment methods of firearms used in adolescent school shootings. JAMA Pediatr 2024;178(1):73–9.

[27] Wintemute GJ, Betz ME, Ranney ML. Yes, you can: physicians, patients, and firearms. Ann Intern Med 2016;165(3):205–13.

[28] Goldstick JE, Carter PM, Walton MA, et al. Development of the SaFETy score: a clinical screening tool for predicting future firearm violence risk. Ann Intern Med 2017;166(10): 707–14.
[29] Hayes DN, Sege R. FiGHTS: a preliminary screening tool for adolescent firearms-carrying. Ann Emerg Med 2003;42(6):798–807.
[30] Carter PM, Cunningham RM. Clinical approaches to the prevention of firearm-related injury. N Engl J Med 2024;391(10):926–40.
[31] Buck-Atkinson J, McCarthy M, Stanley IH, et al. Firearm locking device preferences among firearm owners in the USA: a systematic review. Inj Epidemiol 2023;10(1):33.
[32] Anestis MD, Moceri-Brooks J, Johnson RL, et al. Assessment of firearm storage practices in the US, 2022. JAMA Netw Open 2023;6(3):e231447.
[33] Salhi C, Azrael D, Miller M. Parent and adolescent reports of adolescent access to household firearms in the United States. JAMA Netw Open 2021;4(3):e210989.
[34] Campbell BT, Thaker S, Fallat ME, et al. A multicenter evaluation of a firearm safety intervention in the pediatric outpatient setting. J Pediatr Surg 2020;55(1):140–5.
[35] Ehrlich PF, Pulcini CD, De Souza HG, et al. Mental health care following firearm and motor vehicle-related injuries: differences impacting our treatment strategies. Ann Surg 2022;276(3):463–71.
[36] Nofi CP, Roberts BK, Cornell E, et al. Hospital-based violence intervention programs to reduce firearm injuries in children: a scoping review. J Pediatr Surg 2023;58(11):2212–21.
[37] Flannery DJ, Fox JA, Wallace Mulvey E, et al. Guns, school shooters, and school safety: what we know and directions for change. Sch Psychol Rev 2021;50(2–3):237–53.
[38] CDC. RFA-CE-23-006- firearm injury and death prevention. CDC. Accessed Setember 2024. Available at: https://www.cdc.gov/firearm-violence/php/funded-research/current-awardees-rfa-ce-23-006.html.
[39] Cunningham RM, Carter PM, Ranney ML, et al. Prevention of firearm injuries among children and adolescents: consensus-driven research agenda from the firearm safety among children and teens (FACTS) consortium. JAMA Pediatr 2019;173(8):780–9.
[40] Kivisto AJ, Phalen PL. Effects of risk-based firearm seizure laws in Connecticut and Indiana on suicide rates, 1981-2015. Psychiatr Serv 2018;69(8):855–62.
[41] Miller M, Zhang W, Rowhani-Rahbar A, et al. Child access prevention laws and firearm storage: results from a national survey. Am J Prev Med 2022;62(3):333–40.
[42] Wilson EG, Gregoski MJ, Oddo ER, et al. Are child access prevention laws associated with fewer pediatric firearm injuries? Hosp Pediatr 2024;14(10):823–7.
[43] Hammig B, Bordelon A, Chandler C. Examining media reports of pediatric unintentional firearm injury deaths for prevention messaging concerning secured storage of firearms: U.S., 2021-2022. Inj Epidemiol 2024;11(1):6.
[44] Patrick SW, Loch SF, McNeer E, et al. Voter support for policies associated with child health as national campaign priorities. JAMA Health Forum 2024;5(9):e243305.
[45] Sathya C, Dreier FL, Ranney ML. To prevent gun injury, build better research. Nature 2022;610(7930):30–3.
[46] Talley CL, Campbell BT, Jenkins DH, et al. Recommendations from the American College of Surgeons committee on trauma's firearm strategy team (FAST) workgroup: Chicago consensus I. J Am Coll Surg 2019;228(2):198–206.
[47] Sakran JV, Bornstein SS, Dicker R, et al. Proceedings from the second medical summit on firearm injury prevention, 2022: creating a sustainable healthcare coalition to advance a multidisciplinary public health approach. J Am Coll Surg 2023;236(6):1242–60.

Procalcitonin in Pediatric Emergency Medicine

Niccolò Parri, MD[a], Robert H. Pantell, MD[b],*,
Enitan D. Carrol, MD[c], Walid Abuhammour, MD, MBA[d,e,f],
Javier Benito-Fernández, MD, PhD[g],
Christèle Gras-Le Guen, MD, PhD[h], Alain Gervaix, MD[i,j,k]

[a]Meyer Children's Hospital IRCCS, Florence, Italy; [b]Department of Pediatrics, School of Medicine, University of California San Francisco, 11 Piedmont Street, San Francisco, CA 94117, USA; [c]Department of Clinical Infection, Microbiology and Immunology, University of Liverpool Institute of Infection, Veterinary and Ecological Sciences, Ronald Ross Building, 8 West Derby Street, Liverpool L69 7BE, England, United Kingdom; [d]Mohammad Bin Rashid University - Dubai, United Arab Emirates; [e]The Jordan University- School of Medicine – Amman, Jordan, Dubai, United Arab Emirates; [f]Department of Pediatric Infectious Diseases, Al Jalila Children's Hospital (AJCH) Dubai, Al Jaddaf, United Arab Emirates; [g]Pediatric Emergency Department, Cruces University Hospital, Plaza de Cruces S/n E-48903, Barakaldo, Bizkaia, Spain; [h]Pediatric Emergency Department, Hôpital Mère – Enfant, CHU Nantes, 38 Boulevard Jean Monet, Nantes, France; [i]Department of Gynecology, Geneva University Hospitals & University of Geneva, Geneva, Switzerland; [j]Department of Obstetric, Geneva University Hospitals & University of Geneva, Geneva, Switzerland; [k]Children's Hospital, HUG, Rue Willy Donze 6, Geneva 1205, Switzerland

Keywords
- Procalcitonin • Biomarkers • Febrile infants • Sepsis • Meningitis
- Urinary tract infections • Osteomyelitis

Key points

- Procalcitonin (PCT) is a biomarker that is useful in predicting the risk of invasive bacterial infections in children.
- Clinical prediction models that include clinical appearance, urinalysis, and inflammatory markers, have high sensitivity in detecting urinary tract infections (UTIs), bacteremia, and bacterial meningitis.

Continued

INTRODUCTION

Pediatric emergency visits often stem from suspected infections, particularly in very young children who may not exhibit clear clinical signs. Although only a

*Corresponding author. *E-mail address:* Robert.pantell@ucsf.edu
Twitter: @CarrolEnitan; @JavierBenitoF

https://doi.org/10.1016/j.yapd.2025.01.002

Continued

- Compared with other biomarkers, PCT has the highest area under the curve (AUC) for identifying bacteremia and bacterial meningitis.
- Compared with other biomarkers PCT is superior in UTI to predict pyelonephritis and vesicoureteral reflux and a stronger indicator for pyogenic arthritis and osteomyelitis.
- Quality improvement initiatives and algorithms that include PCT have been documented to significantly lower antibiotic usage, as well as decrease unnecessary lumbar punctures and hospitalizations.

Abbreviations

ANC	absolute neutrophil count
APN	acute pyelonephritis
BMS	Bacterial Meningitis Score
CAP	community-acquired pneumonia
CRP	C-reactive protein
CSF	cerebrospinal fluid
CXR	chest radiograph
ED	emergency department
ESR	erythrocyte sedimentation rate
IBI	invasive bacterial infection
LUS	lung ultrasound
MSE	Meningitis Score for Emergencies
NPV	negative predictive value
OM	osteomyelitis
PCT	procalcitonin
PEWS	Pediatric Early Warning scores
POCTs	point-of-care tests
qSOFA	Quick Sequential Organ Failure Assessment
RA	rheumatoid arthritis
RBUS	Renal bladder ultrasound
RCTs	randomized controlled trials
SA	septic arthritis
SBI	serious bacterial illness
UTIs	urinary tract infections
VCUG	voiding cystourethrogram
VUR	vesicoureteral reflux
WBC	white blood count

small fraction of fever cases are due to bacterial infections that lead to serious morbidity [1], concerns over misdiagnosis, parental anxiety, and public expectations often drive unnecessary antibiotic use, laboratory tests, imaging, and hospitalizations. Despite decreasing prevalence of consequential bacterial infections through advancements in vaccines, technology, and antibiotic stewardship programs, antibiotic prescriptions remain high [2–5]. As most infections are viral, this overuse exposes children to well-known antibiotic-associated drug events such as diarrhea, vomiting, allergic reactions, and emerging microbial resistance to antibiotics.

Continually emerging evidence has documented how antibiotics disrupt and reduce the diversity of a child's microbiome [6]. The establishment of the gut microbiota during the first 2 to 3 years of childhood is essential for the developing immune system and long-term health outcomes. Early and especially repeated microbiota disruption by broad-spectrum antibiotics is associated with an increased risk of early childhood obesity [7], as well as allergic diseases [8], and asthma at school age [9]. Long-term impacts may include among others inflammatory disorders, insulin resistance, and autoimmunity (type 1 diabetes and lupus) [10].

Since the 1970s, considerable research has attempted to distinguish between children at high risk for consequential bacterial infections requiring antimicrobials and potential hospitalizations versus those at low risk who can be safely discharged to home. Older clinical decision models relied on clinical and laboratory features including urinalysis, white blood count (WBC), and absolute neutrophil count (ANC) [11–13]. The newest laboratory aids include centralized molecular tests that can identifying pathogen rapidly but have limitations identifying the causal organism when distinguishing between viral and bacterial infections [14]. Tests in early development are RNA transcriptional profiling and next-generation sequencing of microbial cell-free DNA.

Befinning in the early 1980s host-response biomarkers, like procalcitonin (PCT) and C-reactive protein (CRP), were shown to be more accurate in diagnosing bacteremia than ANC and WBC with respective area under the curves (AUCs) of 0.91, 0.77, 0.61, and 0.48 [15]. PCT rises more rapidly than all other biomarkers (3–6 hours) [16,17], making it particularly useful in early recognition of systemic bacterial infections. Successful antibiotic treatment of the underlying bacterial infection results in a rapid decrease of the PCT concentration with a half-life of 24 hours [18,19]. Randomized controlled trials (RCTs) show the use of PCT for decreasing antibiotic initiation and duration in acute respiratory tract infections [18] and sepsis [19].

The value of PCT in medical decision-making for a variety of clinical situations is discussed in the following sections.

FEVER WITHOUT SOURCE IN INFANTS

Fever without source in infants represents a diagnostic challenge, especially in those aged under 3 months who are at higher risk of infection, accounting for over 180,000 ED visits annually in the United States. While viral causes are common, serious bacterial illness (SBI) comprising UTI, bacteremia, and meningitis occurs in 15% to 20% of infants aged under 60 days, with invasive bacterial infection (IBI), bacteremia, sepsis, and meningitis comprising 1% to 3% [17,20–23]. Bacteremia can rapidly evolve to septic shock, emphasizing the importance of timely evaluation.

To avoid unnecessary interventions and identify young febrile infants at low risk for IBI who may be safely managed as outpatients, the Rochester [11], Boston [12], and Philadelphia [13] criteria were developed in the 1980s and 1990s. While these criteria demonstrate high sensitivity, their modest specificity and requirement for extensive testing limited their clinical utility and widespread adoption. A more recent prediction model, by the Febrile Young Infant Research Collaborative, that did not include PCT demonstrated sensitivity at 98.8%, but with specificity of 31.3% [24]. In a recent study [25], one-third of infants with an IBI were misclassified as low risk by both the modified Boston and Philadelphia fever criteria, and only 4% of those infants identified as high risk actually had an IBI, probably due to well-described changes in the epidemiology and prevalence of IBI since the establishment of the criteria [22,23].

In 2004, the American Academy Of Pediatrics' (AAP's) Pediatric Research in Office Settings national network conducted a prospective observational study of greater than 3000 patients and developed a clinical prediction rule for IBI in febrile infants aged younger than 90 days. This group of experienced pediatricians detected 97.1% of IBI cases and ordered substantially fewer laboratory tests, lumbar punctures, and hospitalizations than existing decision models; the derived rule, relying on assessment of clinical appearance, temperature and age, had comparable sensitivity (94.6%) to the models, with substantially fewer recommendations for hospitalizations and testing, including lumbar punctures [26]. This study eventually led to the AAP creating a guideline generalizable beyond pediatricians with 20 years of clinical experience.

Newer approaches incorporating PCT and CRP have imptoved accuracy in predicting IBIs. PCT has the highest predictive value [27], particularly early in the course of a febrile episode [17,28]. The step-by-step approach, validated in 2016, is a risk stratification algorithm for children aged less than 90 days that includes the sequential evaluation of age, clinical appearance, urinalysis, PCT, CRP, and ANC [20]. This approach was able to risk stratify patients with a higher prevalence of IBI in the high-risk and intermediate-risk groups, compared to the low-risk group. The sensitivity for IBI was 92%. In a head-to-head comparison, the prevalence of potentially missed IBI was higher when using the Lab-score [29,30] or the Rochester criteria than the step-by-step [20]. In 2019, the Febrile Infant Working Group of the Pediatric Emergency Care Applied Research Network derived and validated a prediction rule to identify febrile infants 60 days and younger at low risk for SBIs and IBIs in a prospective multicenter observational study [21]. The prediction rule identified infants at low risk of SBI and IBI using a negative urine analysis result, an ANC of 4000/μL or less, and serum PCT of 0.5 μg/L or less. In contrast to the step-by-step approach, this rule was derived on a different age group (0–60 days), did not exclude infants based on clinical appearance, and included infants with symptoms or signs of respiratory infections. In this cohort of 1681 infants, the rule demonstrated good performance for IBI (sensitivity 96.7%, specificity 61.5%). While sensitivity was comparable to other models, the specificity was moderately higher. One infant with bacteremia and 2 infants with urinary tract infections (UTIs) were misclassified. No patient with bacterial meningitis was missed by the rule.

Until more accurate diagnostic tests, such as novel RNA expression patterns, replace clinical prediction algorithms, it is necessary to have agreed protocols that bring together all current knowledge on the management of young febrile infants [31]. In this sense, the AAP subcommittee on febrile infants published in 2021 its recommendations for the evaluation and management of well-appearing febrile infants aged 8 to 60 days, which includes separate algorithms for infants aged 8 to 21, 22 to 28, and 29-60 days. Unlike previous decision models, it does not indicate mandatory hospitalization of infants in the 22-28 days age group [32]. This document includes management recommendations depending on whether PCT is available or not. When CRP and PCT are not available, the AAP algorithms performed with high sensitivity but modest specificity for detecting IBI [33]. The guideline was tested on nearly 18,000 infants in an AAP Quality Initiative. With substantial adherence to the recommendations, there were significant reductions in lumbar punctures and hospitalizations as well as increased use of oral instead of parenteral antimicrobials [34]. A 2025 study of the guideline's impact on more than 34,000 febrile infants documented an increased use in evaluation of PCT and CRP with a decrease in LPs, hospitalizations, and use of antibiotics [35].

Turning to older infants, in a 2012 cohort of infants (median age 6.7 months), PCT was able to successfully detect IBI (AUC 0.87) compared with CRP (AUC 0.79); for fever less than 8 hours in duration, the figures were 0.97 and 0.76, respectively [30]. The Diafever study is the first RCT in the emergency department (ED) directly comparing age-specific clinical prediction rules, including the biomarker PCT, with routine clinical practice, to identify young febrile infants with low risk for IBI. A total of 4920 patients aged between 6 days and 36 months (median age 2 months) were included. Within 15 days of emergency admission, 26.3% of patients received antibiotic therapy in the intervention group and 38% in the control group, with no significant difference in morbidity. The use of this new algorithm could lead to a significant reduction in antibiotic prescribing in pediatric emergency departments, without increasing morbidity and mortality [36,37].

In summary, for febrile infants, a systematic approach based on the best available serum biomarkers is recommended. While existing models, rules, guidelines, and experienced clinicians demonstrate high sensitivity, their specificity is often low to modest, leading to increased invasive testing, hospitalizations, antimicrobial usage, and costs. Incorporating PCT (≥ 0.5 µg/L), in conjunction with other variables, has been shown to significantly enhance specificity, thereby mitigating iatrogenic medical and social consequences. It is especially useful in infants coming to care within a few hours of fever onset.

SEPSIS

Bacteremia and sepsis are on a continuum, a rapidly progressive and life-threatening infection associated with organ dysfunction [38,39], which if untreated, results in death. Early recognition, appropriate antibiotic therapy, and supportive care are fundamental in improving outcomes of children with suspicion of sepsis. The Surviving Sepsis Campaign International Guidelines

[40] provide an evidence-based approach to the management of septic shock and sepsis-associated organ dysfunction in children [40], with an algorithm for the early resuscitation and management [41].

The 4 Rs of early management of sepsis could be described as (1) Recognize, (2) Risk-stratification, (3) Respond, and (4) Reduce antimicrobial use. Pediatric Early Warning scores (PEWS), Manchester Triage Score, laboratory tests, the Neonatal early onset sepsis calculator [42], and biomarkers (PCT and CRP) can support early recognition of bacterial versus viral infections versus noninfectious inflammatory conditions. Though triage scores are sensitive tools for initial risk stratification of febrile children presenting to the ED, they lack specificity. Combining the biomarker mid regional proadenomedullin (MR-proADM or PCT with PEWS could enhance the identification of high-risk patients, allowing for more targeted interventions and timely management [43]. The Liverpool Quick Sequential Organ Failure Assessment (qSOFA) aims to improve sensitivity and specificity compared to regular qSOFA, by assessing respiratory rate, heart rate, capillary refill time, and AVPU (Alert, Voice, Pain, Unresponsive) scale, but requires further evaluation in other settings prior to recommending more widespread use [44]. In adults, addition of PCT to qSOFA improved early prediction of sepsis, but this has not been evaluated for children [45]. Pre-existing risk factors (age, recent surgery, comorbidity, immunosuppression, and trauma) heighten the suspicion of sepsis. Risk-stratification is important to determine the required level of care, including fluid resuscitation, blood cultures, antibiotics, vasoactive drugs, and antimicrobial stewardship to start antibiotics only if needed, review and rationalize antibiotics and discontinue if needed.

Electronic predictive alert systems based on electronic medical records have provided promising results to identify potential sepsis [46] or severe sepsis in ED and inpatients [43] and to predict sepsis-related mortality [47], ideally combining high sensitivity in predicting sepsis within 48 hours with high predictive value, and a low alert rate [46,47]. The e-POCT, an innovative electronic algorithm using host biomarker (point-of-care tests) (POCTs), including CRP and PCT, significantly lowered antibiotic prescriptions from 94.9% to 11.5% in a randomized controlled study [48]. Future implementation studies are necessary since adherence to the algorithm will be a key factor in making use of e-POCTs advantages.

MENINGITIS

Differentiating bacterial meningitis from aseptic meningitis is a key clinical question. Though most cases of meningitis are aseptic and do not require treatment, bacterial meningitis is a life-threatening condition that requires immediate intravenous broad-spectrum antibiotics to prevent mortality and morbidity. As clinical symptoms do not differ between the two causes, only positive culture of blood and cerebrospinal fluid (CSF) can confirm the definitive diagnosis and children are hospitalized pending results. Combinations of several variables have been used to distinguish the 2 types of meningitis.

The Bacterial Meningitis Score (BMS) combines 5 dichotomous predictors (presence of convulsions, ANC in peripheral blood, ANC in CSF, CSF protein, and CSF Gram stain) to identify children with pleocytosis at low (BMS = 0) or high risk (BMS ≥ 2) of bacterial meningitis. Children at low risk may be followed as outpatients after the administration of a long-acting parenteral antibiotic [49]. In a meta-analysis, PCT measured in blood (≥0.5 µg/L) showed higher diagnostic accuracy for detecting bacterial meningitis than other conventional biomarkers [50]. Adding PCT to the BMS score could significantly increase the specificity of the test [51,52].

In a multicenter cohort study in 25 EDs including 1009 children with CSF pleocytosis (92 bacterial causes), the most important predictors of bacterial meningitis were derived from a retrospective cohort and validated in a prospective cohort. The resulting Meningitis Score for Emergencies (MSE) is derived from the most important predictors: PCT greater than 1.2 µg/L (3 points), CSF protein greater than 80 mg/dL (2 points), CSF ANC greater than 1000 cells/mm^3 (1 point), and CRP greater than 40 mg/L (1 point). An MSE of 1 or greater predicted bacterial meningitis with 100% sensitivity and 77.4% specificity. No children diagnosed with bacterial meningitis had an MSE greater than 2, in contrary to the BMS that missed 2 cases of bacterial meningitis [53].

The MSE, including PCT, can be used to guide initial clinical decision-making in children with CSF pleocytosis without misclassifying children with bacterial meningitis.

URINARY TRACT INFECTIONS

Significant risk factors for UTI in children, apart from sex, are bladder-bowel dysfunction, congenital anomalies of kidneys and the urinary tract, including vesicoureteral reflux (VUR), and the circumcision status in young boys. Oral antibiotic therapy for fewer than 7 to 10 days is adequate for uncomplicated cases. Renal bladder ultrasound (RBUS) examination is advised in all young children with first febrile UTI and in older children with recurrent UTI. Most children with first febrile UTI do not need a voiding cystourethrogram (VCUG); it may be considered in the case of abnormal RBUS examination, atypical causative pathogen, complex clinical course, or known renal scarring [54].

PCT is useful to differentiate cystitis from acute pyelonephritis (APN) in children with febrile UTI. The differentiating between cystitis (35%–40%) and APN (60%–65%) is difficult, but renal scarring is only featured with APN (15% permanent scar) and may lead to future complications [55]. A dimecapto-suuccinic acid (DMSA) scan is the gold standard, but it is invasive and irradiating and not readily available for all patients. Pretest probability may be improved with biomarker evaluation. In a meta-analysis on individual patient data (n = 1011, 60.6% APN), PCT of 0.5 µg/L or greater was shown to be a more robust predictor of DMSA scan-confirmed APN during the early stages of UTI, compared to CRP and white blood cell count (WBC), with an adjusted +

LR 2.5. Using the same cutoff, PCT could predict renal scarring (n = 525, 25.7% renal scarring) with an adjusted + LR 1.6 [56]. In a Cochrane systematic review, the authors came to similar sensitivity (81%) and specificity (76%), making it feasible to rule in APN but not replace the DMSA scan [57]. Negative inflammatory marker levels CRP less than 20 mg/L or PCT less than 0.5 μg/L can be used to rule-out APN [58]. Severity of renal lesions was highly correlated to PCT concentration, but only borderline related to CRP [59]. The risk factors for renal scarring are recurrent UTI, duration of fever, and high-grade VUR, whereas VUR is related to a higher risk of APN and late renal scar [60].

Approximately 20% to 30% of children with a confirmed UTI are diagnosed with VUR, but only about 15% have a grade III or higher that triggers therapeutic consequences. PCT is a strong, independent, and now validated predictor of VUR (OR [odds ratio] of 2.5) that can be used to identify low-risk patients and thus avoid one-third of the unnecessary VCUG in children with a first febrile UTI [61]. PCT of 0.5 μg/L or greater could identify 100% of high-grade VUR, whereas RBUS sensitivity was only 51% but with better specificity (43% vs 72%) [62]. Combination of RBUS with PCT was not clearly superior to using PCT alone [63]. Despite this evidence, the AAP recommends RBUS screening before performing VCUG after first febrile UTI [54].

LOWER RESPIRATORY TRACT INFECTION

Chest radiograph (CXR) is commonly used as a standard for diagnosing community-acquired pneumonia (CAP), but it has limitations such as low sensitivity, inability to differentiate bacterial from viral CAP, or predict clinical course [64–69]. An ideal rule would allow for discrimination of patients with and without radiographic pneumonia, minimizing the need for CXR in most children, unless there is suspicion for CAP-related complications or alternate diagnoses. A model predicting radiographic CAP in children aged 3 months to 18 years was developed, which included age, decreased breath sounds, and duration of fever, but this showed limited performance at intermediate-risk threshold [70].

Biomarkers could improve the models' performance [71]. The incorporation of both CRP and PCT were not inferior to CRP alone [10]. PCT was associated with radiographic pneumonia, and demonstrated modest predictive value for disease severity among children with suspected CAP [72] as well as in children hospitalized with CAP. Its strongest prognostic effect lay in differentiating disease severity [73], which is likely related to the ability of PCT to predict bacterial illness. However, PCT is not as strong a predictor of radiographic pneumonia, as this may be caused by either viral or bacterial etiology. No single test or group of tests can accurately identify the etiology of CAP in a timely manner, and presence of a viral infection does not preclude bacterial coinfection [10]. Given their high NPV, these markers may be helpful in ruling out the most severe outcomes, that is, empyema requiring chest drainage and sepsis [74]. Biomarkers are a valuable tool, particularly, for patients with intermediate or equivocal risk for CAP. While CRP seems to have the best diagnostic performance, PCT can predict outcome, both for disease severity, and for response to empirical beta-lactam treatment [75]. Lung ultrasound (LUS) for the diagnosis of children's pneumonia showed high sensitivity (93%–97%) and specificity (91%–98.2%), with a great variation in ultrasound findings diagnostic of pneumonia, and agreement on reference standard for pneumonia [76,77]. However, differentiation between viral and atypical bacterial CAP was not feasible with LUS [78]. The combination of LUS and PCT presented a better accuracy for bacterial pneumonia in critically ill children compared to LUS or CXR alone, or the combination of CXR and PCT [79]. It is feasible and safe to substitute LUS for CXR, without missing cases of pneumonia or increased rates of adverse effect. Nonetheless, the use of LUS in cases of suspected pneumonia can increase the use of antibiotics by 10% [80].

Diagnostic uncertainty has led to antibiotic overuse in children with viral respiratory tract infections [81–83]. Improved methods for diagnosing pneumonia, especially in determining which children require antimicrobial therapy, are needed [70]. The use of biomarker-guided algorithms can assist with the decision-making for lower respiratory tract infections (LRTIs). Multiple studies including in total over 1000 children with either uncomplicated CAP [84], LRTIs, or pneumonia [85,86] evaluated the impact of an algorithm based on PCT use in adults. PCT-based decision categories for the likelihood of requiring antibiotic treatment of bacterial LRTI were "definitely" (>0.5 µg/L), "probably" (>0.25 µg/L), "probably not"(≤ 0.25 µg/L) and "definitely not" (<0.1 µg/L). Antibiotics can be stopped once the PCT levels fall under the 0.25 µg/L cutoff or with a reduction of up to 90% from peak value. All studies reported on a shorter time of antibiotic exposure with the help of the PCT algorithm (range between -5.6 and -1.8 days depending on severity and complications) and lower initial antibiotic prescription rates (65%–86%) compared to controls. One study did not show decreased prescriptions, but this might be due to the low baseline prescription rates in Switzerland. In one study, adherence to the PCT algorithm resulted in lower rate in antibiotic-related adverse events (3.9% vs 25.2% in controls) [84]. The potential stewardship benefits of PCT when used as intended are monumental.

OSTEOARTICULAR INFECTIONS

Incidence of pediatric osteoarticular infections is estimated to be 9.2 for acute osteomyelitis (OM) and 11.9 to 20.8 for septic arthritis (SA) per 100,000 [87,88]. There are significant differences between developed and developing regions and between age groups [89,90], whereas children aged below 2 years are the most affected. Failure to timely diagnose OM and septic SA can lead to devastating complications, including functional disabilities that occur in 25% to 50% of cases and can even be life-threatening in 5% to 15% of cases [91].

There is no single laboratory marker, which is sensitive and specific in diagnosing these infections accurately. Total WBC, erythrocyte sedimentation rate

(ESR), and CRP are not specific as they can also be elevated in nonpyogenic causes of inflammation [92]. A recent meta-analysis showed that PCT may serve as a biomarker for the diagnosis of OM, but specific optimal cutoffs and specific populations still need to be verified by large studies. No direct evidence was found to support the diagnosis of SA [93].

There are some studies that include children, which have studied the use of PCT to diagnose culture positive SA and OM versus presumed/nonpyogenic (cutoff 0.4 µg/L, 85.2% se, 87.3% sp) [94], and to differentiate acute bacterial SA from acute inflammatory arthritis (cutoff 0.5 µg/L, se 59%, sp 86%). Only synovial fluid WBC had a slightly higher AUC than PCT (0.78 vs 0.82). Combining PCT with other markers (CRP and ESR) did not improve performance [95]. In patients with rheumatoid arthritis (RA) presenting with complications, either noninfectious, nonbacterial infection or bacterial infection, all patients with acute RA flare had negative PCT (<0.1 µg/L). PCT was the only biomarker that could differentiate between the groups, though sensitivity for detecting bacterial infection was low. PCT of less than 0.5 µg/L does not rule out bacterial infection, and physicians should treat appropriately [96]. Elevated PCT has been documented to be a stronger indicator for pyogenic SA and OM than other inflammatory markers. More studies that include clinical variables other than inflammatory markers are needed to determine the added value of PCT in this patient group.

SUMMARY
Antibiotic stewardship
Implementing biomarker-guided algorithms facilitates antibiotic stewardship by aiding in the timely initiation, de-escalation, and discontinuation of antibiotic therapy. This approach can help mitigate the risk of unnecessary antibiotic use, reduce the emergence of antibiotic-resistant strains, and limit disruption of the microbiome.

Severity stratification
Biomarkers, especially PCT, show potential in stratifying the severity of infections. Elevated levels may indicate a higher risk of severe outcomes, allowing for targeted interventions and closer monitoring in pediatric patients identified as high risk.

Reduction of unnecessary procedures and hospitalizations
Lower levels of PCT are especially promising in ruling out infections. Integration of PCT into diagnostic protocols may reduce the need for unnecessary invasive procedures and hospitalizations in cases where bacterial etiology is less likely. This can streamline patient care, minimize discomfort, and optimize resource utilization.

Clinical decision support
Biomarker-guided algorithms provide valuable clinical decision support in pediatric emergency medicine. They assist health care providers in rapidly

assessing the likelihood of bacterial infections, aiding in prompt and appropriate interventions.

RECOMMENDATIONS
Implementation guidelines
For selected pediatric emergency conditions, develop and disseminate clear guidelines indicating where PCT in combination with other biomarkers can improve diagnostic accuracy. Standardized protocols will assist health care professionals in incorporating these tools effectively into their practice.

Educational initiatives
Launch educational initiatives to familiarize health care providers in pediatric emergency settings with the interpretation and application of PCT and other biomarkers. Training programs should include interpretation of algorithms and their application in differentiating bacterial from viral infections and guiding antibiotic decisions.

Research continuation
Encourage ongoing research initiatives to further validate the utility of PCT and other biomarkers in combination with clinical severity scores in diverse pediatric populations and various clinical scenarios. Continuous research will refine protocols and expand the evidence base supporting their use.

CLINICS CARE POINTS

- PCT is a biomarker not generally measurable in serum; levels greater than 0.5 ng/mL are indicative of bacterial infections.
- For detecting bacterial infections, PCT has a greater area under the receiver operating curve than CRP, ANC, or WBC.
- In combination with other clinical and laboratory indicators, PCT has been documented to have the greatest accuracy for detecting IBIs in febrile young infants; it should not be used as the solo predictor.
- PCT is helpful in distinguishing pyelonephritis from cystitis and predicting VUR.
- Antimicrobial usage, invasive testing, and hospitalizations can be decreased by PCT identifying conditions with low risk for bacterial infection and for guiding length of treatment.

DECLARATION OF CONFLICT
This review was developed following a meeting of the authors in September 2023 and conducted with a grant from Thermo Fisher Scientific. None of the authors declare any conflict of interest.

Acknowledgments
The authors thank Dr Beate Walter from B. M. Walter Medical Writing for the assistance in writing of the article.

Disclosure

The authors have nothing to disclose.

References

[1] Nijman RG, Oostenbrink R, Moll HA, et al. A novel framework for phenotyping children with suspected or confirmed infection for future biomarker studies. Front Pediatr 2021;9:688272.

[2] Buckley BS, Henschke N, Bergman H, et al. Impact of vaccination on antibiotic usage: a systematic review and meta-analysis. Clin Microbiol Infect 2019;25(10):1213–25.

[3] Grammatico-Guillon L, Jafarzadeh SR, Laurent E, et al. Gradual decline in outpatient antibiotic prescriptions in paediatrics: a data warehouse–based 11-year cohort study. Acta Paediatr 2021;110(2):611–7.

[4] Vidavalur R, Hussain N. Interstate practice variation and factors associated with antibiotic use for suspected neonatal sepsis in the United States. Am J Perinatol 2024;41(S 01): e1689–97.

[5] Gerber JS, Prasad PA, Fiks AG, et al. Effect of an outpatient antimicrobial stewardship intervention on broad-spectrum antibiotic prescribing by primary care pediatricians: a randomized trial. JAMA 2013;309(22):2345–52.

[6] Ramirez J, Guarner F, Bustos Fernandez L, et al. Antibiotics as major disruptors of gut microbiota. Front Cell Infect Microbiol 2020;10:572912.

[7] Bailey LC, Forrest CB, Zhang P, et al. Association of antibiotics in infancy with early childhood obesity. JAMA Pediatr 2014;168(11):1063–9.

[8] Bisgaard H, Li N, Bonnelykke K, et al. Reduced diversity of the intestinal microbiota during infancy is associated with increased risk of allergic disease at school age. J Allergy Clin Immunol 2011;128(3):646–52.e1-5.

[9] Abrahamsson TR, Jakobsson HE, Andersson AF, et al. Low gut microbiota diversity in early infancy precedes asthma at school age. Clin Exp Allergy 2014;44(6):842–50.

[10] Butel MJ, Waligora-Dupriet AJ, Wydau-Dematteis S. The developing gut microbiota and its consequences for health. J Dev Orig Health Dis 2018;9(6):590–7.

[11] Dagan R, Powell KR, Hall CB, et al. Identification of infants unlikely to have serious bacterial infection although hospitalized for suspected sepsis. J Pediatr 1985;107(6):855–60.

[12] Baskin MN, O'Rourke EJ, Fleisher GR. Outpatient treatment of febrile infants 28 to 89 days of age with intramuscular administration of ceftriaxone. J Pediatr 1992;120(1):22–7.

[13] Baker MD, Bell LM, Avner JR. Outpatient management without antibiotics of fever in selected infants. N Engl J Med 1993;329(20):1437–41.

[14] Shah P, Voice M, Calvo-Bado L, et al. Relationship between molecular pathogen detection and clinical disease in febrile children across Europe: a multicentre, prospective observational study. Lancet Reg Health Eur 2023;32; https://doi.org/10.1016/j.lanepe.2023.100682.

[15] Milcent K, Faesch S, Gras-Le Guen C, et al. Use of procalcitonin assays to predict serious bacterial infection in young febrile infants. JAMA Pediatr 2016;170(1):62–9.

[16] Póvoa P, Coelho L, Dal-Pizzol F, et al. How to use biomarkers of infection or sepsis at the bedside: guide to clinicians. Intensive Care Med 2023;49(2):142–53.

[17] Velasco R, Gomez B, Labiano I, et al. Performance of febrile infant algorithms by duration of fever. Pediatrics 2024; https://doi.org/10.1542/peds.2023-064342.

[18] Schuetz P, Wirz Y, Sager R, et al. Procalcitonin to initiate or discontinue antibiotics in acute respiratory tract infections. Cochrane Database Syst Rev 2017;10(10):CD007498.

[19] Geraerds A, van Herk W, Stocker M, et al. Cost impact of procalcitonin-guided decision making on duration of antibiotic therapy for suspected early-onset sepsis in neonates. Crit Care 2021;25(1):367.

[20] Gomez B, Mintegi S, Bressan S, et al. Validation of the "Step-by-Step" approach in the management of young febrile infants. Pediatrics 2016;138(2); https://doi.org/10.1542/peds.2015-4381.

[21] Kuppermann N, Dayan PS, Levine DA, et al. A clinical prediction rule to identify febrile infants 60 Days and younger at low risk for serious bacterial infections. JAMA Pediatr 2019;173(4):342–51.

[22] Greenhow TL, Hung YY, Herz AM. Changing epidemiology of bacteremia in infants aged 1 week to 3 months. Pediatrics 2012;129(3):e590–6.

[23] Biondi E, Evans R, Mischler M, et al. Epidemiology of bacteremia in febrile infants in the United States. Pediatrics 2013;132(6):990–6.

[24] Aronson PL, Shabanova V, Shapiro ED, et al. A prediction model to identify febrile infants ≤60 Days at low risk of invasive bacterial infection. Pediatrics 2019;144(1); https://doi.org/10.1542/peds.2018-3604.

[25] Lyons TW, Garro AC, Cruz AT, et al. Performance of the modified Boston and Philadelphia criteria for invasive bacterial infections. Pediatrics 2020;145(4); https://doi.org/10.1542/peds.2019-3538.

[26] Pantell RH, Newman TB, Bernzweig J, et al. Management and outcomes of care of fever in early infancy. JAMA 2004;291(10):1203–12.

[27] Norman-Bruce H, Umana E, Mills C, et al. Diagnostic test accuracy of procalcitonin and C-reactive protein for predicting invasive and serious bacterial infections in young febrile infants: a systematic review and meta-analysis. Lancet Child Adolesc Health 2024;8(5):358–68.

[28] Luaces-Cubells C, Mintegi S, García-García JJ, et al. Procalcitonin to detect invasive bacterial infection in non-toxic-appearing infants with fever without apparent source in the emergency department. Pediatr Infect Dis J 2012;31(6):645–7.

[29] Lacour AG, Zamora SA, Gervaix A. A score identifying serious bacterial infections in children with fever without source. Pediatr Infect Dis J 2008;27(7):654–6.

[30] Galetto-Lacour A, Zamora SA, Andreola B, et al. Validation of a laboratory risk index score for the identification of severe bacterial infection in children with fever without source. Arch Dis Child 2010;95(12):968–73.

[31] Kuppermann N, Mahajan P, Ramilo O. Prediction models for febrile infants: time for a unified field theory. Pediatrics 2019;144(1); https://doi.org/10.1542/peds.2019-1375.

[32] Pantell RH, Roberts KB, Adams WG, et al. Evaluation and management of well-appearing febrile infants 8 to 60 Days old. Pediatrics 2021;148(2); https://doi.org/10.1542/peds.2021-052228.

[33] Nguyen THP, Young BR, Alabaster A, et al. Using AAP guidelines for managing febrile infants without C-reactive protein and procalcitonin. Pediatrics 2022; https://doi.org/10.1542/peds.2022-058495.

[34] McDaniel CE, Kerns E, Jennings B, et al. Improving guideline-concordant care for febrile infants through a quality improvement initiative. Pediatrics 2024;153(5); https://doi.org/10.1542/peds.2023-063339.

[35] Dingle E, Pelletier JH, Forbes ML, Rajbhandari P. Resource utilization and cost in management of febrile infants after the 2021 clinical guideline. Pediatrics 2025;155(2):e2024068028.

[36] Hubert G, Launay E, Feildel Fournial C, et al. Assessment of the impact of a new sequential approach to antimicrobial use in young febrile children in the emergency department (DIA-FEVERCHILD): a French prospective multicentric controlled, open, cluster-randomised, parallel-group study protocol. BMJ Open 2020;10(8):e034828.

[37] Malorey D, Launay E, Tavernier E, Gras-Le Guen C. Impact d'un nouvel algorithme dans la prise en charge de la fièvre sans point d'appel du jeune enfant sur la prescription antibiotique aux urgences pédiatriques. Proceedings of the Congress of the French Pediatric Society, May 15, 2024. Nantes, France.

[38] Schlapbach LJ, Watson RS, Sorce LR, et al. International consensus criteria for pediatric sepsis and septic shock. JAMA 2024;331(8):665–74.

[39] Sanchez-Pinto LN, Bennett TD, DeWitt PE, et al. Development and validation of the Phoenix criteria for pediatric sepsis and septic shock. JAMA 2024;331(8):675–86.

[40] Weiss SL, Peters MJ, Alhazzani W, et al. Surviving sepsis campaign international guidelines for the management of septic shock and sepsis-associated organ dysfunction in children. Pediatr Crit Care Med 2020;21(2):e52–106.

[41] Tissieres P, Peters MJ, Kissoon N, et al. Might the surviving sepsis campaign international guidelines be less confusing? Authors' reply. Intensive Care Med 2020;46(8):1658–9.

[42] Kuzniewicz MW, Puopolo KM, Fischer A, et al. A quantitative, risk-based approach to the management of neonatal early-onset sepsis. JAMA Pediatr 2017;171(4):365–71.

[43] Lenihan RAF, Ang J, Pallmann P, et al. Mid-regional pro-adrenomedullin in combination with pediatric early warning scores for risk stratification of febrile children presenting to the emergency department: secondary analysis of a nonprespecified United Kingdom cohort study. Pediatr Crit Care Med 2022;23(12):980–9.

[44] Romaine ST, Potter J, Khanijau A, et al. Accuracy of a modified qSOFA score for predicting critical care admission in febrile children. Pediatrics 2020;146(4); https://doi.org/10.1542/peds.2020-0782.

[45] Bolanaki M. Biomarkers improve diagnostics of sepsis in adult patients with suspected organ dysfunction based on the quick sepsis-related organ failure assessment (qSOFA) score in the emergency department. Crit Care Med 2024; https://doi.org/10.1097/CCM.0000000000006216.

[46] Eisenberg M, Madden K, Christianson JR, et al. Performance of an automated screening algorithm for early detection of pediatric severe sepsis. Pediatr Crit Care Med 2019;20(12):e516–23.

[47] Sepanski RJ, Zaritsky AL, Godambe SA. Identifying children at high risk for infection-related decompensation using a predictive emergency department-based electronic assessment tool. Diagnosis (Berl) 2021;8(4):458–68.

[48] Keitel K, Kagoro F, Samaka J, et al. A novel electronic algorithm using host biomarker point-of-care tests for the management of febrile illnesses in Tanzanian children (e-POCT): a randomized, controlled non-inferiority trial. PLoS Med 2017;14(10):e1002411.

[49] Nigrovic LE, Kuppermann N, Malley R. Development and validation of a multivariable predictive model to distinguish bacterial from aseptic meningitis in children in the post-Haemophilus influenzae era. Pediatrics 2002;110(4):712–9.

[50] Kim H, Roh YH, Yoon SH. Blood procalcitonin level as a diagnostic marker of pediatric bacterial meningitis: a systematic review and meta-analysis. Diagnostics (Basel) 2021;11(5); https://doi.org/10.3390/diagnostics11050846.

[51] Garcia S, Echevarri J, Arana-Arri E, et al. Outpatient management of children at low risk for bacterial meningitis. Emerg Med J 2018;35(6):361–6.

[52] Dubos F, Korczowski B, Aygun DA, et al. Serum procalcitonin level and other biological markers to distinguish between bacterial and aseptic meningitis in children: a European multicenter case cohort study. Arch Pediatr Adolesc Med 2008;162(12):1157–63.

[53] Mintegi S, García S, Martín MJ, et al. Clinical prediction rule for distinguishing bacterial from aseptic meningitis. Pediatrics 2020;146(3); https://doi.org/10.1542/peds.2020-1126.

[54] Mattoo TK, Shaikh N, Nelson CP. Contemporary management of urinary tract infection in children. Pediatrics 2021;147(2); https://doi.org/10.1542/peds.2020-012138.

[55] Gervaix A, Galetto-Lacour A, Gueron T, et al. Usefulness of procalcitonin and C-reactive protein rapid tests for the management of children with urinary tract infection. Pediatr Infect Dis J 2001;20(5):507–11.

[56] Leroy S, Fernandez-Lopez A, Nikfar R, et al. Association of procalcitonin with acute pyelonephritis and renal scars in pediatric UTI. Pediatrics 2013;131(5):870–9.

[57] Shaikh KJ, Osio VA, Leeflang MMG, et al. Procalcitonin, C-reactive protein, and erythrocyte sedimentation rate for the diagnosis of acute pyelonephritis in children. Cochrane Database Syst Rev 2020;9; https://doi.org/10.1002/14651858.CD009185.pub3.

[58] Buettcher M, Trueck J, Niederer-Loher A, et al. Swiss consensus recommendations on urinary tract infections in children. Eur J Pediatr 2021;180(3):663–74.

[59] Benador N, Siegrist C-A, Gendrel D, et al. Procalcitonin is a marker of severity of renal lesions in pyelonephritis. Pediatrics 1998;102(6):1422–5.

[60] Hoberman A, Charron M, Hickey RW, et al. Imaging studies after a first febrile urinary tract infection in young children. N Engl J Med 2003;348(3):195–202.

[61] Leroy S, Romanello C, Galetto-Lacour A, et al. Procalcitonin to reduce the number of unnecessary cystographies in children with a urinary tract infection: a European validation study. J Pediatr 2007;150(1):89–95.

[62] Wallace SS, Zhang W, Mahmood NF, et al. Renal ultrasound for infants younger than 2 Months with a febrile urinary tract infection. AJR Am J Roentgenol 2015;205(4):894–8.

[63] Leroy S, Romanello C, Smolkin V, et al. Prediction of moderate and high grade vesicoureteral reflux after a first febrile urinary tract infection in children: construction and internal validation of a clinical decision rule. J Urol 2012;187(1):265–71.

[64] Ben Shimol S, Dagan R, Givon-Lavi N, et al. Evaluation of the World Health Organization criteria for chest radiographs for pneumonia diagnosis in children. Eur J Pediatr 2012;171(2):369–74.

[65] Shah SN, Bachur RG, Simel DL, et al. Does this child have pneumonia?: the rational clinical examination systematic review. JAMA 2017;318(5):462–71.

[66] Swingler GH. Observer variation in chest radiography of acute lower respiratory infections in children: a systematic review. BMC Med Imaging 2001;1(1):1.

[67] Virkki R, Juven T, Rikalainen H, et al. Differentiation of bacterial and viral pneumonia in children. Thorax 2002;57(5):438–41.

[68] Elemraid MA, Muller M, Spencer DA, et al. Accuracy of the interpretation of chest radiographs for the diagnosis of paediatric pneumonia. PLoS One 2014;9(8):e106051.

[69] Lynch T, Bialy L, Kellner JD, et al. A systematic review on the diagnosis of pediatric bacterial pneumonia: when gold is bronze. PLoS One 2010;5(8):e11989.

[70] Ramgopal S, Ambroggio L, Lorenz D, et al. A prediction model for pediatric radiographic pneumonia. Pediatrics 2022;149(1); https://doi.org/10.1542/peds.2021-051405.

[71] Ramgopal S, Lorenz D, Navanandan N, et al. Validation of prediction models for pneumonia among children in the emergency department. Pediatrics 2022;150(1); https://doi.org/10.1542/peds.2021-055641.

[72] Florin TA, Ambroggio L, Brokamp C, et al. Biomarkers and disease severity in children with community-acquired pneumonia. Pediatrics 2020;145(6); https://doi.org/10.1542/peds.2019-3728.

[73] Sartori LF, Zhu Y, Grijalva CG, et al. Pneumonia severity in children: utility of procalcitonin in risk stratification. Hosp Pediatr 2021;11(3):215–22.

[74] Florin TA, Ambroggio L, Brokamp C, et al. Reliability of examination findings in suspected community-acquired pneumonia. Pediatrics 2017;140(3); https://doi.org/10.1542/peds.2017-0310.

[75] Cohen JF, Leis A, Lecarpentier T, et al. Procalcitonin predicts response to beta-lactam treatment in hospitalized children with community-acquired pneumonia. PLoS One 2012;7(5):e36927.

[76] Balk DS, Lee C, Schafer J, et al. Lung ultrasound compared to chest X-ray for diagnosis of pediatric pneumonia: a meta-analysis. Pediatr Pulmonol 2018;53(8):1130–9.

[77] Orso D, Ban A, Guglielmo N. Lung ultrasound in diagnosing pneumonia in childhood: a systematic review and meta-analysis. J Ultrasound 2018;21(3):183–95.

[78] Elabbas A, Choudhary R, Gullapalli D, et al. Lung ultrasonography beyond the diagnosis of pediatrics pneumonia. Cureus 2022;14(2):e22460.

[79] Guitart C, Rodríguez-Fanjul J, Bobillo-Perez S, et al. An algorithm combining procalcitonin and lung ultrasound improves the diagnosis of bacterial pneumonia in critically ill children: the PROLUSP study, a randomized clinical trial. Pediatr Pulmonol 2022;57(3):711–23.

[80] Jones BP, Tay ET, Elikashvili I, et al. Feasibility and safety of substituting lung ultrasonography for chest radiography when diagnosing pneumonia in children: a randomized controlled trial. Chest 2016;150(1):131–8.

[81] Hersh AL, Shapiro DJ, Pavia AT, et al. Antibiotic prescribing in ambulatory pediatrics in the United States. Pediatrics 2011;128(6):1053–61.

[82] Nyquist AC, Gonzales R, Steiner JF, et al. Antibiotic prescribing for children with colds, upper respiratory tract infections, and bronchitis. JAMA 1998;279(11):875–7.

[83] Gonzales R, Malone DC, Maselli JH, et al. Excessive antibiotic use for acute respiratory infections in the United States. Clin Infect Dis 2001;33(6):757–62.

[84] Esposito S, Tagliabue C, Picciolli I, et al. Procalcitonin measurements for guiding antibiotic treatment in pediatric pneumonia. Respir Med 2011;105(12):1939–45.

[85] Baer G, Baumann P, Buettcher M, et al. Procalcitonin guidance to reduce antibiotic treatment of lower respiratory tract infection in children and adolescents (ProPAED): a randomized controlled trial. PLoS One 2013;8(8):e68419.

[86] Wu G, Wu G, Wu S, et al. Comparison of procalcitonin guidance-administered antibiotics with standard guidelines on antibiotic therapy in children with lower respiratory tract infections: a retrospective study in China. Med Princ Pract 2017;26(4):316–20.

[87] Walter N, Bärtl S, Alt V, et al. The epidemiology of osteomyelitis in children. Children 2021;8(11):1000.

[88] Kim J, Lee MU, Kim T-H. Nationwide epidemiologic study for pediatric osteomyelitis and septic arthritis in South Korea: a cross-sectional study of national health insurance review and assessment service. Medicine 2019;98(17):e15355.

[89] Riise ØR, Kirkhus E, Handeland KS, et al. Childhood osteomyelitis-incidence and differentiation from other acute onset musculoskeletal features in a population-based study. BMC Pediatr 2008;8:45.

[90] Montgomery NI, Epps HR. Pediatric septic arthritis. Orthop Clin North Am 2017;48(2): 209–16.

[91] Hatherill M, Tibby SM, Sykes K, et al. Diagnostic markers of infection: comparison of procalcitonin with C reactive protein and leucocyte count. Arch Dis Child 1999;81(5): 417–21.

[92] Mathews CJ, Weston VC, Jones A, et al. Bacterial septic arthritis in adults. Lancet 2010;375(9717):846–55.

[93] Zhang HT, Li C, Huang YZ, et al. Meta-analysis of serum procalcitonin diagnostic test accuracy for osteomyelitis and septic arthritis in children. J Pediatr Orthop B 2023;32(5):481–9.

[94] Maharajan K, Patro DK, Menon J, et al. Serum Procalcitonin is a sensitive and specific marker in the diagnosis of septic arthritis and acute osteomyelitis. J Orthop Surg Res 2013;8(1):19.

[95] Paosong S, Narongroeknawin P, Pakchotanon R, et al. Serum procalcitonin as a diagnostic aid in patients with acute bacterial septic arthritis. Int J Rheum Dis 2015;18(3):352–9.

[96] Sato H, Tanabe N, Murasawa A, et al. Procalcitonin is a specific marker for detecting bacterial infection in patients with rheumatoid arthritis. J Rheumatol 2012;39(8):1517–23.

Advances in Pediatrics 72 (2025) 41–56

ADVANCES IN PEDIATRICS

ELSEVIER
MOSBY

Seizures and Shaking in Newborns and Babies

Megan Langille, MD

David Geffen School of Medicine at UCLA, Harbor- UCLA, 1000 West Carson Street, Box 468, Torrance, CA 90509, USA

Keywords

- Neonatal seizures • Shaking • Seizure mimickers • Babies • Infants
- Abnormal movement

Key points

- Newborns and babies can present with movements that look like seizures but are nonepileptic and may not require any treatment besides reassurance.
- Over and under diagnosis of seizures should be avoided so that the management plan is appropriate.
- Movements more concerning for seizures may include *vital sign changes, stereotyped, occur across different setting/situations, are not stimulus induced/ trigger, involve head/eye movement, and cannot be stopped with repositioning.*
- Note any risk factors for seizures-birth history concerning for hypoxic-ischemic encephalopathy/prematurity/neonatal intensive care unit stay, genetic condition/diagnosis, developmental delay, and prior seizures.
- If seizures are suspected in a newborn or baby, the appropriate work up should follow, including electroencephalography and imaging.

INTRODUCTION

Seizures occur throughout all stages of childhood, but in the neonatal and infant period differentiating seizures from mimickers represents a unique challenge. Babies make many movements that could be mistaken for seizures, some even stereotyped and repetitive [1]. While these movements can represent serious conditions that require treatment, others are benign and call for only reassurance to the caregivers. Accurate diagnosis is essential to identify

E-mail address: mlangille@dhs.lacounty.gov

https://doi.org/10.1016/j.yapd.2025.01.001

seizures and to perform proper evaluation and prompt initiation of antiseizure medications (ASM). Proper diagnosis can spare a baby inappropriate use of ASM in nonepileptic conditions which could have harmful side effects.

Even for an experienced clinician it can be difficult to say if a neonate in the neonatal intensive care unit (NICU) is having a seizure or not based solely on witnessing the event. This can lead to both under and over diagnosis of seizures [2,3]. If the event is recurring, then capture on electroencephalography (EEG) can definitively characterize the episode. For many older infants and children, however, a thorough history of the event from an eyewitness with description of activity before, during, and after the event can be very useful. A video of the event, especially if recorded while the parent repositions or tries to interrupt the event can help clarify the diagnosis and guide work up. There are many possible nonepileptic conditions which may mimic seizures, these are outlined in Box 1.

Features more suggestive of a seizure (Box 2) include vital sign changes, abnormal eye/head movements, or movements that are not suppressible with position change [4]. It is important to ask if anything triggers an event or if the event is associated with certain activities or situations. Mimickers are more likely to have a trigger or association with location, activity, or emotion.

Another important consideration is a child's risk factors for seizures (Box 3), such as preterm birth, perinatal hypoxic-ischemic encephalopathy (HIE) or neurologic injury, autism, macro/microcephaly, developmental delay, or regression of development. If risk factors are present, then the potential yield of a seizure work up is increased.

Box 1 details common movements/conditions mistaken for seizures and divided by age of onset. We will focus on the neonatal, infant, and early childhood period, but of course mimickers can occur in all age groups.

SEIZURE MIMICKERS IN BABIES AND YOUNG CHILDREN
Neonatal Onset
Jitteriness
Jitteriness refers to recurrent tremor and the terms are often used interchangeably to denote involuntary, rhythmic, and oscillatory movement of equal

Box 1: Seizure mimics across childhood

Seizure Mimics Across Childhood		
Neonate		
Jitteriness		
Myoclonus		
Startle		
Neonatal extreme pain syndrome		
Benign neonatal sleep myoclonus		
Infancy		
	Early	**Late**
	Benign torticollis of infancy	
	Benign myoclonus of infancy	
	Alternating Hemiplegia of childhood	
	Sandifer Syndrome	
	Cardiac arrhythmia/syncope	
		Breath holding
		Shudder attacks
Toddler		
		Self stimulation behavior
		Breath Holding spells
		Benign Positional Vertigo
School age		
		Tics
		Stereotypies
		Parasomnias
		Vasovagal syncope
Adolescent		
		Hemiplegic migraine
		Narcolepsy/cataplexy
		Postural orthostatic hypotension (POTS)

amplitude around a fixed axis, with either fine or course quality. Jitteriness of the newborn is common and can be confused for seizures because it is a repetitive movement, but there are important distinctions.

Characteristics. The affected limb(s) may change laterality from event to event. Movement is increased or triggered when infant is unwrapped, upset, or startled. Movement is suppressed when baby is wrapped, soothed, or limb is repositioned or gently held. It is not associated with eye movements, or vital sign changes [4,5].

Epidemiology. Two-thirds of healthy neonates have some fine tremor in the first 3 days of life [6]. Neonatal tremor may be due to immaturity of spinal inhibitory interneurons causing an excessive muscle stretch reflex, and resolution occurs as baby grows [7]. While it can be physiologic, jitteriness is seen with drug withdrawal, metabolic derangements like hypoglycemia, hypocalcemia, infection or sepsis, brain injury like HIE, intracranial hemorrhage, or hyperthyroidism, and hypothermia [6,8].

What to expect. Studies have shown infants with jitteriness or tremor do well long-term with normal neurodevelopment unless there is history of perinatal

Box 2: Features of suggestive of seizure versus alternative diagnosis

Supportive of seizure	Less likely in seizures
Head/eye movements	Movements are random/nonrhythmic,
Stereotyped events	events look different each time
Change in vital signs	No Change in vital signs
Nonsuppressible	Suppressible with repositioning
Occur across different settings	Triggered by emotion, location, or
with no clear trigger	activity
Change in awareness	Aware and interactive during event
during event	Long events (over 10 min) with no
+ risk factor for seizure/epilepsy	postictal period
(see box 3)	

complications. Thirty percent of jittery neonates with a history of perinatal complications like HIE have abnormal neurodevelopment on follow-up [1,9].

Myoclonus

Myoclonus is a brief, sudden, shock-like jerking movement of a limb. It is irregular and arrhythmic with a higher amplitude than a tremor. Myoclonus can be a single or repetitive movement and can be localized to a body part or generalized. Myoclonus can originate from the cortex, brainstem, or spinal cord [10]. Myoclonus can be epileptic, but this is uncommon in the neonate [1,4].

Characteristics. Nonepileptic myoclonus can be suppressed with restraint or repositioning of affected body part and may be triggered by a stimulus unlike epileptic myoclonus. Nonepileptic neonatal myoclonus can be benign or could indicate an injury to the central nervous system (CNS). Neonates with pathologic myoclonus will have an abnormal neurologic examination, and EEG testing [5].

Epidemiology. Pathologic neonatal myoclonus can be seen with severe injuries like high-grade intraventricular hemorrhage, HIE, and glycine encephalopathy

Box 3: Screen for risk factors for seizures/epilepsy

Developmental delay/developmental regression, autism spectrum disorder

Prior seizure

Neonatal intensive care unit stay/premature birth/hypoxic-ischemic encephalopathy

Family history of epilepsy

Prior neruologic injury

[11]. Transient and benign myoclonus has been reported in premature neonates after benzodiazepine exposure [12].

What to expect. Myoclonus in the setting of a neonate with perinatal complications and/or an abnormal neurologic examination should prompt further work up for CNS injury, including an EEG and imaging.

Benign neonatal sleep myoclonus
Characteristics. Rhythmic myoclonic jerks seen only during sleep and usually bilateral and repetitive in contrast to adult sleep myoclonus which is typically a singular and unilateral jerk movement [13]. Episodes of synchronous or asynchronous myoclonus can be prolonged up to 1 hour if the child is not woken and this can lead to concern for status epilepticus [14]. It is distinguished from seizures because it only occurs during sleep and stops as soon as the baby is awakened. It is typically seen in healthy and full-term infants. Unlike other seizure mimics restraining or holding the shaking limb(s) could worsen the movement. If an EEG is obtained, it will be normal without discharges during the movement. Movement can be provoked during an EEG by rocking the baby gently in head-to-toe direction and gradually increasing speed [15].

Epidemiology. Benign neonatal sleep myoclonus begins in the first few days of life and occurs in 0.8 to 3/1000 newborns. One proposal for the underlying mechanism causing the movement is immaturity of serotonergic pathways in the brainstem which would normally suppress movement during sleep [16].

What to expect. Stops spontaneously at around 4 months of age.

Startle disease or neonatal hyperekplexia
Characteristics. A rare disorder with generalized rigidity of muscles and nocturnal myoclonus and an exaggerated startle reaction to sound, touch, and even visual stimuli. The startle movement involves facial grimacing and blinking followed by flexion of the trunk. Babies can have a more dramatic startle response characterized by generalized tonic spasm with tonic flexion of limbs and trunk with clenching of fists. Apnea can occur with these movements due to chest wall tightness. Babies remain awake and aware during the movements. Startle can be triggered by light tap to glabella and does not habituate with repeat taps [17].

Epidemiology. Symptoms begin shortly after birth in a neonate without a history of perinatal complications. It is a familial condition inherited in autosomal recessive manner associated with gene mutations in GLRA1, GLRB, and SLC6A5 [18].

What to expect. Clonazepam can help lessen startle response. EEG may be done to help rule out seizures, and genetic testing to aid in diagnosis and counseling. Generalized stiffness decreases around a year of age, while startle responses persist often until adolescents or even continue through adulthood. Some children have mild intellectual disability [17].

Infant Onset

Benign paroxysmal torticollis of infancy

Recurrent episodes of painless head tilting likely secondary to cervical dystonia.

Characteristics. Episodes of torticollis that can last minutes and sometimes even weeks. May shift in laterality between attacks and are accompanied by pallor, vomiting, ataxia, and irritability [5].

Epidemiology. Begins in the first few months of life. May indicate a propensity to have migraines later in life and usually there is a strong family history of migraines (55%) [19]. Gross or fine motor delays may develop but are likely to resolve completely with therapy and follow-up.

What to expect. Episodes completely resolve by school age, usually head tilt is less prominent after infancy, but may be replaced with benign positional vertigo, cyclic vomiting, and then later migraine headaches. Treatment is not necessary for brief episodes, but an association exists between longer episodes and developmental delay. Benign paroxysmal torticollis of infancy is a rare condition so the literature on treatment is sparse. Topiramate can be an effective management option. Antiinflammatory and antinausea medications can also be considered [19].

Benign myoclonus of infancy

Characteristics. Presents as brief jerking movements with flexion or extension of trunk, limbs, and head. Movements appear similar to infantile spasms, but only occur when the baby is awake while infantile spasms would also occur during sleep and there is no association of benign myoclonus of infancy with developmental regression or underlying medical conditions.

Epidemiology. Benign myoclonus of infancy usually presents between 3 and 15 months but can begin even in the neonatal period. The condition occurs in healthy babies without risk factors for epilepsy.

What to expect. May need EEG to rule out seizures/infantile spasms. Events will remit and are not associated with any neurodevelopmental delay. If the myoclonus begins earlier in infancy, events are likely to stop by 9 months of age, however, if onset is later in infancy, then events are likely to persist to 2 years of age [20].

Alternating hemiplegia of childhood

Characteristics. Intermittent, alternating episodes of hemiplegia lasting minutes to 2 weeks. Triggers are multiple and include irregular sleep, diet, water exposure, cold, and certain physical activities. The weak side can change during an episode or from one episode to the next. Besides paralysis, children can experience choreoathetosis, dystonia, nystagmus, and dyspnea. Also, they may have sudden flushing or pallor, and this can be during an episode of weakness or occur separately. Symptoms abate completely during sleep but can restart after awakening.

Cognitive function is also affected, with nearly all affected individuals having some degree of developmental delay and intellectual disability [21].

Epidemiology. Average age of onset is between 3.5 and 8 months. This is a rare diagnosis with an incidence of 1:1,000,000 children [22]. Mutations in ATPA3 gene are most common. It may initially worsen, but overtime decreases overall.

What to expect. EEG and imaging are done to rule out stroke and vasculopathy. There is no cure; medication may lessen severity and frequency of episodes.

Sandifer syndrome
Characteristics. Episodes of abnormal posturing can include back arching, posturing/stiffening of limbs, neck, arms, and/or turning/tilting of the head. Babies are awake and alert during the movement but are often upset, fussy, and/ or crying. There should be a clear pattern of movement following feeds.

Epidemiology. Occurs in children under 2 who have gastroesophageal reflux disorder (GERD) or hiatal hernia. May be seen in neurologic abnormalities. There is an association with severe hypotonia and feeding difficulties like frequent spit ups.

What to do next. If movement always follows feeding, then baby should be evaluated for GERD. If movements occur before feeds or in a more sporadic manner, then neurology referral and work up for seizures is prudent. Sandifer syndrome is likely to resolve over time, treatment should focus on GERD management—medications, change in feeding quantity, or formula or position, gastrointestinal (GI) referral may be needed, and some children may undergo Nissen fundoplication [23].

Syncope
Characteristics. Can occur at any age including in infancy and in young children. Syncope can present with sudden loss of consciousness as well as pallor, loss of tone, or tonic posturing. These can be symptoms prior to the event like dizziness, nausea, heart palpitations, or tunnel vision. Children may have posturing or shaking briefly after the syncopal event. Loss of urine can also occur during syncope or seizures. After syncope, a child may be more fatigued but should not have frank confusion or alteration as one might see during a postictal period. Also, movements in a seizure tend to last longer, and in terms of loss of tone, a person who has syncope will be more likely to brace themselves for a fall compared to someone experiencing a seizure.

Epidemiology. Majority of syncope in children is vasovagal in nature, but if syncope occurs in young children, then a work up for an arrythmia should be considered.

What to expect. Work up and prognosis will depend on the exact etiology for syncope.

Breath-holding spells
Characteristics. Are associated with either pallor or cyanosis. Usually there are triggers, but it is an involuntary event. A classic example is a child hurts themselves

is upset and crying and the breath-holding spells occurs after an expiration. A child may have stiffness or involuntary convulsions or a transient loss of consciousness, which can lead to confusion with seizures. They are often precipitated by fright, pain, and crying.

Epidemiology. *Breath holding spells* effect 0.1% to 4.6% of children. They typically have no seizure risk factors or other health concerns. They usually start between 6 and 18 months and reach a peak around 12 to 14 months. Sometimes, there is a family history of breath-holding spells [24].

What to expect. Check for iron deficiency or anemia, some evidence suggest children may have fewer and less severe episodes with supplementation even if they are not deficient [25]. Some genetic syndromes have an association with breath-holding spells and with particularly early and severe episodes. There is no role for antiseizure medication. Many children will not need treatment, but glycopyrrolate and atropine have been used for severe and frequent episodes.

Shudder attacks
Episodes begin in late infancy and often concern for seizure arises because episodes do appear as stereotyped shaking/stiffening.

Characteristics. Brief and sudden onset of involuntary stiffening with shoulder shaking, and upper extremities, sometimes trunk and sometimes facial expression changes which lasts several seconds up to 15 seconds duration. Babies are awake and aware during the whole episode, they do not occur in sleep. Often movement is triggered by excitement, eating, or frustration. A classic scenario is a baby is in a highchair and when they see their food they will have a brief shudder attack. However, episodes can occur anytime throughout the day and may happen many times and seemingly without a trigger, although they tend to be more frequent at mealtime.

Epidemiology. Occur in otherwise healthy children without risk factors for epilepsy. Many mechanisms have been proposed but it is unclear what causes shudder attacks and no clear association with future neurologic issues has been substantiated.

What to expect. Benign movement that resolves without intervention over time, and does not require medication. Antiseizure medication does not reduce episodes and has no role in treatment [26].

Early Childhood Onset
Self-stimulation behavior
Previously called infantile masturbation, events with rhythmic hip flexion and adduction with legs crossing, may occur more when in highchair or car seat, or child may lay/lean on wall/table. Parents may describe eyes as "glazed over" or distant expression but child is completely conscious and will interact. Parents can interrupt the event, but child may be mad or resume the movement once able. Child may grunt, flush, or sweat. History alone often is enough

to make diagnosis and need no further work up. It is helpful if the parent has videoed the episode.

Benign paroxysmal vertigo
Events occur abruptly in children 2 to 5 years of age with vertigo, nystagmus, and ataxia. Often a child may look scared, grab onto parent, and stop moving during the event. In a very young child, it may be difficult for them to communicate what they feel. Benign paroxysmal vertigo (BPV) occurs in 2% of children and some will have a history of benign paroxysmal torticollis of infancy (BPTI) as an infant. BPV is also thought to be a migraine precursor. BPV can be brought on by stress, lack of sleep, hunger, lights, and change in schedule/travel.

Parasomnias
Examples of parasomnias with features easy to confuse wiith seizures include night terrors, confusional arousals, and sleepwalking. Parasomnias occur in the first few hours of sleep (non-rapid eye movement [REM] sleep). Episodes last at least 3 to 5 minutes and may occur intermittently. Parasomnias can be distinguished from frontal lobe seizures which typically are frequent and happen throughout the night. Episodes of frontal lobe seizures are shorter lasting less than 2 minutes.

Tics
Tics are involuntary, sudden, rapid movements or vocalizations (sniffing, coughing, throat clearing, or words) that can be repetitive. They can be simple or complex. Tics are nonrhythmic in contrast to seizures. Children with tics may report feeling an urge to make the movement that alleviates the urge once the movement is made. They can temporarily suppress the tic but this leads to discomfort and distress. Tics remit during sleep and are interruptible. The frequency/severity of tics has a waxing and waning quality. Common triggers are stress, excitement, fatigue, and illness. Often a tic occurs for a period of time and then a new tic "replaces" the first, one but old and new tics can co-occur. Tics tend to decrease when a child is concentrating or absorbed in an activity [27]. Tics generally begin between 3 and 8 years of age. Almost a quarter of children (24%) will have transient tics which eventually subside. Tourette's syndrome (TS) requires a combination of vocal and motor tics for 1 year. One-third of those with TS will continue to have tics in adulthood, a third will have resolution of tics, and a third will have improvement of tics. Education of caregivers is important to reinforce that tics are not dangerous or cause bodily harm to the child. In fact, children are often unaware of their tics unless someone else brings it up. If the tics are bothering the child or creating social difficulties, then behavioral intervention is first line for a child who can cooperate. Medications can be considered next including guanfacine, clonidine, and topiramate. It is important to screen for attention deficit hyperactivity disorder, anxiety, and obsessive-compulsive disorder which can run together with tics particularly in those with TS.

Stereotypies
These are rhythmic, involuntary movements (body rocking, head rocking/bobbing, hand flapping/wrist shaking) that can be interrupted. The child is aware/awake the whole time. Usually these movements begin by 3 years of age, and while they can be seen in neurotypical children they are more likely in children with autism or atypical neurodevelopment. Stereotypies can present in babies as head bobbing, shivering movements [28]. Children are not bothered or even aware of the movements. Movements may come out more when the child is concentrating or excited. They are distinguished from seizures because they are interruptible and have triggers that cause or exacerbate episodes.

Adolescent Onset
Postural orthostatic tachycardia syndrome
POTS are episodes of light headedness, vision blurring, and chest discomfort. Prolonged standing can trigger or precede the event; laying or sitting down can resolve symptoms, but the child may experience postevent fatigue.

Narcolepsy/cataplexy
Daytime sleepiness, cataplexy, or loss of tone in response to strong emotion like startle/fear are hallmarks. Teens can have sleep paralysis and hypnagogic hallucinations.

Hemiplegic migraine
Classified as migraines with an aura and focal weakness. Sometimes speech disturbance, visual symptoms, and paresthesia may also occur as aura prior to migrainous headache. Weakness has been reported to last for weeks in some patients. If there is a family history, then genetic investigation may reveal mutations in CACNA1A, ATP1A2, or SCN1A. This is a rare condition.

Neonatal and infantile epilepsies
Neonatal and infantile-onset seizures can have many underlying etiologies but most often there is a history compatible with brain injury like HIE or ischemic stroke or hemorrhage and work up including EEG and neuroimaging and labs for reversible metabolic derangements aid in proper diagnosis. Once structural or metabolic conditions are properly ruled out, genetic neonatal epilepsies should be considered. Some are benign and require no or limited treatment and others are severe and will require lifelong treatment and have poor long-term neurodevelopmental prognosis. Box 4 highlights features of genetic epilepsy disorders [29].

Self-limited familial or nonfamilial epilepsy
- *Self-limited neonatal (familial) epilepsy*
- *Self-limited infantile (familial) epilepsy*
- *Self-limited neonatal infantile (familial) epilepsy*

The term self-limited (familial) epilepsy applies to babies with the onset of seizures as a neonate or infant, and the seizures remit over time with normal

Box 4: Neonatal and infantile epilepsy syndromes

Diagnosis	Associated seizure type	Onset	Involved genes	Prognosis	NOTES/alternate names
Self-limited neonatal familial epilepsy	Focal motor seizures, may have apnea or autonomic changes, often are frequent when they first occur.	Usually 2–3 d of life, can be up to 3 mo of age	KCNQ2, KCNQ3, SCN2A	Normal development seizure typically remit by 6 mo, often by 6 wk some children may go onto have epilepsy.	Often are started on medication but able to wean off.
Self-limited familial infantile epilepsy	Focal motor seizures, brief	3–20 mo, 6 mo most common	PRRT2, SCN8A	Seizure remission by age 2 is typical, may have risk of seizures later in life.	
Self-limited familial neonatal-infantile epilepsy	Sequential focal motor seizures, ± apnea/cyanosis	Birth–23 mo 13 wk most common	SCN2A	Seizure remission by age 2 is typical. May have risk of seizures later in life.	Requires family members with both neonatal and infantile onset.
Genetic epilepsy febrile seizure +(GEFS+)	Variable, generalized tonic-clonic, or focal seizure.	6 mo+	SCN1A	Children do very well, normal development but may have occasional febrile or afebrile seizures into adolescence.	
Myoclonic epilepsy in infancy	Myoclonic seizures, often triggered by noise/touch.	6 mo–2 y	SLC2A1, HCN4	Seizures remit by age 6; minority may have other seizure types later in life. Some will have cognitive/motor delay later in childhood.	

(continued on next page)

(continued)

Diagnosis	Associated seizure type	Onset	Involved genes	Prognosis	NOTES/alternate names
Early infantile epileptic encephalopathy	Epileptic spams and tonic seizures	2 wk-3 mo	ARX, CDKL5, SLC25A22, STXBP1, KCNQ2, SPTAN1, SCN2A	Severe neurodevelopmental disabilities, intractable seizures, early mortality.	Ohtahara syndrome Electroencephalography shows burst suppression magnetic resonance imaging may show lesion.
Early myoclonic encephalopathy	Multifocal myoclonus	Birth to months	STXBP1, TBC1D24, GABRA1	Severe neurodevelopmental disabilities, early mortality	
Epilepsy in infancy with migrating focal seizures	Focal clonic/tonic seizures	Days to months	SLC25A22, TBC1D24, KCNT1, SCN1A, SCN2A, PLCB1, QARS	Severe neurodevelopmental disabilities, refractory seizures	
Infantile spasms	Spasms occurring in clusters, arms, and trunk flex, can rarely have extensor spams with opisthotonic posture.	3–12 mo	variable	Neurodevelopmental delay/disabilities common esp with incomplete response to medication, spasms may be replaced with multiple types of treatment refractory seizures.	West syndrome/Infantile Epileptic Spasms Syndrome Diverse underlying etiology
Dravet Syndrome	Seizures triggered by fever/heat, prone to prolonged seizures	6–18 mo	SCN1A	Early development is normal, over time speech delay and further neurodevelopmental disabilities and refractory seizures become apparent.	Severe myoclonic epilepsy of infancy. May present with febrile seizures first.

neurodevelopment. All are autosomal dominant disorders with pathologic variants in several key genes. Importantly, neuroimaging and laboratory studies are normal and often the family history is positive for self-limited seizures in other family members including parents. If there is no family history, it is possible the child represents a de novo variant. Also, incomplete penetrance has been described in all associated genes so parents could be asymptomatic carriers [29].

Gene testing is helpful to determine the best medication choice and may aid in determining the prognosis as some gene variants are associated with epilepsy later in life.

Generalized epilepsy with febrile seizures
Generalized epilepsy with febrile seizures plus (GEFS+) is a group of genetic epilepsy syndromes which often present during the first year of life. The most common and mildest phenotype of the GEFS + spectrum is simple febrile seizures, which begin in infancy and usually stop by age 5. When the febrile seizures continue after age 5 or other types of seizure develop, the condition is called febrile seizures plus (FS+). Seizures in FS + usually end in early adolescence. GEFS+ is associated with an autosomal dominant pattern and is caused by variations in SCN1B which encodes the beta 1 subunit of sodium channels. At the more severe end of the spectrum is Dravet syndrome described later.

Within a family with GEFS+, the phenotype can vary widely from person to person. Each person even within the same family can have different combinations of febrile seizures and epilepsy/seizure types. For example, one family member may have only febrile seizures, while another also has afebrile seizures, or another has febrile seizures but well beyond the typical age range, sometimes into adolescence. While GEFS+ is usually diagnosed in families, it can occur in individuals with no history of the condition in their family.

Ohtahara syndrome/early infantile epileptic encephalopathy
Ohtahara or early infantile epileptic encephalopathy is a rare cause of seizures in neonates and infants. Often the first seizure is around 2 weeks of age but can present as late as 3 months of age. Spasms or tonic seizures occur out of sleep and while baby is awake and can recur even hundreds of times per day [30].

Most often associated with structural brain abnormalities some pathogenic variations in various genes have been described (see Box 4). The EEG pattern will show burst suppression. As children grow, other seizure types may develop. Seizures are difficult to control, highly refractory to medication, and babies have high early in life mortality rates. Those who survive will have a high seizure burden, and severe neurodevelopmental disabilities. As they grow, there can be progression to a Lennox Gastault phenotype where assistance for activities of daily living and refractory seizures are characteristic.

Infantile spasms/infantile epileptic spasm syndrome
Infantile spasm or IESS are terms that include babies and children who might not fit into West syndrome criteria, but often the terms are used interchangeably. West syndrome was named after Dr William West who had a child with

infantile spasms and in his letter to Lancet in 1841 wrote a still classic description including characteristics of the spasms, onset in the first year of life and developmental delay, and disability [31,32]. A characteristic abnormal EEG pattern-(hypsarrhythmia), and regression/plateau in development as well as ramping up of events to many times a day in clusters are common. Etiology is diverse and includes structural abnormalities, genetic syndromes, as well as acquired postnatal injuries, traumatic brain injury, survivors of submersion injuries, and survivors of serious CNS infections. Pathophysiology is still poorly understood. Differential diagnoses include less serious conditions like colic, GERD, or benign neonatal sleep myoclonus. More severe conditions like other types of seizures/encephalopathy may also be on the differential. An EEG is helpful to distinguish, but if done very soon after start of spasms can be negative and so should be repeated. Prognosis is poor for many, especially if a child has an underlying condition with neurodevelopmental disabilities. Shorter time from onset of spasms to diagnosis and treatment initiation can have a more favorable outcome underscoring the importance of prompt diagnosis.

Dravet syndrome
Dravet syndrome, known in the past as severe myoclonic epilepsy of infancy, is a rare developmental and epileptic encephalopathy characterized by febrile seizures in the first year of life that become frequent, recurrent, and treatment-resistant seizures both with and without fever. Eighty percent of patients have a pathogenic variant in the sodium channel gene SCN1A. Dravet syndrome is sometimes considered on spectrum with GEFS+.

In about half of cases, the first seizure is in the setting of a fever so the diagnosis of febrile seizure may be given initially until seizures become more frequent and occur when the child is afebrile. Seizures also tend to be prolonged. Triggers for seizures include heat like hot baths, immunizations, sunlight, exercise, or stress/excitement.

Complications include developmental delay/disability, sleeping issues, and risk of mortality from sudden unexpected death of epileptic person.

SUMMARY
Babies and small children can have movements that are mimickers for seizures but are nonepileptic and call only for reassurance. It is important over and under diagnosis of seizures be avoided so that the management plan is appropriate.

A thorough description of the event and the child's medical history help guide the work up and treatment decisions. Features more suggestive of seizure are *vital sign changes, stereotyped, occur across different setting/situations, involve head/eye movement, cannot be stopped with repositioning, and are not stimulus induced/trigger.*

If a child's medical history is positive for risk factors for seizures, then further work up may be necessary. Risk factors include birth history concerning for HIE/prematurity/NICU stay, genetic condition/diagnosis, developmental delay, and prior seizures.

EEG and imaging may be necessary when seizure disorder is suspected and can clarify diagnosis. There are many neonatal and infantile epilepsies to consider on the differential and treatment and prognosis varies depending on diagnosis.

CLINICS CARE POINTS

- Determining whether an event is seizure or not based on witnessing the event in neonates is unreliable and can lead to both under and over diagnosis.
- A thorough history of the event from an eyewitness with description of activity before, during and after the event can be very useful.
- A video of the event, especially if one event is recorded while parent repositions or tries to interrupt event.
- Movements which mimics seizures will change across the age spectrum from newborn to infant, toddler and adolscent/adult.

References
[1] Huntsman RJ, Lowry NJ, Sankaran K. Nonepileptic motor phenomena in the neonate. Paediatr Child Health 2008;13(8):680–4.
[2] Malone A, Ryan CA, Fitzgerald A, et al. Interobserver agreement in neonatal seizure identification. Epilepsia 2009;50(09):2097–101.
[3] Murray DM, Boylan GB, Ali I, et al. Defining the gap between electrographic seizure burden, clinical expression and staff recognition of neonatal seizures. Arch Dis Child Fetal Neonatal Ed 2008;93(03):F187–91.
[4] Volpe JJ. Neonatal seizures: neurology of the newborn. 4th edition. Philadelphia (PA): WB Saunders Elsevier; 2001.
[5] Stainman R, Kossoff E. Seizure mimics in children: an age-based approach. Curr Probl Pediatr Adolesc Health Care 2020;50:100894.
[6] Armentrout DC, Caple J. The jittery newborn. J Pediatri Health Care 2001;15:147–9.
[7] Shuper A, Zalzberg J, Weitz R, et al. Jitteriness beyond the neonatal period: a benign pattern of movement in infancy. J Child Neurol 1991;6:243–5.
[8] Rossman NP, Donelly JH, Bruan MA. The jittery newborn and infant: a review. Dev Behav Pediatr 1984;5:263–73.
[9] Futagi Y, Suzuki Y, Toribe Y, et al. Neurologic outcomes of infants with tremor within the first year of life. Pediatri Neurol 1999;21:557–61.
[10] Cohen R, Shuper A, Straussberg R. Familial benign neonatal sleep myoclonus. Pediatr Neurol 2007;36:334–7.
[11] Sher MS. Pathological myoclonus of the newborn: electrographic and clinical correlations. Pediatr Neurol 1985;1:342–8.
[12] Lee DS, Wong HA, Knoppert DC. Myoclonus associated with lorazepam therapy in very low birth weight infants. Biol Neonate 1994;6:311–5.
[13] Turanli G, Senbil N, Altunbasak S, et al. Benign neonatal sleep myoclonus mimicking status epilepticus. J Child Neurol 2004;19:62–3.
[14] Ramelli GP, Sozzo AB, Vella S, et al. Benign neonatal sleep myoclonus: an under recognized, non epileptic condition. Acta pedatr 2005;94:962–3.
[15] Alfonso L, Papazian O, Aicardi J, et al. A simple maneuver to provoke benign neonatal sleep myoclonus. Pedatrics 1995;96:1161–3.
[16] Nagy E, Hollody K. Parosxymal non epileptic events in infancy: five cases with typical features. Epileptic Disord 2019;21:458–62.

[17] Scarcella A, Coppola G. Neonatal sporadic hyperekplexia: a rare and often unrecognized entity. Brain Dev 1997;19:226–8.

[18] Dreissen YEM, Bakker MJ, Koelmann JHTM, et al. Exaggerated startle reactions. Clin Neurophysiol 2012;123:34–44.

[19] Gelfand AA. Episodic syndromes of childhood associated with migraine. Curr Opin Neurol 2018;31:281–5.

[20] Fine A, Wirrell E. Seizures in children. Peds in Review 2020;41(7):321–46.

[21] Capuano A, Garone G, Tiralongo G, et al. Alternating hemiplegia of childhood: understanding the genotype-phenotype relationship of ATP1A3 variations. Appl Clin Genet 2020;13:71–81.

[22] Lagman-Bartolome AM, Lay C. Pediatric migraine variants: a review of epidemiology, diagnosis, treatment, and outcome. Curr Neurol Neurosci Rep 2015;15(6):34.

[23] Mindlina I. Diagnosis and management of Sandifer syndrome in children with intractable neurological symptoms. Eur J Pediatr 2020;179(2):243–50.

[24] Leung AKC, Leung AAM, Wong AHC, et al. Breath-holding spells in pediatrics: a narrative review of the current evidence. Curr Pediatr Rev 2019;15(1):22–9.

[25] Zehetner AA, Orr N, Buckmaster A, et al. Iron supplementation for breath-holding attacks in children. Cochrane Database Syst Rev 2010;5:CD008132.

[26] Wang JJ, Goldman RD. Shuddering attacks: a benign phenomenon in children. Can Fam Physician 2021;67(2):107–8.

[27] Singer HS. Tics and tourette syndrome. Contin Lifelong Learn Neurol 2019;25:936–58.

[28] Mackenzie K. Stereotypic movement disorders. Semin Pediatr Neurol 2018;25:19–24.

[29] Millevert C, Weckhuysen S. ILAE Genetics Commission. ILAE Genetic Literacy Series: self-limited familial epilepsy syndromes with onset in neonatal age and infancy. Epileptic Disord 2023;25(4):445–53.

[30] Beal JC, Cherian K, Moshe SL. Early-onset epileptic encephalopathies: ohtahara syndrome and early myoclonic encephalopathy. Pediatr Neurol 2012;47(5):317–23.

[31] Eling P, Renier WO, Pomper J, et al. The mystery of the Doctor's son, or the riddle of West syndrome. Neurology 2002;58(6):953–5.

[32] Cardenal-Muñoz E, Auvin S, Villanueva V, et al. Guidance on Dravet syndrome from infant to adult care: road map for treatment planning in Europe. Epilepsia Open 2022;7(1): 11–26.

Advances in Pediatrics 72 (2025) 57–68

ADVANCES IN PEDIATRICS

The Ouchless Pediatric Emergency Department

Sergey Kunkov, MD, MS, MBA

Department of Pediatrics, Texas Tech University Health Sciences Center, 3601 4th Street, Stop 9406, Lubbock, TX 79430, USA

Keywords
• Pain • Children • Emergency • Ouchless

Key points

- *Multidisciplinary approach*: Combine pharmacologic, nonpharmacologic, and environmental strategies to reduce pain and anxiety, promoting humane and accessible care in pediatric emergency departments (PEDs).
- *Nonpharmacologic techniques*: Use distraction (eg, storytelling, toys, virtual reality) and cognitive-behavioral strategies, tailored to developmental needs, as cost-effective first-line defenses against pain and anxiety.
- *Pharmacologic interventions*: Employ topical anesthetics, intranasal medications, or sedation protocols for rapid relief when nonpharmacologic methods are insufficient, focusing on minimal invasiveness and safety.
- *Environmental modifications*: Create sensory-friendly, child-centered PED settings with dimmable lighting, interactive play areas, and quiet spaces to reduce anxiety, especially in sensory-sensitive children.
- *Parental involvement*: Engage parents and child life specialists to provide emotional support, manage procedural distress, reduce sedation needs, and improve overall pediatric care experiences.

INTRODUCTION

Pediatric emergency medicine has increasingly embraced the concept of "ouchless care," an approach that focuses on preventing or reducing pain and anxiety during emergency medical treatment. This model addresses not only the physical discomfort of the child but also the emotional and psychological components of their experience in the emergency department (ED). Given the developmental sensitivity of children, unaddressed pain can lead to long-term physical and psychological sequelae, including increased pain perception in future medical encounters and avoidance of health care [1].

E-mail address: sergey.kunkov@ttuhsc.edu

https://doi.org/10.1016/j.yapd.2025.02.001

Abbreviations
ED   emergency department
IV   intravenous
VR   virtual reality

THE HISTORY AND EVOLUTION OF THE OUCHLESS APPROACH IN PEDIATRIC EMERGENCY CARE

The "ouchless approach" in pediatric emergency care has evolved over decades, rooted in growing recognition of the physical and emotional impact of pain and anxiety on children. Its development has been shaped by shifts in medical understanding, cultural attitudes toward pediatric pain, and technological innovations. What began as an acknowledgment of children's unique needs has blossomed into a comprehensive framework that integrates medical, psychological, and environmental strategies to improve the care experience.

THE EARLY DAYS: OVERLOOKING PEDIATRIC PAIN

For much of medical history, pediatric pain was underestimated or outright ignored. Until the midtwentieth century, many believed that children, particularly neonates, had underdeveloped nervous systems and lacked the capacity to feel or remember pain. This misconception led to inadequate pain management in children undergoing medical procedures, including surgeries performed without anesthesia [2].

The turning point came in the 1980s, with groundbreaking research disproving these myths [2,3].

Studies demonstrated that infants and children possess fully developed pain receptors and that untreated pain could have both immediate and long-term consequences, including heightened pain sensitivity and psychological trauma [4]. These findings catalyzed a shift in attitudes, making pediatric pain management a growing priority.

"Ouchless APPROACH" COMING OF AGE

The Dr Neil Schechter and colleagues' [5] article in Pediatrics in 1997, "The Ouchless Place: No Pain, Children's Gain," was the first description of a multidisciplinary pain interest group building a comprehensive program of uniform assessment and treatment of pain in children within a single medical center. This was also the first mentioning of the "ouchless" approach in the medical literature. In 2001, Joint Commission on the Accreditation of Healthcare Organizations issued a report stating that during the hospitals' accreditation process, they will also be evaluated on the adequacy of their pain control measures [6].

Nevertheless, the progress was hard, and over the next decade, there were multiple studies documenting inadequate pain control in children both in the United States and in Europe [7,8].

In 2008 Dr Schechter published a follow-up report "From the Ouchless Place to Comfort Central: The Evolution of a Concept" depicting evolution of the concept and recognizing that while a true ouch (or pain)-free place is difficult to create, organizational efforts to maximize comfort in children should be undertaken in a systematic manner [9].

Over the past 10 to 15 years, multiple children's hospitals' EDs adopted ouchless approach [10–12]. "Ouchless" pediatric medicine was also featured in national media [13], raising awareness of the pain management challenges in sick and injured children and approaches to fast and safe pain relief in emergency situations.

RATIONALE FOR AN OUCHLESS APPROACH

Creating an "ouchless" pediatric emergency department (PED) is more than just a patient-centered approach; it is a transformative philosophy under which pediatric pain and anxiety, both of which are historically underrecognized, are prospectively and aggressively addressed. Implementing an ouchless PED approach combines a spectrum of evidence-based methods to reduce the physical and emotional trauma associated with medical interventions in children. Recent research emphasizes that heightened preprocedural anxiety can lead to diminished procedural success, especially with sedation [14,15].

Another important element of the ouchless approach includes formulating diagnostic and treatment plan prior to any pain-inducing or anxiety-inducing interventions, whenever possible, so that they can be "bundled" (such as drawing blood for tests and placing IV catheter all at once) or minimized (such as choosing oral route for rehydration vs intravenous [IV] placement [16], or administering intranasal analgesic prior to proceeding with imaging studies for a patient with a deformed extremity after trauma [17]).

Through nonpharmacologic interventions, pharmacologic analgesia, procedural sedation, and environmental modifications, this approach aims to make pediatric emergency care more humane, effective, and accessible.

The physiologic and psychological impacts of pain and distress in pediatric patients are well-documented [18]. Beyond the immediate trauma, untreated pain can have long-term effects on a child's perception of health care, potentially causing health care avoidance and poor adherence to treatments [19]. Reducing pain and distress not only improves cooperation during current visits but also positively shapes a child's health care interactions throughout life. Studies demonstrate the link between preprocedural anxiety and the success of procedural sedation, noting that anxiety mitigation plays a critical role in sedation efficacy and procedural cooperation [14].

NONPHARMACOLOGIC INTERVENTIONS

Nonpharmacologic interventions serve as the first line of defense in reducing pain and anxiety in pediatric patients. These approaches are particularly advantageous as they are often low-cost, minimally invasive, and can be effectively tailored to each child's developmental needs. Moreover, these techniques can be taught to clinicians providing pediatric emergency care and applied in the settings were dedicated child life specialist or psychologist may not be readily available.

Cognitive-behavioral techniques

Cognitive-behavioral techniques such as distraction, guided imagery, and positive reinforcement have proven effective in managing procedural pain. These methods work by redirecting a child's focus away from the procedure, thereby reducing perceived pain and discomfort.

Distraction

Distraction can be active, when the child is an active participant in distracting activity (such as an interactive game on a tablet), or passive, when the child is the observer or a passive participant of an activity (such as observing a nurse blowing bubbles).

Distraction techniques, which can range from storytelling and interactive toys to mobile games, have been shown to reduce pain scores by up to 40% in pediatric patients undergoing procedures [20]. Low-tech interventions, such as imitation of blowing bubbles during immunization administration were shown to be an effective distraction to reduce pain perception [21].

Novel distraction techniques utilizing technology show promise as a great nonpharmacological approach to pain reduction during interventions.

Positioning

Allowing children to choose their position during medical procedures and involving parents or caregivers in the process can significantly enhance the child's comfort and reduce pain and anxiety. Upright positioning during procedures, such as IV access, decreases distress in children and improves satisfaction among family members, without negatively affecting procedural success rates [22].

Parental presence and support

The role of parental presence during pediatric procedures is increasingly recognized as a critical component of reducing procedural distress. A meta-analysis published in 2018 revealed that children with a caregiver present during procedures exhibited lower levels of anxiety, increased cooperation, and shorter procedure times [23]. However, health care professionals must also consider the potential anxiety of the parents, as their stress can inadvertently heighten the child's distress. Training parents in coping techniques and involving them in distraction methods can further enhance procedural outcomes.

Child life specialists

Child life specialists are essential in an ouchless PED, particularly for children undergoing complex procedures. These trained professionals use age-appropriate education, relaxation techniques, and play therapy to help children understand and cope with medical procedures. By helping children to process their experiences, child life specialists can reduce the need for pharmacologic sedation, improve procedural cooperation, and decrease overall ED length of stay by approximately 15% [24]. The American Academy of Pediatrics endorses the use of child life services in the ED, emphasizing their role in enhancing the quality of pediatric care through reduced trauma and anxiety [25].

The use of cold and vibration devices

Cold and vibration devices have emerged as effective tools in minimizing pain and anxiety during minor invasive procedures in PEDs. Examples include the Buzzy device, a small handheld device that combines a vibrating motor with a detachable ice pack, often used during needle-related procedures like IV insertions, blood draws, and immunizations. The Buzzy device is applied just above the procedural site, where its vibration and cooling mechanisms disrupt pain signals to the brain. Similarly, products like the CoolSense Pain Numbing Applicator use instant cooling to desensitize the skin before injections.

These devices are portable, easy to use, and effective in managing pain and anxiety, making them an ideal addition to a PED focused on creating an "ouchless" environment. These devices combine localized cooling with gentle vibration to desensitize the skin and distract the child, thereby reducing the perception of pain. The application of cold numbs the superficial nerve endings, reducing pain transmission, while vibration stimulates mechanoreceptors, overriding pain signals through the gate control theory of pain [26]. Together, these modalities provide a synergistic effect that is particularly beneficial in procedures such as venipuncture, IV insertion, and immunizations.

Studies have demonstrated the efficacy of cold and vibration devices in reducing pain during needle-related procedures. A randomized controlled trial by Baxter and colleagues [27] found that the use of a cold and vibration device significantly decreased pain scores in children undergoing IV cannulation compared to standard care.

Virtual reality

Virtual reality (VR) is an emerging tool in pediatric pain management, offering a nonpharmacological approach to reducing pain and anxiety in children [28]. VR studies showed the effectiveness of VR in reducing pain perception during burn dressing changes, IV placements, and other painful procedures [29].

By immersing children in engaging and interactive virtual environments, VR helps distract them from discomfort and reduces their perception of pain.

The mechanism behind VR's efficacy lies in its ability to engage multiple senses and occupy the child's cognitive resources, thereby diminishing their focus on pain. This effect aligns with the Gate Control Theory of Pain, which suggests that nonpainful stimuli can "close the gate" to painful signals [26].

In a study involving children requiring IV placement for imaging procedures, participants were randomly assigned to either a VR distraction group or a standard care group. The VR group used a head-mounted display featuring an engaging game during the procedure. Results indicated that children in the VR group experienced lower pain and anxiety levels compared to the standard care group, highlighting the effectiveness of VR as a distraction tool during painful procedure [30].

In PEDs, VR has been used successfully during procedures such as blood draws, suturing, and fracture reductions. Many institutions now incorporate VR into their "ouchless" care programs, alongside pharmacologic and behavioral strategies. While VR is a promising tool, barriers such as cost, accessibility, and staff training need to be addressed for widespread implementation. Further research is necessary to optimize VR protocols, evaluate long-term outcomes, and integrate VR seamlessly into pediatric health care settings.

Emerging technology
Using humanoid robots for IV insertion in children was also shown to be an effective distraction technique [31].

PHARMACOLOGIC APPROACHES
Pharmacologic interventions are vital in an ouchless PED, particularly for children who cannot be adequately managed with nonpharmacologic methods alone. The use of pharmacologic analgesia and sedation should be carefully tailored to the child's needs, with an emphasis on rapid onset, minimal invasiveness, and safety.

Topical anesthetics
Topical anesthetics, such as lidocaine-prilocaine cream, or liposomal lidocaine cream, are often used to numb the skin before IV placement or phlebotomy. A systematic review found that pretreating the site with topical anesthetics significantly reduces reported pain scores in pediatric patients, providing both a practical and effective solution for minor yet painful procedures [32]. Liposomal lidocaine increased cannulation success on the first attempt when compared with placebo and decreased time of insertion as well as pain scores [33].

A mixture of lidocaine, epinephrine, and tetracaine is very effective when applied to lacerations [34].

Moreover, when topical anesthetics are coupled with distraction techniques, studies have shown even greater reductions in pain perception [34,35].

Intranasal medications
Intranasal administration of analgesics and sedatives, such as fentanyl and midazolam, provides a needle-free option that is especially beneficial for children with high anxiety or needle phobia. Intranasal fentanyl provides rapid pain relief—typically within 10 minutes of administration—making it an ideal choice for acute pain management in the PED [36,37]. It can also be a good management choice for children with orthopedic trauma prior to imaging studies, providing not only fast pain relief but also potentially resulting in better imaging quality.

Intranasal midazolam has also been shown to be effective for anxiolysis and mild sedation, enabling better cooperation for short procedures without the need for IV access [38].

Sucrose/breastfeeding for neonates

Oral administration of 24% or 25% sucrose during painful procedures to neonate or infant is a simple and effective method of dealing with the patient's discomfort [39,40]. Breastfeeding or dipping a pacifier in an expressed breast milk can produce similar results [41].

Sedation protocols

Procedural sedation is essential for certain painful or prolonged procedures. Schreiber and colleagues [14] highlight the importance of reducing preprocedural anxiety to increase sedation success rates and reduce the likelihood of adverse reactions. A tiered sedation protocol allows for the appropriate selection of sedatives based on the level of procedure invasiveness and the child's anxiety. Through presedation education and appropriate medication selection, health care providers can achieve a safer and more effective sedation experience [42].

ENVIRONMENTAL MODIFICATIONS

The physical environment of the PED can greatly influence a child's anxiety and pain perception. Environmental modifications aimed at creating a calming, child-friendly atmosphere are an integral part of the ouchless approach.

Sensory-friendly spaces

A sensory-friendly ED design incorporates elements that reduce sensory overload, such as dimmable lighting, soundproofing, and visually soothing decor. Research suggests that children with autism spectrum disorder and sensory processing difficulties, in particular, benefit from these modifications, experiencing reduced anxiety and improved cooperation during visits [43]. Furthermore, sensory-friendly spaces have been shown to improve behavioral outcomes for pediatric patients as a whole, reducing the need for physical or pharmacologic restraints [1].

Minimized waiting times

Extended waiting times can exacerbate anxiety and fear in pediatric patients. Studies show that long waits not only increase child distress but also negatively impact parental satisfaction and their perception of care quality. Implementing expedited triage for pediatric cases, as well as dedicating fast-track lanes for simpler complaints, has been shown to reduce waiting times by as much as 50% [21]. The use of patient pagers or text message updates can further reassure families and improve their overall ED experience.

Child-centered design

Child-centered design elements such as wall murals, aquariums, interactive play areas, and access to digital entertainment devices can serve as effective distractions. Hospitals that have invested in these design modifications report higher satisfaction rates among pediatric patients and their families [44]. These spaces can also facilitate positive associations with health care, reducing the risk of long-term medical anxiety and avoidance.

IMPLEMENTING THE OUCHLESS APPROACH IN EMERGENCY CARE

Staff training

Effective implementation of an ouchless PED requires that all ED staff, including physicians, nurses, and support staff, receive specialized training in pediatric pain management and nonpharmacologic techniques. Studies demonstrate that staff trained in both pharmacologic and nonpharmacologic pain management approaches are more confident in managing pediatric pain and anxiety, reducing the need for sedation by 25% in some cases [16]. Interdisciplinary training workshops and simulation exercises have proven effective in building team cohesion and improving procedural outcomes.

Evidence suggests that pediatric emergency nurses can accurately predict the need for IV placement while triaging patients [45]. Empowering pediatric emergency nurses in making decisions for topical anesthetic cream placements and creating standing protocols would expedite care and reduce discomfort for such patients, who tend to be sicker than the rest of the patients.

Integrated care models

An integrated care model combines pharmacologic, nonpharmacologic, and environmental strategies in a cohesive plan tailored to each pediatric patient. Research indicates that integrated models are associated with improved patient and family satisfaction, reduced sedation rates, and shorter ED lengths of stay. These models also improve staff efficiency and enable a more consistent delivery of child-centered care [37].

Case studies

Case study 1: managing acute anxiety in a young patient

A 4 year old patient presented to the PED with a laceration requiring suturing. The child exhibited severe anxiety and refused to be still, which made it challenging for the team to proceed with the wound closure. The child life specialist intervened, using storytelling and a favorite cartoon on a tablet to distract the child. Meanwhile, a topical anesthetic was applied to the wound site. After 15 minutes of distraction and topical analgesia, the procedure was completed without additional sedation, demonstrating the efficacy of combining nonpharmacologic methods with minimal pharmacologic intervention.

Case study 2: comfort positioning during laceration repair

A 4 year old girl required suturing for a chin laceration. Instead of the traditional supine position, the medical team employed a "comfort positioning" technique, seating the child upright on her caregiver's lap. This position provided emotional support and reduced the child's anxiety, resulting in a more cooperative patient and a smoother procedure. Comfort positioning has been shown to decrease distress in pediatric patients during various medical interventions.

Case study 3: minimizing pain in a fracture management
A 7 year old boy presented to the PED with a forearm deformity sustained during a fall. To manage his acute pain without the need for IV access, clinicians administered intranasal fentanyl. Within minutes, the patient reported significant pain relief, facilitating easier positioning for radiographic imaging and eventual casting.

This case exemplifies the efficacy of intranasal fentanyl as a rapid, noninvasive analgesic option in pediatric emergencies.

Case study 4: virtual reality for intravenous placement
An anxious 10 year old girl was given a VR set, and liposomal lidocaine cream was applied to the site before IV placement for sedation prior to brain MRI. She was distracted and engaged with the VR set enough for almost painless IV placement.

Case study 5: unsuccessful spinal puncture at the outside hospital
A 1 month old boy is transferred from an outside facility for fever and irritability. Two attempts at spinal puncture there were unsuccessful due to "infant's excessive movement." No analgesia or topical anesthetics were used.

At the receiving pediatric ED, liposomal lidocaine cream was applied to L4 area of the infant's spine. After 20 minutes, it was removed, the infant was positioned in left lateral decubitus position, and 24% sucrose was administered orally. Subcutaneous lidocaine was injected at the site of the planned spinal puncture. Spinal fluid was then obtained on the first attempt.

SUMMARY
The ouchless PED approach emphasizes a holistic, multidisciplinary approach to reducing pain and anxiety in pediatric emergency care. By incorporating pharmacologic and nonpharmacologic techniques, environmental modifications, and family-centered care strategies, the ouchless model improves the quality of pediatric care, enhances patient and family satisfaction, and reduces long-term health care aversion. With continued research and broader implementation, the ouchless approach has the potential to become a standard of care in pediatric emergency medicine.

CLINICS CARE POINTS

- Preemptive Pain Management: Use topical anesthetics (eg, liposomal lidocaine cream) for procedures such as IV placement or lumbar punctures. Apply these agents early to allow sufficient time for efficacy. Administer oral sucrose for infants during minor procedures to reduce procedural pain.

- Non-Pharmacological Interventions: Engage children with distraction techniques (eg, toys, tablets, virtual reality) to shift their focus away from the procedure. Incorporate child life specialists to provide age-appropriate psychological support during distressing situations.

- Parental Involvement: Encourage parents to stay with their child during procedures when appropriate, as their presence can provide comfort and reduce anxiety. Educate parents about coping strategies, such as guided breathing exercises, to support their child effectively.

- Sedation for Painful Procedures: Use procedural sedation protocols with agents like intranasal fentanyl or intranasal midazolam for moderate pain or anxiety relief. Always assess and document the child's pain using validated scales, such as FLACC (Face, Legs, Activity, Cry, Consolability) for younger children or a numeric pain scale for older children.

- Creating a Child-Friendly Environment: Design treatment areas to be visually appealing and calming (eg, colorful walls, cartoon posters) to reduce fear and anxiety.

- Minimize unnecessary noise and chaos in the emergency department to promote a sense of safety.

- Trauma-Informed Care: Screen for past traumatic experiences that may influence a child's response to care. Communicate clearly and at the child's developmental level to build trust and reduce fear.

Pitfalls

- Over-reliance on single interventions without integrating multidisciplinary strategies may reduce overall effectiveness in pain and anxiety management.

- Failing to tailor distraction techniques to the child's developmental needs may lead to increased distress and reduced intervention success.

- Overuse or underuse of sedation or pharmacologic interventions can compromise safety or create negative healthcare experiences. Ignoring environmental factors, such as noise or overstimulation, may worsen anxiety, especially in sensory-sensitive children.

- Minimizing the role of parents or child life specialists can increase distress and decrease coping during procedures.

DECLARATION OF AI AND AI-ASSISTED TECHNOLOGIES IN THE WRITING PROCESS

During the preparation of this article, the author used Gen AI. After using this tool/service, the author reviewed and edited the content as needed and takes full responsibility for the content of the publication.

Disclosure

The author has nothing to disclose.

References

[1] Kammerer E, Eszczuk J, Caldwell K, et al. A qualitative study of the pain experiences of children and their parents at a Canadian children's hospital. Children (Basel) 2022;9(12): 1796.

[2] Anand KJS, Hickey PR. Pain and its effects in the human neonate and fetus. N Engl J Med 1987;317(21):1321–9.

[3] Owens ME, Todt EH. Pain in infancy: neonatal reaction to a heel lance. Pain 1984;20(1): 77–86.

[4] Grunau RE, Craig KD. Pain expression in neonates: facial action and cry. Pain 1987;28(3): 395–410.

[5] Schechter NL, Blankson V, Pachter LM, et al. The ouchless place: No pain, children's Gain. Pediatrics 1997;99(6):890–4.

[6] Phillips DM. JCAHO pain management standards are unveiled. Joint Commission on Accreditation of Healthcare Organizations. JAMA 2000;284(4):428–9.

[7] Banos JE, Barajas C, Martin ML, et al. A survey of postoperative pain treatment in children of 3–14 years. Eur J Pain 1999;3(3):275–82.

[8] Ljungman G, Gordh T, Sorensen S, et al. Pain in paediatric oncology: interviews with children, adolescents and their parents. ActaPaediatr 1999;88(6):623–30.

[9] Schechter NL. From the ouchless place to comfort central: the evolution of a concept. Pediatrics 2008;122(Supplement 3):S154–60.

[10] Available at: https://www.stlouischildrens.org/conditions-treatments/emergency-room/ouchless-emergency-care. Accessed January 20, 2025.

[11] Available at: https://renaissance.stonybrookmedicine.edu/pediatrics/fellowship/emergency-medicine/about. Accessed January 20, 2025.

[12] Available at: https://www.shoremedicalcenter.org/centers/emergency/pediatrics. Accessed January 20, 2025.

[13] Landro L. New devices take the pain out of hospital visits. Wall St J 2015.

[14] Schreiber KM, Cunningham SJ, Kunkov S, et al. The association of preprocedural anxiety and the success of procedural sedation in children. American Journal of Emergency Medicine 2006;24(4):397–401.

[15] Heden L, von Essen L, Ljungman G. Children's self-reports of fear and pain levels during needle procedures. NursingOpen 2019;7(1):376–82.

[16] Spandorfer PA, Alessandrini EA, Joffe MD, et al. Oral versus intravenous rehydration of moderately dehydrated children: a randomized, controlled trial. Pediatrics 2005;115(2):295–301.

[17] Borland ML, Jacobs I, King B, et al. A randomized controlled trial comparing intranasal fentanyl to intravenous morphine for managing acute pain in children in the emergency department. Ann Emerg Med 2007;49(3):335–40.

[18] Howard RF. Current status of pain management in children. J Am Med Assoc 2003;290:2464–9.

[19] Weisman SJ, Bernstein B, Schechter NL. Consequences of inadequate analgesia during painful procedures in children. Arch Pediatr Adolesc Med 1998;152(2):147–9.

[20] Kleiber C, Harper DC. Effects of distraction on children's pain and distress during medical procedures: a meta-analysis. Nurs Res 1999;48(1):44–9.

[21] French GM, Painter EC, Coury DL. Blowing away shot pain: a technique for pain management during immunization. Pediatrics 1994;93(3):384–8.

[22] Sparks LA, Setlik J, Luhman J. Parental holding and positioning to decrease IV distress in young children: a randomized controlled trial. J Pediatr Nurs 2007;22(6):440–7.

[23] Broome ME, Bates TA, Lillis PP, et al. Children's medical fears, coping behaviors and pain perception during a lumbar puncture. Oncol Nurs Forum 1990;17(3):361–7.

[24] AAP Committee on Hospital Care, Jewell J, Jackson M, et al. Child life services. Pediatrics 2021;147(1):e202004026.

[25] Kleiber C, Sorenson M, Whiteside K, et al. Topical anesthetics for intravenous insertion in children: a randomized equivalency study. Pediatrics 2002;110(4):758–61.

[26] Mendell L. Constructing and deconstructing the gate theory of pain. Pain 2013;155(2):210–6.

[27] Baxter AL, Cohen LL, McElvery HL, et al. An evaluation of a vibrating cold device for reducing pain in pediatric venipuncture. Pain Med 2017;18(10):1905–11.

[28] Arane K, Behboudi A, Goldman RD. Virtual reality for pain and anxiety management in children. Can Fam Physician 2017;63(12):932–4.

[29] Gold JI, Kim SH, Kant AJ, et al. Effectiveness of virtual reality for pediatric pain distraction during IV placement. Cyberpsychol Behav 2006;9(2):207–12.

[30] Schlechter A, Whitaker W, Iyer S, et al. Virtual reality distraction during pediatric intravenous line placement in the emergency department: a prospective randomized comparison study. Am J Emerg Med 2021;44:296–9.

[31] Ali S, Sivakumar M, Beran T, et al. Study protocol for a randomised controlled trial of humanoid robot-based distraction for venipuncture pain in children. BMJ Open 2018;8:e023366.

[32] Borland M, Jacobs I, Gilhoed G. Intranasal fentanyl reduces acute pain in children in the emergency department: a safety and efficacy study. Emerg Med 2002;14(3):275–80.

[33] Taddio A, Soin HK, Schuh S, et al. Liposomal lidocaine to improve procedural success rates and reduce procedural pain among children: a randomized controlled trial. CMAJ 2005;172(13):1691–9.

[34] Martin HA. The power of lidocaine, epinephrine, and tetracaine (LET) and a child life specialist when suturing lacerations in children. J Emerg Nurs 2017;43(2):169–70.

[35] Peavey E, Knox R, Reyers E. Inclusive design for patients with autism spectrum disorders. Healthc Des 2020.

[36] Alsabri L, Hafez AH, Singer E, et al. Efficacy and safety of intranasal fentanyl in pediatric emergencies: a systematic review and meta-analysis. Pediatr Emerg Care 2024;40(10): 748–52.

[37] Saunders M, Adelgais K, Nelson D. Use of intranasal fentanyl for the relief of pediatric orthopedic trauma pain. Acad Emerg Med 2010;17:1155–61.

[38] Foster M, Cox K. Intranasal fentanyl and midazolam use in a pediatric emergency department. Paediatr Child Health 2014;(6):e105.

[39] American Academy of Pediatrics, and Fetus and Newborn Committee, American Academy of Pediatrics Section on Surgery, Canadian Paediatric Society Fetus and Newborn Committee, Batton DG, Barrington KJ, Wallman C, et al. Prevention and management of pain in the neonate: an update. Pediatrics 2006;118(5):2231–41.

[40] Slater R, Cornelissen L, Fabrizi L, et al. Oral sucrose as an analgesic drug for procedural pain in newborn infants: a randomised controlled trial. Lancet 2010;376(9748):1225–32.

[41] Shah PS, Herbozo C, Aliwalas LL, et al. Breastfeeding or breast milk for procedural pain in neonates. Cochrane Database Syst Rev 2012;12:CD004950.

[42] Wilson S, Cote C, American Academy of Pediatrics, American Academy of Pediatric Dentistry. Guidelines for monitoring and management of pediatric patients before, during, and after sedation for diagnostic and therapeutic procedures. Pediatrics 2019;143(6):e20191000.

[43] Chumpitazi C, Chang C, Atanelov Z, et al. Managing acute pain in children presenting to the emergency department without opioids. J Am Coll Emerg Physicians Open 2022;3(2):e12664.

[44] Litwin S, Clarke L, Copeland J, et al. Designing a child family and healthcare provider center procedure room in the tertiary care children's Hospital. Health Environments Research and Design Journal 2023;16(3):195–209.

[45] Fein JA, Gorelick MH. The decision to use topical anesthetic for intravenous insertion in the pediatric emergency department. Acad Emerg Med 2006;13:264–8.

Advances in Pediatrics 72 (2025) 69–92

ADVANCES IN PEDIATRICS

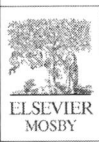

Vascular and Gastrointestinal Access in Children

Andrew C. Sayce, MD, DPhil[a], Stefan Scholz, MD, PhD[b],*

[a]Department of Surgery, University of Pittsburgh Medical Center, Pittsburgh, PA, USA; [b]Division of Pediatric General and Thoracic Surgery, UPMC Children's Hospital, University of Pittsburgh, Pittsburgh, PA, USA

Keywords
- Vascular access • Pediatric • Ultrasound • Enteral access • Gastrostomy

Key points
- A diversity of techniques has evolved to establish and maintain vascular and enteral access. Clinical judgment must drive decision-making for selection of technique.
- Vascular access has evolved from landmark-based to image-guided approaches.
- The mode of vascular or enteral access must incorporate duration of access need and patient physiology.
- Open, laparoscopic, percutaneous, and endoscopic techniques are all reasonable in the appropriate patient context.
- Complications are relatively rare, but the high frequency of interventions necessitates attention to diagnosis and early management to limit harm.

INTRODUCTION

Safe and reliable delivery of appropriate fluid, nutrition, and medication is a largely an assumed component of modern medicine. From the first description of intravenous (IV) infusion in the seventeenth century [1], a diverse repertoire of robust techniques for establishing and maintaining vascular access has been developed. Similarly, enteral supplementation (eg, supplemental supply of nutrients/medication to the gastrointestinal tract [GI]) has developed over millennia as our understanding of anatomy and technical resources have expanded from

*Corresponding author. E-mail address: stefan.scholz@chp.edu

https://doi.org/10.1016/j.yapd.2025.03.005

Abbreviations

ACS	American College of Surgeons
CLABSI	central line-associated bloodstream infection
CVC	central venous catheter
CVL	central venous line
G	gastrostomy
GERD	gastroesophageal reflux disease
GI	gastrointestinal
GJ	gastro-jejunostomy
IJ	internal jugular
IO	intraosseous
IV	intravenous
J	jejunostomy
NG	nasogastric
NICU	neonatal intensive care unit
OG	orogastric
PEG	percutaneous endoscopic gastrostomy
PICC	peripherally inserted central catheter
PICU	pediatric intensive care unit
UGI	upper gastrointestinal contrast study
VAT	vascular access team

enemas used in Ancient Egypt to minimally invasive surgical techniques for gastrostomy (G) and fundoplication available today.

For many medical providers, consideration of access need only extend to order entry for peripheral IV catheter placement and/or basic techniques for peripheral venipuncture. In the pediatric population, such peripheral access may prove challenging due to patient anatomy (eg, patients weighing <2 kg) or psychosocial factors (eg, patient fear) of the procedure. For the pediatric surgeon, in particular, it is essential to understand the available options beyond peripheral IV placement.

In consideration of vascular access, one must always initially question whether there is an enteral alternative with an abundance of evidence to support preference of direct enteral nutrition whenever feasible. Prolonged parenteral feeding results in atrophy and increased permeability of the gut mucosa. The lack of peristalsis results in the stagnation of bowel contents and changes in the intestinal microflora.

This preference for enteral delivery can generally be extended to delivery of fluid, electrolytes, and medications; however, the clinical context of a patient and pharmacokinetics and pharmacodynamics must be considered. For example, vancomycin delivered orally does not cross the intestinal epithelial barrier and is approved for oral administration in treating pseudomembranous colitis caused by *Clostridioides difficile*, but has no efficacy in this clinical context if delivered IV. In contrast, with methicillin-resistant *Staphylococcus aureus* infection, IV vancomycin is a highly effective therapy. This example is used to highlight the importance of clinical knowledge and judgment in the decision for access and route of administration of therapy.

Vascular access is a fundamental procedure in pediatric medicine, but pediatric patients present unique challenges due to their small vessel size, and associated increased risk of complications, as well as limited choice of venous access sites. Achieving safe and effective vascular access requires careful planning, appropriate equipment selection, and technical expertise.

This review provides an overview of vascular as well as enteral access in children, focusing on indications, techniques, and postoperative management. We provide detailed descriptions of vascular followed by enteral access considerations. The following Discussion and Clinical Care Points highlight overarching evidence-based information related to techniques and use of access devices.

VASCULAR ACCESS
History
Although the practice of bloodletting was popular for millennia, the first IV infusion required critical developments in understanding vascular anatomy. Leonardo Da Vinci is generally credited with providing the first detailed anatomic description and drawing of the human heart in 1510; however, it was not until William Harvey presented Excercitatio anatomica de motus cordis et sanguinis in 1616 (and published in 1628) that the pattern of blood flow within the human body was understood [2]. Until this point, the liver, rather than the heart, was widely assumed to be the origin of blood and blood flow. Shortly thereafter, the first IV infusion in humans was described by Johann Elsholtz in Clysmatica nova in 1665 [1]. From this first description of vascular access, sites, techniques, and technologies for establishing and maintaining IV delivery exploded. The development of hollow needles and glass syringes in the early 1900s made IV therapy more practical. In the 1950s, Dr Sven-Ivar Seldinger introduced the Seldinger technique, revolutionizing central venous catheterization by enabling wire-guided placement of catheters [3]. The 1960s saw the introduction of peripherally inserted central catheter (PICC) lines and the use of Teflon-coated catheters to reduce thrombosis risk. The Hickman and Broviac catheters, developed in the 1970s and 1980s, allowed long-term central venous access for chemotherapy and parenteral nutrition [4]. The introduction of ultrasound-guided vascular access in the 1990s improved success rates and reduced complications. Advances in catheter materials (eg, antimicrobial-impregnated and heparin-coated catheters) have further reduced infection risks. The development of totally implantable venous access devices (eg, Port-a-Caths) has improved the quality of life for patients requiring long-term IV therapy. The evolution of vascular access techniques has significantly improved patient outcomes, making central venous catheterization safer and more effective for patients.

Indications for vascular access
Vascular access in children is performed for various medical and surgical indications:

- IV fluid administration in dehydration, shock, and perioperative care.

- Parenteral nutrition in children with GI dysfunction or malabsorption syndromes.
- Long-term antibiotic therapy for conditions such as osteomyelitis or endocarditis.
- Chemotherapy in pediatric oncology patients requiring repeated cycles of cytotoxic drugs.
- Hemodialysis or plasmapheresis in children with end-stage renal disease or autoimmune disorders.
- Frequent blood sampling in neonates and critically ill children to minimize venipuncture trauma.
- Emergency access for rapid resuscitation during cardiac arrest or severe trauma.

Contraindications for vascular access

While vascular access is often necessary, certain contraindications must be considered:

- Infection at the intended access site (eg, cellulitis and abscess).
- Severe coagulopathy increasing the risk of hemorrhagic complications.
- Vascular anomalies or previous thrombosis limiting available sites.
- Patient instability where alternative access (eg, intraosseous [IO]) may be faster and safer.

Preprocedural planning

Effective planning for vascular access in pediatric patients is essential for success. As with all procedures, this begins with a thorough review of the patient's medical history, focusing on prior access complications, venous anatomy (eg, known variants and presence of thrombosis), and anticipated clinical needs. Detailed considerations include

- Access goals: Is short-term or long-term therapy anticipated? For example, does the patient require short-term peripheral IV access for rehydration or do they require delivery of chemotherapy for weeks to months and, therefore, require a tunneled central catheter? What needs to be delivered? For example, does the patient need caustic medications such as vasopressors or hyperosmolar solutions that would necessitate central delivery? Do frequent imaging studies need to be performed such that a catheter appropriate for rapid infusion (eg, Powerport) of contrast is necessary? What level of simultaneous access is required which will determine number of lines/ports?
- Patient factors:
  o How can psychosocial aspects such as pain and fear be mitigated? Is the child likely to interfere with establishing or continuing access, and if so, what can be done to limit this interference?
  o Coagulation status: Complete review of coagulation studies (complete blood count, partial thromboplastic time [PTT], and International Normalized Ratio [INR]) is crucial. This may not be available in the emergent setting; however, coagulation status should be known in advance whenever possible and abnormalities corrected where possible. Image-guided access and attempts by experienced providers are suggested in the setting of uncorrected coagulopathy.

○ Access history: Review of prior central line placements or recent peripheral access attempts can inform target selection. For example, peripheral venipuncture should not be attempted distal to a recently failed cannulation site in which the vein was injured. Similarly, scarring or stenosis from previous central access may necessitate alternative central cannulation site selection.

A thorough consideration of the "Preprocedural planning access" section will help guide site, catheter selection, positioning, premedication, and securement of one's planned catheter. Failure to anticipate answers to these questions leads to inadequate delivery of treatment.

Peripheral access

Peripheral venous access is the mainstay of vascular access during most hospital admissions and appropriate for IV hydration, most medication administration, and blood sampling. It is technically straightforward and safer than central access and can be performed at the bedside without anesthesia, although topical analgesics can be helpful, especially for children. In US hospitals, peripheral IV access is often obtained by skilled members of the patient care team, such as nurses on the vascular access team or anesthesia providers [5].

Pediatric veins are small in caliber and often difficult to see and feel, especially in a dehydrated child or infant who is fasting for an operation. Obtaining peripheral IV access in this setting can be challenging. Ultrasound can help the identification of vascular anatomy and guide catheter placement to increase success [6]. Other technological advancements include transilluminators for infants and near-infrared vein finders for older children. Although all those modalities require advanced training, improved vein visibility can lead to increased success at access.

Invariably, it is essential for this procedure to be familiar with the anatomic locations amenable to peripheral IV insertions:

- Superficial veins of the forearm and the dorsal hand: Often good targets for peripheral venous access. The antecubital fossa should not be crossed with the catheter unless the arm is immobilized since the catheter can kink.
- Greater and lesser saphenous veins and its extension on the dorsum of the foot (medial and lateral marginal veins) [7]: Often a good target, especially anterior to the medial malleolus, best visualized with the foot held in plantar flexion. The distal saphenous vein is a good target for an emergent peripheral cut-down for direct venipuncture. However, maintenance of peripheral IV access in children and adolescents is often not practical.
- Scalp: Limited to neonates.
- External jugular vein: Good size and visibility but often challenging to access percutaneously due to excessive mobility and compressibility.

Central venous access

Central venous access is required for secure or long-term access for vasoactive medications, hyperosmolar fluid (including total parenteral nutrition [TPN]), and cytotoxic medications, such as chemotherapy. Clear communication (and documentation) between the primary provider and the proceduralist (pediatric surgeon, interventional radiologist, and critical care pediatrician) is essential to ensure placement of the correct access catheter (number of lumens, size, and location).

Please see Table 1 for the different types of central venous catheters and their use.

Central line placement technique

Before placement, the interventionalist needs to decide where to place the catheter. Central access is typically obtained via the internal jugular (IJ) vein, subclavian vein, or femoral vein of either side. The IJ is the most used site and offers a straight route to the right atrium, easy visibility with ultrasound, but the line position may change with turning of the head, especially in small infants. The subclavian vein offers a fixed position with good stability and comfort, but ultrasound guidance may not be possible. This access should not be used for hemodialysis catheters due to higher rate of stenosis that would preclude arteriovenous (AV)-fistula creation on the same side. Femoral vein access can be technically less challenging with easy landmarks (femoral artery) and under ultrasound guidance. Line infections of this access site do not seem to be higher although femoral access is not usually used for tunneled and cuffed long-term catheters except occasionally in newborns and infants who are not ambulatory [8].

As mentioned previously, the Swedish radiologist Sven-Ivar Seldinger published a novel technique for vascular access involving a needle, a wire, and a catheter in 1953 [3]. The Seldinger technique has become the standard approach for percutaneous vascular access. The actual standard today is performing central vascular access using the ultrasound-guided Seldinger technique by pediatric surgeons, interventional radiologists, and pediatricians. Applicable ultrasound techniques include in-line and transverse approaches depending on the location and the size of the patient. Percutaneous venous access in infants and children should be obtained with a 21 g or 22 gauge needle that allows passage of a 0.018 inch coaxial wire with a flexible tip to minimize damage to the access vein itself and the surrounding structures (eg, use a dedicated microaccess kit). In small children and infants, any curved-tip wire should be avoided since the radius of the curvature is often too large for the child's vein. The microaccess kit also contains a 3 French dilator with a 4Fr sheath that facilitates change of the small access wire to a more robust 0.035 inch wire that can be used to dilate the tract for the placement of larger catheters in bigger patients, if so desired [9]. Central venous access can be obtained using anatomic landmarks. This approach should be considered as historic today since ultrasound guidance has made access procedures safer and easier, particularly for children [10,11].

The American College of Surgeons (ACS) supports the use of real-time ultrasound guidance for the placement of central venous catheters. The ACS encourages health care systems to provide for the appropriate education, training, and resources required [12]. For our small patients, a high-frequency (7.5–20 MHz) linear array transducer provides the best resolution for the

Table 1
Types of central venous access

Line		Duration of Use	Requires Operating Room	Example Uses	Advantages	Limitations
Nontunneled	PICC (Fig. 1)	Months	No	Prolonged antibiotic Administration TPN Short-term chemotherapy	Easier to insert and remove by trained nurses Lower cost	Increased risk of infection and thrombosis Requires weekly care by trained family providers or visiting nurses
	Percutaneous central venous line (CVL)	Weeks	No	Vasopressor, hyperosmolar fluid or medication administration as inpatient	Lower risk of infection and thrombosis Longer duration	—
	Percutaneous hemodialysis line	Weeks	No	Acute hemodialysis	—	—

(continued on next page)

Table 1 (continued)

	Line	Duration of Use	Requires Operating Room	Example Uses	Advantages	Limitations
Tunneled	Cuffed CVL (Hickman, Broviac, Fig. 2)	Months to years, regular use	Yes (but lower infection rates) neonatal intensive care unit (NICU)	Prolonged outpatient parenteral nutrition Chemotherapy	Lower risk of infection More durable access	Insertion needs pediatric surgery or IR, and anesthesia Higher cost
	Port (Fig. 3)	Months to years, intermittent use	Yes	Chemotherapy	More durable access for longer use Lower risk of infection and thrombosis Comfortable and cosmetic	Insertion needs pediatric surgery or IR, and anesthesia Smallest ports may be too large for infants/young children Higher cost Limited flows Need for special training and equipment for access Freq flushes and heparin locks Access requires skin puncture, which may not be tolerated in infants/young children

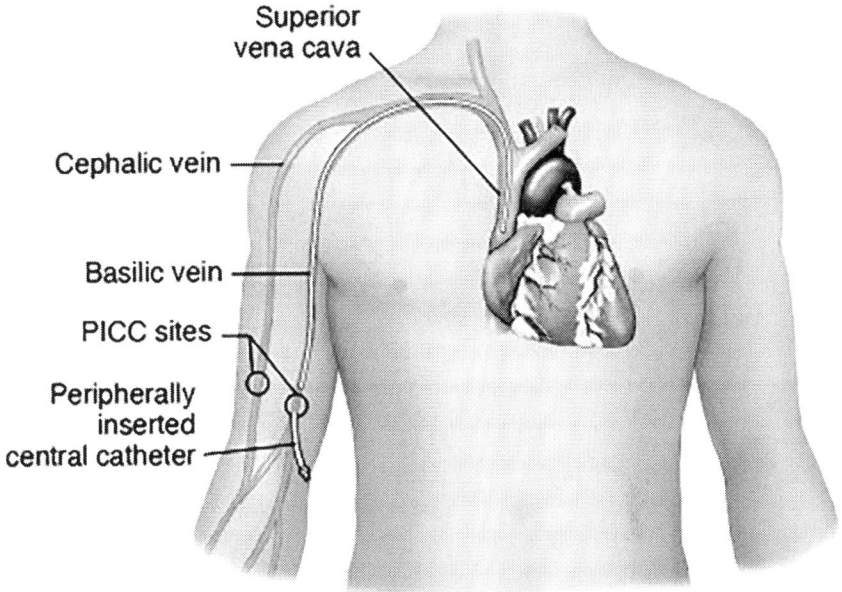

Fig. 1. Peripherally inserted central catheter (PICC) can be inserted using the basilic or cephalic vein. These catheters are thin, flexible tubings that gets inserted into a vein in the upper arm and threaded into the superior vena cava near the heart as shown in the pictorial. Benefits include stable venous access for extended periods of time, reduction of repeated needle sticks and ability to administer parenteral nutrition or concentrated medications that may irritate smaller veins, such as chemotherapy. Chintamani, Dr. L. Gopichandran, Mrinalini Mani, Lewis's Adult Health Nursing I & II with Integrated Pathophysiology and Geriatrics, 5th Edition, 2024, Elsevier India.

placement of the needle and wire in more superficial vessels (Fig. 4). In the operating room, fluoroscopy is an essential tool for safe CVL placement. Guidewire and dilator/peel-away sheath placement can be seen in real-time. Appropriate catheter position is confirmed at the end of the procedure. In the NICU and pediatric intensive care units (PICU), fluoroscopy cannot be used due to radiation restrictions. It is, therefore, even more important to master ultrasound guidance for these procedures. Final positioning is usually checked by a confirming chest radiograph. Generally, the central line can be used directly after placement.

Today, vascular cut-down techniques have been largely replaced by percutaneous access, but are still utilized by pediatric surgeons for vascular access in the smallest patient in the NICU or for extracorporeal membrane oxygenation access [5]. The major central veins are often accessed via the external jugular, facial, and saphenous veins by pediatric surgeons in a cut-down approach, especially in infants, to place small cuffed and tunneled Broviac catheters.

- Central line placements in neonatal and pediatric patients can be technically demanding and suboptimal positioning of the catheter tip can spark controversy between primary providers and proceduralists that may lead to the need

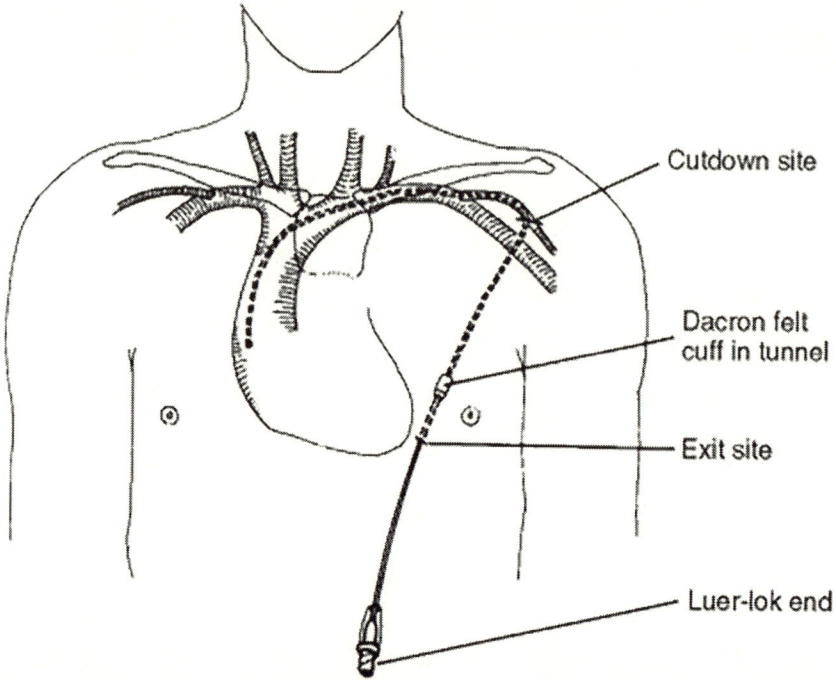

Fig. 2. Diagrammatic representation of Broviac catheter in proper position, with tip in right atrium. The cuff is placed under the skin close to the exit site of the catheter at the beginning of the subcutaneous tunnel, well away from access to a central vein, such as the internal jugular vein or the subclavian vein. The cuff helps prevent infections by acting as a physical barrier and promote tissue ingrowth to secure the catheter and reduce bacterial migration. Overall, the path of the catheter is similar to that of the implantable port in Figure 3. (*From* Bennion RS, Wilson SE: Hemodialysis and vascular access. In Moore WS, ed: Vascular surgery: a comprehensive review, Philadelphia, 1991, WB Saunders).

for revision or removal of the catheter in the operating room. Ideal position of the catheter tip is directly at the cavo-atrial junction. More proximal tip placement is associated with subsequent tip migration into other venous locations while deep central lines may result in extension of thrombus to the tricuspid valve, potentially requiring operative intervention.

PICCs are long, thin, and flexible catheters that are functionally central venous catheters but are inserted peripherally. They can be as small as 1.9 French (26 gauge) for preterm infants and can be placed through a peel-away sheath introduced with a 23 gauge needle in modified Seldinger technique. Please see Table 1 for more details. A common target for PICC placement is the basilic vein since it allows easy catheter passage into the subclavian vein and superior vena cava.

Vascular access is minimally invasive and well tolerated. Pain is generally mild, and there are few limitations on routine activity. Routine flushing with saline or heparinized solutions is necessary to prevent occlusion. Strict hand

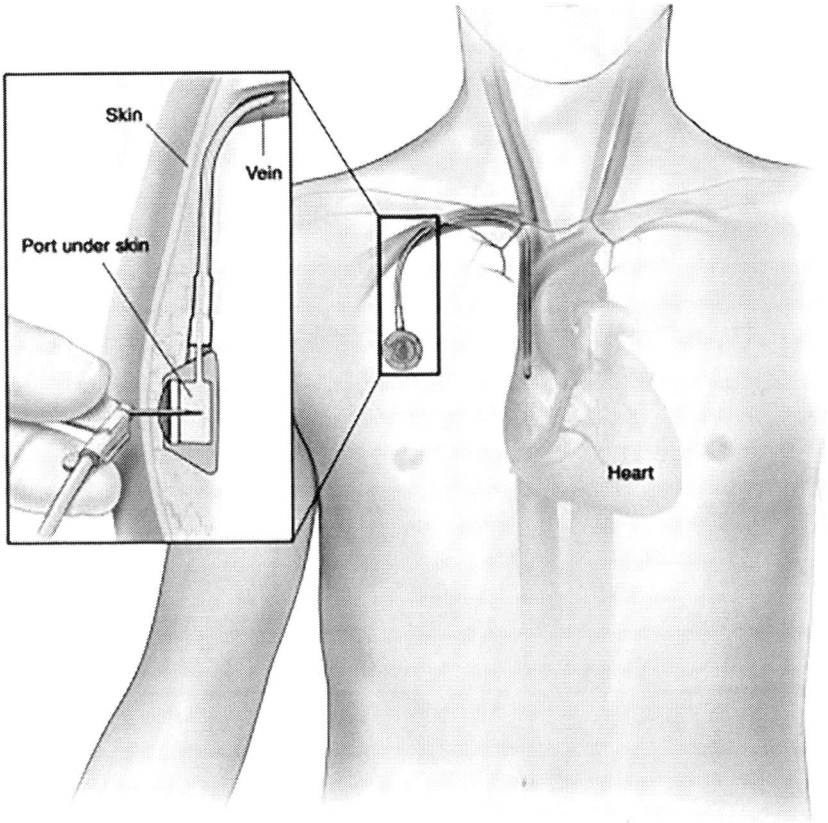

Fig. 3. An implantable port, also known as a port-a-cath or central venous catheter, is a medical device implanted under the skin that provides long-term access to a large vein. Its septum can be accessed by a special Huber needle that prevents leakage from the port. It is used for administering medications, chemotherapy, blood transfusions, and drawing repeated blood samples. A port reduces the need for multiple needle sticks and allows for long-term administration of medications while minimizing infectious compliucations. The Port pictured above allows high pressure infusion of contrast or other fluids when necessary. (© 2011 Terese Winslow LLC).

hygiene and sterile dressing changes should be adhered to in order to minimize catheter-related bloodstream infections. Before discharge home, families should be trained in catheter care, signs of infection, and flushing protocols.

The IO route provides rapid vascular access in a crisis. This route is mostly utilized for infants and small children in an emergent trauma setting where peripheral vascular access cannot be obtained. This may be also used effectively in older patients.

Removal
Peripheral IVs and CVLs are discontinued prior to hospital discharge. PICCs and cuffed CVLs (Hickman and Broviac) are removed when no longer needed.

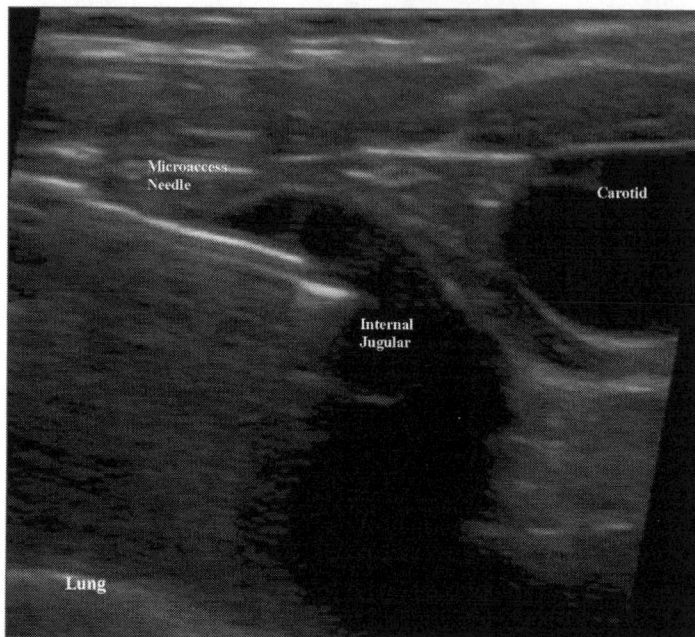

Fig. 4. Placement of the microaccess needle under ultrasound guidance using the in-line technique. With this approach, the needle can be seen in its entire length and the tip can be directed safely into the lumen of the internal jugular vein for central catheter insertion (see above, the tip of the needle is in the lumen of the vessel). Utilizing the Seldinger technique, a wire is forwarded through the needle into the vessel that can guide advancement of a sheath or a central line.

- Peripheral intravenous catheters (PIVs), percutaneous CVLs, and PICC lines can easily be removed by pulling them out. For supradiaphragmatic central lines, the patient should bear down during pulling. Gentle pressure can be held to ensure hemostasis and a gauze dressing is placed.
- Cuffed CVLs require local anesthesia at the insertion site (small children often also require sedation or general anesthesia) because the cuff induces scar formation and must be dissected free from the catheter, which can cause pain.
- Port removal requires general anesthesia in children because the port and its tubing must be surgically removed from its subcutaneous pocket.

Complications and management
Early complications.

- Arterial injury: Central veins are accompanied by major arteries, and vascular access attempts may result in arterial injury. The risk can be minimized by using a small access needle with ultrasound guidance that allows clear visualization of the surrounding anatomy. In case of arterial injury, a micropuncture needle can be withdrawn and holding pressure is usually adequate for hemostasis. If a large bore needle has caused the arterial injury, especially in the neck, consideration should be given to leaving it in placed to plug the hole and additional imaging obtained as this injury may need direct surgical repair of the arteriotomy. In case of injury to the femoral artery, holding pressure may suffice.

- Pneumothorax: IJ and subclavian access attempts carry the risk of lung puncture and subsequent pneumothorax, and a chest radiograph should be obtained after the procedure.

Late complications.

- Line malfunction and damage: Cuffed CVLs can break due to the exposed portion of the catheter and the activity level of children. Silastic catheters can often be repaired using available kits or may need operative replacement.
- Line thrombosis and occlusion: Line thrombosis can occur in critically ill children, such as patients with trauma, and those with malignancy. Tissue plasminogen activator is one option to reverse thrombosis. Ethanol (70%) and hydrochloric acid may clear occlusions caused by lipid or mineral deposits. If not successful, catheter removal and replacement are necessary.
- Perforation: Perforation of the superior vena cava or right atrium by a central venous catheter is a rare, but serious, complication. The catheter material (silastic vs polyurethane) does not affect the perforation risk. PICC lines carry a higher incidence than CVLs inserted via the IJ or subclavian. Access through the right IJ provides the least risk due to its straight course because the side of the catheter contacts and rubs the vessel wall and not the tip. Perforation below the pericardial reflection can cause cardiac tamponade and above the reflection exsanguination into the pleural space. Whipping of the catheter during heart beats can cause wall erosion and perforation; ideally, the catheter tip should be placed near the cavo-atrial junction to limit risk [5,9].
- Vessel thrombosis or stenosis: Thrombosis due to central venous catheters is common, especially in small infants and children with trauma or cancer. Treatment involves the removal of the offending line and anticoagulation. Permanent stenosis, most common in the subclavian vein, is rare and often the cause of multiple central lines over years.
- Infection:
  - Exit-site infection on the skin at the exit site of the catheter caused by a skin pathogen. Antibiotics and local wound care usually resolve this.
  - Tunnel or pocket infection is more serious than an exit-site infection with typical signs of erythema, induration, tenderness, and pus from the exit site. Line removal becomes necessary in most cases.
  - Central line-associated bloodstream infection (CLABSI) is the most serious of the catheter-related infections that leads to systemic sepsis and possible mortality. External signs may not be present and risk factors include neutropenia, TPN, and intestinal failure. Strategies for preventing CLABSI in children include chlorhexidine skin preparation and chlorhexidine-impregnated dressings as well as the use of heparin and antibiotic-impregnated central venous catheters or use of ethanol lock or vancomycin lock therapy [13]. More recently, taurolidine as a catheter locking solution was found to significantly reduce CRBSI in pediatric patients but better evidence is still needed [14].

If CLABSI is suspected, peripheral and central blood cultures should be promptly drawn prior to initiating empiric antibiotics. Antibiotics may be a sufficient treatment, but if the bacteremia has not cleared after 48 to 72 hours, the catheter should be removed. Some resistant organisms, such as *S aureus* or *Bacillus cereus* as well as fungi, may necessitate line removal. A new catheter should not be placed until 48 hours after the first negative blood culture and should be placed at a new insertion site.

SUMMARY

Vascular access in children is a critical yet challenging procedure requiring careful selection of catheter type and access approach. Most procedures can be performed percutaneously with the Seldinger technique. The use of ultrasound and fluoroscopy guidance has significantly improved safety and efficacy. In particular, using ultrasound guidance can decrease complications associated with vascular access but requires patience and experience. Postprocedural care, including catheter maintenance and infection prevention, is essential to ensure long-term success. Today's proceduralists should be comfortable performing these procedures and should be able to diagnose and treat the common complications.

Pediatric enteral access

Introduction

Enteral access is a critical intervention in pediatric patients with feeding difficulties due to congenital anomalies, neurologic disorders, prematurity, or GI conditions. The selection of an appropriate access method is guided by the patient's underlying pathology, expected duration of feeding support, and anatomic considerations. While nasogastric (NG) and orogastric (OG) tubes are common for short-term feeding, surgical options such as G, gastro-jejunostomy (GJ), and jejunostomy (J) are preferred for long-term nutritional support. Advances in endoscopic, laparoscopic, and fluoroscopic techniques have improved safety and efficiency in pediatric enteral access.

History of pediatric enteral access

The concept of enteral feeding dates back centuries. The first documented attempts at enteral feeding involved nutrient-rich enemas in ancient Egypt and Greece. In the eighteenth and nineteenth centuries, John Hunter (1793) introduced the use of orogastric and NG tubes for enteral feeding, marking the beginning of modern enteral access. NG tubes became widely used in neonatal care in the early twentieth century, particularly for preterm infants who could not coordinate sucking and swallowing. The development of percutaneous endoscopic gastrostomy (PEG) in 1980 by Michael Gauderer and colleagues [15], a pediatric surgeon, revolutionized long-term enteral access in children. The adoption of laparoscopic and fluoroscopic techniques has minimized procedural risks and improved patient outcomes [16]. The Feeding Tube Awareness Foundation reports that 100,000 American children currently rely on feeding tubes for nutrition [17,18].

Box 1: Conditions that most frequently are associated with need for feeding access

Cardiac and neurologic anomalies (cerebral palsy, seizure disorder, and muscular dystrophy)

Severe developmental delay

Prematurity with immature suck–swallow reflex

Inborn errors of metabolism

Intestinal failure and malabsorption syndromes

Pancreatitis

Vocal cord paralysis

Chronic aspiration

Severe oral aversion

Oncologic conditions and other chronic illness requiring prolonged nutritional support

Congenital anomalies (cleft palate and esophageal atresia)

Gastric decompression (eg, following fundoplication)

Conditions precluding oral feeding (maxillofacial or esophageal surgery, head/face trauma, or tumors)

Indications for enteral access

Enteral access should be considered in patients with functioning intestines who are at risk for failure to thrive by not maintaining adequate caloric intake and hydration. The decision to place a short-term or long-term feeding access device is largely based on clinical considerations.

Most common *anatomic and physiologic* indications include cardiac and neurologic anomalies (Box 1).

Contraindications for enteral nutrition and its access such as bowel obstruction or severe ileus, uncorrectable coagulopathy increasing bleeding risk, severe peritonitis, or intra-abdominal sepsis should be considered.

Patient evaluation and selection of access route

An initial nutritional assessment should be obtained, and the swallowing function may be studied with a barium swallow test. If the patient cannot swallow, the care team should determine if the patient will tolerate NG feeds. If it is safe, an NG feeding trial can be attempted. NG feeding (or in infants OG feedings) may be the optimal route for short-term enteral access. In infants, orogastric feeding tubes can be placed. However, all of the aforementioned feeding tubes are prone to dislodgement and the need for replacement. They are uncomfortable, unsightly, can cause epistaxis or sinusitis and possibly hinder the patient from participating in routine activities. NG tubes may make eating and swallowing uncomfortable. Percutaneous G and J tubes avoid or greatly minimize these problems, especially if a low-profile button is placed instead of a longer

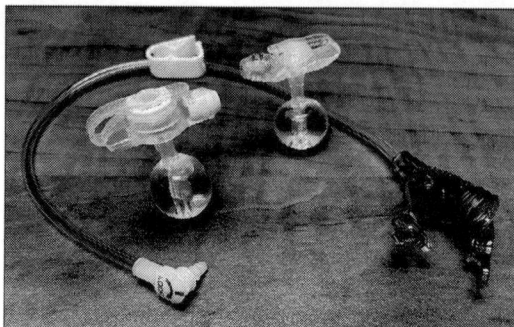

Fig. 5. Two available gastrostomy button models. The internal retention balloon keeps the button securely anchored within the stomach and can be deflated through the balloon valve with a 5 mL syringe for button change. The feeding port features a 1 way valve and a safety lid to prevent leaking and can be accessed with the appropriate connection tubing.

tube. Disadvantages of the placement of feeding buttons include the need for a surgical procedure, even with low complication rate, the need for stoma site care, potential stoma site infections, early dislodgement of the button with the need for a reoperation, leaking from the site, and granulation tissue or scar formation after removal. If the NG feeding trial is successful and enteral access is expected to be required for an extended period, then a surgically placed G button should be considered [19] (Fig. 5).

If the patient tolerates NG feedings, an upper gastrointestinal contrast study (UGI) is not needed since the incidence of malrotation is very low overall and no functional distal obstruction is present [20]. In patients with congenital heart disease, who have a higher incidence of malrotation, an UGI could be obtained. Alternatively, an abdominal ultrasound can also diagnose malrotation reliably. In case of malrotation, a Ladd's procedure may be added to the laparoscopic placement of a G button.

If a patient does not tolerate NG feedings or NG feedings cannot be performed, an UGI should be performed to rule out distal obstruction or structural abnormality. If none is found, gastroesophageal reflux disease (GERD) needs also to be considered. The UGI can also diagnose a hiatal or paraesophageal hernia and suggest GERD but cannot quantify this. In younger patients, GERD is often only clinically diagnosed and a fundoplication or, alternatively, a GJ could be performed in addition to G (Fig. 6). A 24 hour impedance and/or pH-probe can be placed to quantify GERD, but this is usually reserved for older patients. If distal obstruction or a structural abnormality of the gastroesophageal junction is identified, this should be surgically corrected when placing a G button. If severe GERD is encountered, consideration should be given to combining a G with a fundoplication or to GJ placement.

Preoperative preparation
Prior to placement of a G button, the indication for the surgical procedure and possible complications are discussed with the family. It is important to set

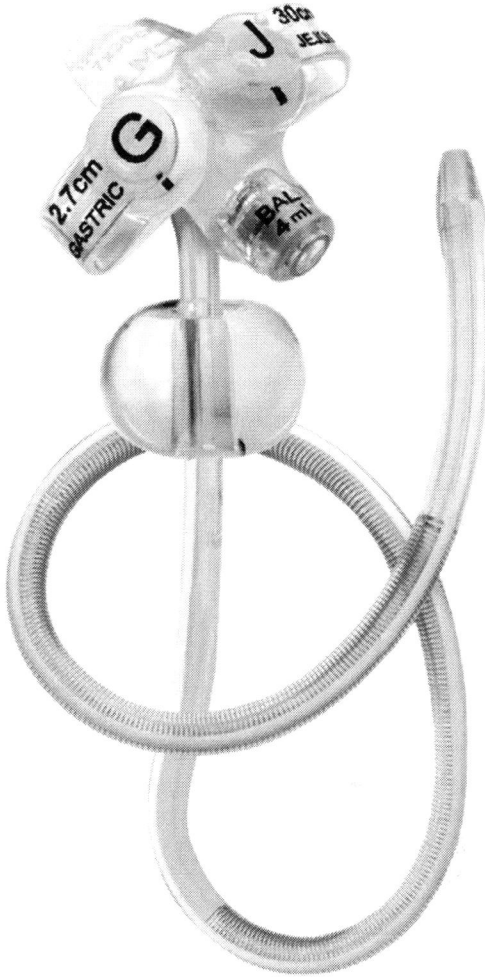

Fig. 6. G-JET Button—low-profile gastric and jejunal balloon feeding tube. Gastric (G) and jejunal (J) feeding ports. These GJ buttons come in multiple lengths and sizes to adjust to the pediatric patient. Image provided courtesy of Applied Medical Technology, Inc.

expectations for the postoperative period as well as long-term management. Education and training of the family regarding function, use, and care of the G button should be started prior to placement. Unless the patient has other comorbidities, additional laboratory tests are not needed.

Enteral access procedures and techniques
There are 3 main techniques of placing a G button (or tube) that all have advantages and disadvantages. For children, placement of feeding buttons is usually chosen for its low profile and better acceptance of patients and parents. In the case of older patients with a very thick abdominal wall (more

than 6 cm), a long feeding tube will be chosen since the length of the tract would exceed the length of the available buttons. Adult surgeons routinely choose feeding tubes and do not place buttons. In some institutions, primary G buttons or tubes are placed by interventional radiologists utilizing fluoroscopic techniques.

A primary GJ button or tube can also be placed in the operating room or the interventional radiology (IR) suit depending on indication and local protocols. In patients with GERD and intolerance of gastric feedings or significant aspiration risk, G buttons are often combined with a laparoscopic fundoplication (most often Nissen fundoplication in the United States). Primary J tubes and buttons are reserved for patients that do not have a stomach or do not tolerate any form of gastric nutrition. J tubes are rarely placed surgically in pediatric clinical practice and require more specialized laparoscopic or open techniques for placement.

Laparoscopic placement of gastrostomy button/tube. Laparoscopic-assisted placement of a G button has become the routine procedure for most pediatric patients today. The laparoscopic approach is preferred by most pediatric surgeons because it has been shown to be safer than the traditional open gastrostomy [21]. In addition, this is a minimally invasive procedure that can be performed directly under laparoscopic vision through the umbilicus effectively leaving no scars and causing minimal intraoperative and postoperative pain that can be well controlled through routine modalities such as intraoperative regional pain blocks (bilateral rectus sheath block in combination with left subcostal transversus abdominis plane block) and postoperative tylenol administration. Relative contraindications such as previous laparotomy with peritoneal adhesions, decreased cardiac function, or congenital anomalies can generally be negotiated with low insufflation and routine laparoscopic lysis of adhesions [22]. The surgical technique requires transabdominal suspension of the stomach to the abdominal wall that is achieved with direct placement of percutaneous gastric retention sutures or placement of T-fasteners into the stomach under direct vision with the laparoscope and/or an endoscope. After the stomach has been suspended, the Seldinger technique [3] is used to place a hollow needle and then a wire into the stomach. The small abdominal wall opening, and the G are then dilated over the wire under laparoscopic vision with ascending dilators up to 16 to 20 French. The final tract length is measured and a 14 French G button (available sizes 10–18 French) of that length is placed over the wire into the gastric lumen and its balloon inflated for retention. If a component is external, the retention sutures or the T-fasteners are removed after approximately 2 to 5 days, depending on practice. The G button is then left in place for at least 2 to 3 months to allow adequate healing of the gastro-cutaneous fistula before the first button change is performed and taught to the parents. Longer G tubes can be placed in a similar manner in larger patients. G buttons are typically changed by the parents every 3 to 6 months or as necessary.

Open placement of gastrostomy button/tube. G button (or tube) placement in an open approach is most often added to concomitant open exploratory laparotomy performed for another reason. A Stamm G is usually performed whereby the stomach is sutured to the peritoneal surface of the abdominal wall through retention sutures place through the posterior rectus sheath. A gastric purse-string suture is added around the new button or tube to narrow the G around the new button. This technique adds safety to the G placement and makes intra-abdominal leakage and early dislodgment very unlikely, even if the balloon unintentionally deflates soon after the procedure.

Percutaneous endoscopic gastrostomy tube. Publication of the PEG technique by a team around Michael Gauderer [15], a pediatric surgeon, in 1980 changed the way feeding tubes were placed when most tubes were placed by an open approach in children and adults. His publication remains the most cited pediatric surgery article to date. This technique does not require entry into the peritoneal cavity and additional incisions are not needed. Today, the procedure is the most used technique for placing feeding tubes in adults and can be performed with minimal anesthesia, most commonly in the intensive care units, even in fragile patients. The basic procedure requires upper gastroscopy with insufflation of the stomach and apposition to the abdominal wall. A transcutaneous hollow needle is placed into the stomach after insufflation and ensuring that the light inside the insufflated stomach is visualized on the abdomen. A looped wire is placed through the needle and is then pulled out of the mouth by retracting the endoscope. A long feeding tube with a cone tip is then secured to the looped wire and pulled through the mouth and the esophagus into the stomach and through the gastric and abdominal wall. The tube remains secured in the gastric lumen with a soft disk preventing easy dislodgment (Fig. 7). After the tract has matured, at least 6 weeks later, this tube can also be changed to a G button or ballooned tube

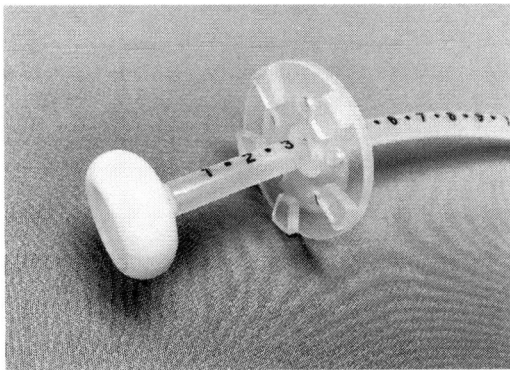

Fig. 7. Percutaneous endoscopic gastrostomy (PEG) tube. The internal bumper keeps the tube in the stomach, the external retention disc is placed on the tube after it is pulled through the stomach and the abdominal wall. The disc can be adjusted to the patient's abdominal wall thickness and prevents further migration into the duodenum. A common complication of after PEG placement is to adjust the retention disc too tight on the abdominal wall leading to erosion and breakdown.

depending on patient body habitus and preference. PEGs are mostly placed in older children and teenagers in Children's Hospitals since they have thicker abdominal walls. On the other hand, PEGs may have a higher complication rate since the needle can unknowingly traverse the colon or other hollow viscera. The outside disk may migrate allowing the inner mushroom disk to migrate further into the duodenum, resulting in gastric outlet obstruction. Alternatively, the outer disk may be too tight, thus compressing the abdominal wall and causing erosion. Adequate distance should be always kept between the inside gastric "mushroom" and the outside disk.

Ultrasound-guided gastrostomy tube placement. In the setting of a hostile abdomen, such as due to adhesions from prior operations, an alternative approach is to fill the stomach with saline via an NG tube and to use ultrasound for the placement of T-fasteners followed by a Seldinger approach to needle-wire-dilation of a tract and placement of a G button over the wire (similar to the laparoscopic placement described previously). Upper endoscopy may help to guide tube placement once the T-fasteners are in place. A preoperative CT may help to ensure that the stomach is in an appropriate location for access.

Laparoscopic placement of primary gastro-jejunostomy buttons/tubes. In patients with intolerance of gastric feedings, primary GJ buttons and tubes can be placed laparoscopically as an alternative to G button combined with a fundoplication. The technique comprises the steps for an initial placement of a G button. However, instead of placing the G button, a wire is placed through the gastrotomy site and through the pylorus into the duodenum and jejunum under fluoroscopy. The wire is then used to forward a GJ button or tube over the wire into the jejunum. Placement is then confirmed with contrast under fluoroscopic guidance. Small children of weight less than 6 to 10 kg are at higher risk for intestinal perforation from a GJ button or tube [23].

An established G can secondarily be converted to a GJ if gastric feedings are not tolerated, even despite a fundoplication. Reasons include duodenal dysmotility, intractable GERD, and poor gastric emptying. Techniques utilize either fluoroscopy or the endoscope and are performed by pediatric surgeons, interventional radiologists, or gastroenterologists.

Placement of jejunostomy button/tube. Direct J buttons and tubes are rarely placed and are usually reserved for long-term feeding access after failures of gastric access with possible previous fundoplication or when the stomach is not available for access, for example, after gastric replacement of the esophagus. J tubes or buttons can be placed open or using minimally invasive approaches. With an open approach, a Witzel tunnel, wherein the jejunum is approximated to itself for a few centimeters over the top of the tube and J tube site, is created around the jejunostomy and the tube to avoid leakage, a technique used more commonly by adult surgeons. These are nonballoon tubes that are prone to "falling out," but replacement is similarly relatively simple. When performed laparoscopically, a loop J or a Roux-en-Y limb is surgically created such that a tube with a balloon may be placed to prevent dislodgement, often leading to higher satisfaction among parents and patients.

Complications and management. Major complications are uncommon with enteral access procedures. Overall, PEGs can have complications rates up to 10% in the children while reported complication rates for laparoscopic G can range up to 4% [24]. PEGs can inadvertently be placed through the colon while laparoscopic G carries the risk of injury to the stomach, particularly in very small patients with fragile tissues. The tip of the tube or button may be misplaced behind the stomach when the backwall of the stomach is perforated with the needle and the wire or into the gastric submucosal space with inadvertent infusion of feeds into the wall of the stomach.

Early dislodgement of the G carries the risk that the tube is placed into the peritoneal cavity if the gastro-cutaneous fistula has not sufficiently matured. Feeding the peritoneal cavity may lead to sepsis and a surgical emergency with possible mortality if not recognized early enough. A contrast study to confirm intraluminal placement should be used liberally or the G may be replaced in the operating room under laparoscopic and/or endoscopic guidance.

Granulation tissue on the cutaneous aspect of the G site is common, especially in the first months after initial placement. This can usually be controlled by cautery with silver nitrate sticks or with steroid cream. Most times, G tube granulation will resolve with application of these techniques. Other problems include infections or abscesses of the abdominal wall that are less common. Erosion into the abdominal wall and breakdown of the site and its surrounding skin are caused by buttons that have an inadequate stem length (Fig. 8).

Leakage of the fistulous tract is a common problem and may be caused by a button that is too short or by a dilated G site that is the result of increased

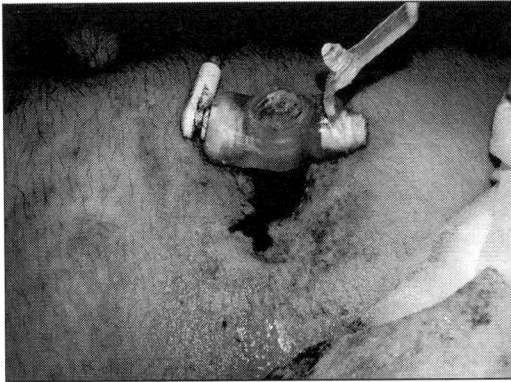

Fig. 8. A patient with a gastro-jejunostomy button that was poorly cared for. The button was too tight and eroded into the abdominal wall tissue creating tissue breakdown and a friable and bleeding wound. Acidic gastric juice has been leaking over the surrounding abdominal wall skin causing skin irritation and erosion.

movement of a button or tube. Enteral access tubes may become clogged if thick formulas or medications are given, the longer and thinner the tube the more often this occurs. Numerous liquids have been tried to reopen a clogged tube including warm water, carbonated beverages, such as cola or ginger ale, or cranberry juice. Additives, such as meat tenderizer, papain, or Castile soap can be mixed with the warm water. Finally, G tubes can migrate into the pylorus resulting in gastric outlet obstruction or partially retract into the subcutaneous tissues, mimicking G site infection because of profound erythema and tenderness.

GJ tubes can cause small bowel to small bowel intussusception causing obstruction that can be resolved by removing the tube. More frequently, the jejunal portion of the tube can retract and dislodge back into the stomach or the tube can fall out. This is a frequent cause for return to the hospital and for pediatric surgical or interventional radiology procedures to change and reposition the jejunal portion of the tube. Etiologies of retraction of the GJ tube into the stomach include retching, poor peristalsis, looping of the tube in the stomach, and inadequate length of the tube [19].

Dedicated J tubes can cause volvulus of the small intestines around the access site that can lead to bowel obstruction and ischemia. This necessitates surgical exploration and correction with resection or additional suture pexy if the bowel is reducible and viable.

There are 2 reasons why a GJ tube with jejunal feedings may not be the best long-term solution for feeding access. The first is that jejunal feedings do not allow boluses and must be given continuously via a pump, which is a distinct disadvantage of J feedings over G tube feedings from the point of view of quality of life for parents and families. The second is that GJ tube displacement, the tube falling out or the tip retracting into the stomach, is relatively frequent and, unlike a G or J tube, requires a trip to the hospital/emergency department/clinic so that the tube can be replaced in IR or the operating room (OR). Thus, it is advisable to have a discussion of options with the family as to long-term plans for durable feeding access, be that fundoplication or another approach to allow G tube feedings or J tube placement, in those patients in whom long-term GJ tube feeding access is expected to be required.

Follow-up. After the placement of a G feeding button, patients usually stay in the hospital for 1 to 2 days. Most pediatric centers have dedicated teams and protocols for patient and family teaching that starts in the preoperative period and continues with follow-up. The clinical team needs to develop a relationship with the family since they will be followed for years for nutritional management as well as changing/upsizing the feeding button and managing complications and, possibly, removal sometime in the future.

Removal. Enteric access removal is performed when the access device is no longer required. Often, this consists of weight gain without supplemental tube feeding for a number of weeks/months. The device usually can be simply removed in clinic with placement of a dressing with a barrier cream to retard leakage. The tract can be cauterized with silver nitrate sticks to remove its inner lining and to facilitate complete closure. If large amounts of leakage persist for more than 1 to 2 weeks or small amounts of leakage for greater than 6 weeks, closure of the site may be required either operatively or endoscopically.

SUMMARY

Pediatric enteral access has evolved significantly with the adoption of minimally invasive techniques, reducing morbidity, and improving patient outcomes. Proper selection of the access method is crucial, balancing risks and benefits based on the child's specific needs.

CLINICS CARE POINTS

- The requirement and selection of vascular or enteral access must be targeted to the specific clinical situation of the child to allow proper selection of access method balancing risks and benefits.
- Evidence has accumulated that vascular access should be obtained in an ultrasound-guided fashion.
- Short- and long-term complications are common overall due to the large number of access procedures and must be minimized as much as possible.
- Patients should be evaluated repeatedly for the possibility to discontinue vascular or enteral access.
- Most patients can successfully use a gastrostomy button for routine enteral access, in some cases combined with an anti-reflux procedure.

Disclosure
The authors have nothing to disclose.

References

[1] Escholtz JS. Clysmatica nova: sive ratio, qua in venam sectam medicamenta immitti possint, ut eodem modo, ac si per os assumta fuissent, operentur: addita etiam omnibus seculis inaudita sanguinis transfusione. 2. Coloniae Brandenburgicae : Ex officina Georgi Schultzi, impensis Danielis Reichelii; 1667.

[2] Harvey W, De Landau H, Burndy L. Exercitatio Anatomica de Motv Cordis et Sangvinis in Animalibvs. Sumptibus F. Fitzeri; 1628. doi:10.5479/sil.126677.39088002685501.

[3] Seldinger SI. Catheter replacement of the needle in percutaneous arteriography; a new technique. Acta Radiol 1953;39(5):368–76.

[4] Hickman RO, Buckner CD, Clift RA, et al. A modified right atrial catheter for access to the venous system in marrow transplant recipients. Surg Gynecol Obstet 1979;148(6):871–5.

[5] Vascular Access Procedures | Operative Pediatric Surgery, 2e | AccessSurgery | McGraw Hill Medical. Available at: https://accesssurgery.mhmedical.com/content.aspx?sectionid=53539574&bookid=959&Resultclick=2. Accessed February 17, 2025.

[6] Tang L, Wang F, Li Y, et al. Ultrasound guidance for radial artery catheterization: an updated meta-analysis of randomized controlled trials. PLoS One 2014;9(11):e111527; https://doi.org/10.1371/journal.pone.0111527.

[7] Ricci S, Moro L, Antonelli Incalzi R. The foot venous system: anatomy, physiology and relevance to clinical practice. Dermatol Surg 2014;40(3):225–33.

[8] Arvaniti K, Lathyris D, Blot S, et al. Cumulative evidence of randomized controlled and observational studies on catheter-related infection risk of central venous catheter insertion site in ICU patients: a pairwise and network meta-analysis. Crit Care Med 2017;45(4):e437–48.

[9] Church JT, Jarboe MD. Vascular access in the pediatric population. Emerg Pediatr Surg 2017;97(1):113–28.

[10] Brass P, Hellmich M, Kolodziej L, et al. Ultrasound guidance versus anatomical landmarks for subclavian or femoral vein catheterization. Cochrane Database Syst Rev 2015;1(1): CD011447.

[11] Bruzoni M, Slater BJ, Wall J, et al. A prospective randomized trial of ultrasound- vs landmark-guided central venous access in the pediatric population. J Am Coll Surg 2013;216(5): 939–43.

[12] Revised recommendations for use of real-time ultrasound guidance for placement of central venous catheters. ACS. Available at: https://www.facs.org/about-acs/statements/use-of-real-time-ultrasound-guidance-for-placement-of-central-venous-catheters/. Accessed February 17, 2025.

[13] Huang EY, Chen C, Abdullah F, et al. Strategies for the prevention of central venous catheter infections: an American pediatric surgical association outcomes and clinical trials committee systematic review. J Pediatr Surg 2011;46(10):2000–11.

[14] Sun Y, Wan G, Liang L. Taurolidine lock solution for catheter-related bloodstream infections in pediatric patients: a meta-analysis. PLoS One 2020;15(4):e0231110; https://doi.org/10.1371/journal.pone.0231110.

[15] Gauderer MW, Ponsky JL, Izant RJ. Gastrostomy without laparotomy: a percutaneous endoscopic technique. J Pediatr Surg 1980;15(6):872–5.

[16] McSweeney ME, Smithers CJ. Advances in pediatric gastrostomy placement. Gastrointest Endosc Clin N Am 2016;26(1):169–85.

[17] What is FTD? The feeding tube foundation. Available at: https://www.feedingtubefoundation.org/what-is-ftd. Accessed February 18, 2025.

[18] Liu K, Abudusalamu A, Yang J, et al. Effectiveness of early enteral feeding on health outcomes in preterm infants: an overview of systematic reviews. Eur J Clin Nutr 2023;77(6): 628–36.

[19] Jarboe MD, Speck KE, Demehri F, et al, Pediatric surgery NaT - enteral access, Available at: https://www.pedsurglibrary.com/apsa/view/Pediatric-Surgery-NaT/829032/all/Enteral_Access.

[20] Abbas PI, Naik-Mathuria BJ, Akinkuotu AC, et al. Routine gastrostomy tube placement in children: does preoperative screening upper gastrointestinal contrast study alter the operative plan? J Pediatr Surg 2015;50(5):715–7.

[21] Sulkowski JP, De Roo AC, Nielsen J, et al. A comparison of pediatric gastrostomy tube placement techniques. Pediatr Surg Int 2016;32(3):269–75.

[22] Gillory LA, Megison ML, Harmon CM, et al. Laparoscopic surgery in children with congenital heart disease. J Pediatr Surg 2012;47(6):1084–8.

[23] Massoumi RL, Abdelhafeez AH, Christensen MA, et al. Gastrojejunostomy tube bowel perforations in low-weight infants. JPEN J Parenter Enteral Nutr 2016;40(8):1177–82.

[24] Liu R, Jiwane A, Varjavandi A, et al. Comparison of percutaneous endoscopic, laparoscopic and open gastrostomy insertion in children. Pediatr Surg Int 2013;29(6):613–21.

Advances in Pediatrics 72 (2025) 93–102

ADVANCES IN PEDIATRICS

Pediatric Lymphadenopathy

Danielle Cameron, MD, MPH[a,b],
Alyssa Stetson, MD, MPH[b,c], Jennifer Blase, MD, PhD[d],
Christopher B. Weldon, MD, PhD[a,e,f,*]

[a]Harvard Medical School; [b]Division of Pediatric Surgery Mass General for Children, Department of Surgery Mass General Brigham; [c]University of Cincinnati; [d]C.S. Mott Children's Hospital, University of Michigan; [e]Boston Children's Hospital; [f]Dana-Farber Cancer Institute

Keywords
- Lymphadenopathy • Pediatric lymphadenopathy • Cervical lymphadenopathy
- Soft tissue masses • Malignancy evaluation

Key points

- History and physical are fundamental to guiding evaluation of soft tissue masses in children.
- Cervical lymphadenopathy (LAD) is often ultimately classified as benign idiopathic, but providers should be alert for concerning features associated with malignancy:
  - Lymph node characteristics: supraclavicular location, large size, or fixed, matted, or nontender on examination.
  - Patient signs and symptoms: systemic "B" symptoms, generalized LAD, or dyspnea.
  - Imaging: abnormal lymph nodes on ultrasound, mediastinal mass, mediastinal LAD.
- The differential for soft tissue neoplasms is extensive, but it can be narrowed based on mass location, the history, and the exam.

INTRODUCTION

A child with soft tissue swelling can alarm parents and represent a diagnostic challenge for providers. While a common cause of soft tissue swelling is lymphadenopathy (LAD), the differential for soft tissue swelling is broad and includes many diagnoses that mimic LAD. This article focuses on the presentation and

*Corresponding author. Harvard Medcial School, Boston Children's Hostpial, Department of Surgery, 300 Longowwd Avenue, Fegan 3, Boston, MA 02115. E-mail address: Christopher.weldon@childrens.harvard.edu

https://doi.org/10.1016/j.yapd.2025.03.008
0065-3101/25/© 2025 Elsevier Inc. All rights reserved, including those for text and data mining, AI training, and similar technologies.

Abbreviations

AFB   acid-fast bacilli
CMV   cytomegalovirus
CNB   core needle biopsy
CT   chest tomography
CXR   chest radiograph
EBV   Epstein-Barr virus
ESR   erythrocyte sedimentation rate
FNAB   fine needle aspiration biopsy
HIV   human immunodeficiency virus
KD   Kawasaki disease
LAD   lymphadenopathy
LN   lymph node
NHL   non-Hodgkin's lymphoma
RMS   rhabdomyosarcoma

diagnostic work up of LAD in the pediatric patient. However, it would be prudent to point out a few diagnostic challenges associated with cervical masses that frequently mimic LAD: torticollis is often associated with a mass in the body of the sternocleidomastoid muscle and may be mistaken for a lymph node. Likewise, thyroid nodules may be difficult to distinguish from lymph nodes. Finally, it may be difficult to discern a thyroglossal duct cyst in the midline upper neck adjacent to the hyoid bone and a lymph node (LN) (Fig. 1). Abscesses, dermoid cysts, pilomatrixomas, salivary gland tumors, lipomas, and vascular/lymphatic malformations may also mimic lymph nodes at times.

LYMPHADENOPATHY

LAD is defined as a LN greater than 1 cm in transverse dimension, although LNs up to 1.5 cm may be normal in the inguinal region but up to only 0.5 cm in the auricular, preauricular, and epitrochlear regions [1–3]. LAD is

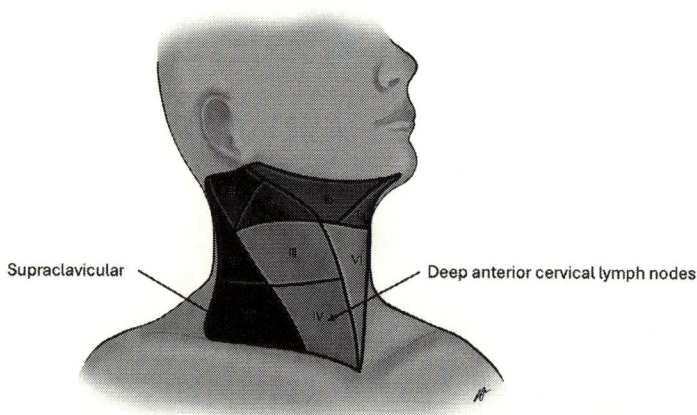

Supraclavicular   Deep anterior cervical lymph nodes

Fig. 1. LN zones of the neck. (*Illustrated by* Lucy Nam, MD.)

extremely common in children, with palpable LNs present in 41% of children 2 to 5 years and 90% of children 4 to 8 years [1,2,4]. Palpable, nonenlarged lymph nodes do not specifically denote underlying pathology. Peripheral LAD is classified as isolated versus diffuse based on whether greater than 2 noncontiguous nodal basins are involved, and, importantly, as acute if present for less than 2 weeks, subacute if present for 2 to 6 weeks, or chronic if present for greater than 6 weeks [1]. Cervical LAD is the most common location in children [4]. Approximately two-thirds of patients with cervical LAD have benign, idiopathic LAD [2]. The most common etiologies of enlarged lymph nodes in the cervical region are Epstein-Barr virus (EBV) infections, malignancy, and granulomatous disease [2,5].

The differential diagnosis for LAD can be categorized as idiopathic, infectious, malignant, immunologic, or iatrogenic. LAD can only be deemed "benign, idiopathic" after a thorough investigation. The key feature to the diagnostic work-up is a thorough history and physical as this simple undertaking can often reveal the cause—or substantially narrow the differential—eliminating the need for further testing.

History and physical examination

A detailed history and physical are essential when a patient presents with soft tissue swelling suggestive of LAD. Indications for other diagnostic measures should be determined after this evaluation, and non-LAD causes should be considered. The history should focus on patient characteristics and exposures, and LN characteristics (Table 1) [1,2,4,6]. All associated details of the history must be identified, including issues with dentition, recent skin infections, rashes, bites (especially ticks), abscesses, trauma, and immunizations. The history should also seek symptoms consistent with recent viral or other illnesses, travel history, or exposure to animals (especially cats). Finally, one should ascertain the presence of other medical conditions, including immunologic compromise or symptoms of immunologic diseases such as fevers, rashes, myalgias, and myositis.

The physical examination should include an assessment of characteristics of the lesion, anatomic location, and local and systemic signs (Table 2) [1,2,4,6].

Table 1

Elements of the history that distinguish lower and higher risk for malignancy in the setting of lymphadenopathy

	Lower risk for malignancy	Higher risk for malignancy
History		
Age	Childhood	Adolescence
Duration	Acute/Subacute	Chronic (>4–6 wk)
B Symptoms	Absent	Present
Dyspnea	No	Yes
Change in size	Stable	Increasing in size
Concurrent or prior malignancy	No	Yes

B Symptoms, fever, weight loss, night sweats.

Table 2
Physical examination factors for identifying lymph nodes at higher risk for malignancy

	Lower risk for malignancy	Higher risk for malignancy
Physical examination		
Size	<2 cm	>2 cm
Location	Nonsupraclavicular	Supraclavicular
Lymph node sites	1 site	≥3 sites
Mobility	Mobile	Fixed to underlying structures
Tenderness	Yes	No
Fluctuance/erythema	Yes	No
Pallor/petechia	No	Yes

Upon completion of the history and physical, a focused differential diagnosis can be created to guide any required testing and/or develop a surveillance plan.

Malignancy
Malignancy is the greatest concern when patients present with new LAD, but it is rare [4,7–10]. Malignancy should be considered for any LN that is grossly enlarged or persistent for more than 4 to 6 weeks [1]. Patients with supraclavicular LAD have the highest risk of malignancy [1,5,7]. This anatomic variant denotes significant LAD involvement ascending from the mediastinum identified medially by the clavicular head extending laterally on the clavicle [11].

The most common causes of malignant cervical LAD before age 6 are acute leukemia, neuroblastoma, rhabdomyosarcoma (RMS), and non-Hodgkin's lymphoma (NHL). After age 6, the most common causes are Hodgkin's lymphoma, NHL, and RMS [2]. However, local cancers such as melanoma, salivary gland neoplasms, and thyroid cancer can also cause LAD [2].

Nonmalignant causes
Infection. Infectious cervical LAD is most often viral, with EBV and cytomegalovirus (CMV) the most frequently identified pathogens [5]. EBV alone is responsible for approximately 9% of cervical LAD [5]. Human immunodeficiency virus (HIV) can also cause LAD; patients typically presenting with cervical, axillary, and occipital nodes in association with systemic symptoms for greater than 1 week [1]. Otherwise, viral LAD is generally self-resolving, and thus other etiologies should be considered if it persists past 4 to 7 days [1].

Approximately 4% of cervical LAD is secondary to bacterial infection, with common pathogens including *Streptococcus*, *Staphylococcus aureus* (especially methicillin-resistant *S aureus*), *Bartonella henselae*, *Mycobacterium avium* complex, and *Mycobacterium tuberculosis* [5]. *Bartonella*, which causes cat-scratch disease, is responsible for approximately 0.6% of all cervical LAD, but can also rarely cause generalized LAD [4,5]. Patients with bacterial LAD often have signs of infection in the region of the LNs such as pharyngitis, otitis media, tonsillitis in the case of cervical LAD, or a local wound infection [2]. Compared with viral LAD, bacterial LAD is more likely to be isolated or present as lymphadenitis [1].

An unusual, but intriguing cause of LAD is atypical mycobacterium. Persistent LN masses are typically observed in the submandibular region. Biopsy often results in nonhealing, draining wounds and is only corrected by excision of the LN mass. Antituberculosis antibiotics may or may not have utility.

Lyme disease should be considered in endemic areas as it can cause significant LAD, especially in the regional LN basins near the bite [12]. While other tick-borne diseases such as ehrlichiosis, anaplasmosis, rocky mountain spotted fever, and babesiosis can also cause LAD they are less commonly associated [13–16]. Certain bacterial pathogens, namely atypical mycobacterium, tuberculosis, and *Bartonella henselae*, can cause subacute or chronic LAD [2]. *Toxoplasma Gondii* infection can also present with LAD [17].

Immunologic disease. An unusual cause of LAD is secondary to an immunologic etiology including Kawasaki disease (KD), Kikuchi-Fujimoto syndrome, and systemic lupus erythematous. These diseases have additional clinical characteristics that can point the provider to the correct diagnosis [1,11]. In the case of KD, one may observe persistent fever, conjunctivitis, erythema of the oral mucosa, and erythema or swelling of hands and feet [18].

Drug or vaccination reactions. Many drugs can cause an acute reaction with associated LAD. Common pharmacologic triggers are phenytoin, isoniazid, and allopurinol, as well as antimicrobials, especially vancomycin, pyrimethamine, and trimethoprim-sulfamethoxazole [2,19]. Patients will typically have other systemic symptoms such as fever, rash, jaundice, cytopenia, or hepatosplenomegaly (HSM) [1]. Eosinophilia is also common [19].

Certain immunomodulatory drugs, particularly thiopurine analogues and antitumor necrosis factor medications, are associated with an increased risk of lymphoma. The data regarding cyclosporine and methotrexate are less conclusive [20].

Finally, any vaccination causes local trauma, and thus LN basins draining the affected anatomic location can respond to this insult with LAD.

Laboratory and imaging data
Following construction of the differential diagnosis, adjuncts to the visit can help elucidate the underlying cause. These tests are generally a combination of imaging and laboratory tests (Table 3).

Laboratory tests. A complete blood count with differential and peripheral blood smear can narrow the differential diagnosis. An elevated white blood count can suggest an infectious cause, while cytopenia can indicate viral, immunologic, or a malignant hematologic etiology [2]. Systemic lupus erythematosus may cause lymphopenia. Thrombocytosis is often reactive but may also be secondary to KD [2]. EBV can present with elevated atypical lymphocytes or monocytes, while blasts with pancytopenia are concerning for a hematologic malignancy [2].

Inflammatory markers (erythrocyte sedimentation rate [ESR] and C-reactive protein [CRP]) should be sent. Persistently elevated ESR or CRP are concerning for malignancy. An elevated uric acid and lactate dehydrogenase can be secondary to high cell turnover, indicating malignancy [2]. Liver function tests are useful to evaluate for systemic conditions including EBV [2].

Table 3
Laboratory data identifying lymph nodes at higher risk for malignancy

	Lower risk for malignancy	Higher risk for malignancy
Laboratory data		
Anemia	No	Yes
Leukopenia	No	Yes
Thrombocytopenia	No	Yes
White blood count differential	Atypical lymphocytes	Blasts
Positive tests for infection	Yes	No
Uric acid/Lactate Dehydrogenase	Normal	High

Specific diagnostic tests are available for certain infectious etiologies including tuberculosis, CMV, EBV, *Bartonella henselae*, toxoplasmosis, Lyme, HIV, Ehrlichia, anaplasmosis, and streptococcus [21].

Imaging. Ultrasound is the first-line modality for masses suspicious for LAD due to its low cost, availability, lack of required sedation, ability to identify surrounding masses and to discern lymph nodes concerning for malignancy (Table 4) [2,6]. These factors also make ultrasound ideal for surveillance of suspicious lesions [22]. However, it is operator dependent, cannot always visualize the complete mass, and is not effective in all parts of the body (chest, parts of the abdomen and pelvis) [2,6].

Lymph nodes should be evaluated for architecture and size in 3 dimensions. Normal LNs are ovoid with homogenous echotexture, smooth borders, and a clearly distinguishable fatty hilum [3]. Abnormal LNs will appear fixed, round, and hypervascular with irregular borders, changes in the appearance of the cortex and/or hilum, and loss of a central fatty hilum [1,23]. A more circular LN shape with a long:short ratio of <2 is predictive of malignancy [24]. An enlarged transverse dimension is most prognostic for lymphoma [3]. Finally, in addition to characterizing abnormal LNs, ultrasound can also be used to identify LN mimics.

Table 4
Imaging results which identify lymph nodes at higher risk for malignancy

	Lower risk for malignancy	Higher risk for malignancy
Imaging		
Ultrasound	Ovoid with homogenous echotexture, smooth borders, and a distinguishable fatty hilum	Fixed, round, and hypervascular, irregular borders, cortex and/or hilum changes, and loss of a central fatty hilum. Long:short ratio <2
Chest X ray	Normal; signs of infection	Mediastinal widening/mass

Chest radiograph (CXR) can assist with determining the etiology of LAD if there is a concern for systemic illness, pneumonic process, and/or mediastinal LAD. CXR may demonstrate signs of pulmonary infection such as pleural effusion, atelectasis, consolidation, or empyema [25]. Mediastinal widening, presence of a mass, or LNs can also be identified. In this case, CXR can be essential in guiding cross-sectional imaging.

In the setting of a mediastinal mass or significant LAD, chest tomography (CT) is helpful to stratify perioperative risk and evaluate for tracheal compression. Additional testing such as pulmonary function tests and echocardiogram may be necessary to assess for impaired respiratory mechanics, presence of a pericardial effusion, and compression on the heart or great vessels. These results, in addition to those of a chest CT, can be utilized to define sedation risk if anesthesia is warranted for a biopsy [26,27].

MRI and nuclear medicine tests are rarely needed for the evaluation of pediatric soft tissue masses at diagnosis. The most common indications are inability to fully visualize the mass due to intracranial or intraspinal extension, concern for other lesions, or identifying metastatic lesions [2,6].

Biopsy. Biopsy should be performed if a mass is suspicious for malignancy or persists without a known diagnosis. [1,2]. Surgical biopsies—incisional (partial LN sampling) or excisional (whole LN removal)—are the gold standard for LN sampling. Incisional biopsy can be user-dependent and may not generate adequate tissue if only part of the LN is excised [28]. Furthermore, they generally require the same degree of anesthesia as an excisional biopsy, and as such, excisional biopsy is preferred to guarantee an adequate tissue sample. If multiple LNs are present, the largest or most abnormal LN should be excised [2]. Regardless of surgical biopsy type, an intraoperative pathologic assessment is warranted to ensure sufficient tissue was acquired.

If surgical biopsy is not possible, then small specimen biopsies can be performed, including fine needle aspiration biopsy (FNAB) or core needle biopsy (CNB). FNAB and CNB can both procure samples that are sufficient to test cell morphology, immunophenotyping, and microbiology [1]. Advantages of these procedures are improved cosmesis, and they may avoid general anesthesia. However, FNAB lacks the ability to evaluate LN architecture, and thus will not be able to distinguish between malignant lymphoid lesions and reactive hyperplasia [29]. Utilization of FNAB and CNB is dependent on institutional preference and the pathologist's experience in cytopathological evaluation.

Once the biopsy is obtained, the sample should be sent *fresh* for the studies outlined in Box 1: histology, Gram stain, bacterial culture, acid-fast bacilli (AFB) culture and smear, AFB polymerase chain reaction test, and fungal smear and culture [2]. If there is concern for lymphoma, the LN should be sent for immunohistochemistry which can identify cell lineage and phase of maturation, detect specific alterations in genes, visualize the extent of cell proliferation, and identify targets for therapy. This process depends on sufficient samples and proper fixation, and so an expert pathologist should be available to guide the process [30].

Box 1: Typical tests for lymph node biopsy samples

Histology
Bacterial culture and Gram stain
Acid-fast bacilli (AFB) culture and smear
AFB polymerase chain reaction test
Fungal culture and smear
Lymphoma immunohistochemistry and flow cytometry

SUMMARY

Children frequently present for evaluation with soft tissue swelling and LAD. The differential is broad and includes benign and malignant etiologies of LAD, soft tissue neoplasms, and non-neoplastic etiologies. History and physical examination are essential to narrowing the differential diagnosis and guiding next steps in evaluation and management.

CLINICS CARE POINTS

- History and physical are fundamental to guiding evaluation of soft tissue masses in children.
- Cervical lymphadenopathy (LAD) is often ultimately classified as benign idiopathic, but providers should be alert for concerning features associated with malignancy:
  - Lymph node characteristics: supraclavicular location, large size, or fixed, matted, or nontender on examination.
  - Signs and symptoms: systemic "B" symptoms, generalized LAD, or dyspnea.
  - Imaging: abnormal LNs on ultrasound, mediastinal mass, or LAD.
- The differential for LN mimics in children is extensive but can be narrowed based on location of the mass.

Acknowledgements

The authors would like to acknowledge Lucy Nam, MD for medical illustration (see Fig. 1).

Disclosure

The authors have nothing to disclose.

References

[1] Grant CN, Aldrink J, Lautz TB, et al. Lymphadenopathy in children: a streamlined approach for the surgeon - a report from the APSA Cancer Committee. J Pediatr Surg 2021;56(2): 274–81.
[2] Chang SSY, Xiong M, How CH, et al. An approach to cervical lymphadenopathy in children. Singapore Med J 2020;61(11):569–77.

[3] Ahuja AT, Ying M, Ho SY, et al. Ultrasound of malignant cervical lymph nodes. Cancer Imaging 2008;8(1):48–56.

[4] Berce V, Rataj N, Dorič M, et al. Association between the clinical, laboratory and ultrasound characteristics and the etiology of peripheral lymphadenopathy in children. Children (Basel) 2023;10(10):1589.

[5] Deosthali A, Donches K, DelVecchio M, et al. Etiologies of pediatric cervical lymphadenopathy: a systematic review of 2687 subjects. Glob Pediatr Health 2019;6:2333794X19865440.

[6] Navarro OM. Pearls and pitfalls in the imaging of soft-tissue masses in children. Semin Ultrasound CT MR 2020;41(5):498–512.

[7] Soldes OS, Younger JG, Hirschl RB. Predictors of malignancy in childhood peripheral lymphadenopathy. J Pediatr Surg 1999;34(10):1447–52.

[8] Bozlak S, Varkal MA, Yildiz I, et al. Cervical lymphadenopathies in children: a prospective clinical cohort study. Int J Pediatr Otorhinolaryngol 2016;82:81–7.

[9] Ingolfsdottir M, Balle V, Hahn CH. Evaluation of cervical lymphadenopathy in children: advantages and drawbacks of diagnostic methods. Dan Med J 2013;60(8):A4667.

[10] Locke R, Comfort R, Kubba H. When does an enlarged cervical lymph node in a child need excision? A systematic review. Int J Pediatr Otorhinolaryngol 2014;78(3):393–401.

[11] Soares L, Rebelo Matos A, Mello Vieira M, et al. Generalized lymphadenopathy as the first manifestation of systemic lupus erythematosus. Cureus 2022;14(10):e30089.

[12] Tunev SS, Hastey CJ, Hodzic E, et al. Lymphoadenopathy during lyme borreliosis is caused by spirochete migration-induced specific B cell activation. PLoS Pathog 2011;7(5): e1002066.

[13] Akel T, Mobarakai N. Hematologic manifestations of babesiosis. Ann Clin Microbiol Antimicrob 2017;16(1):6.

[14] Schutze GE, Buckingham SC, Marshall GS, et al. Human monocytic ehrlichiosis in children. Pediatr Infect Dis J 2007;26(6):475–9.

[15] Chochlakis D, Ioannou I, Tselentis Y, et al. Human anaplasmosis and Anaplasma ovis variant. Emerg Infect Dis 2010;16(6):1031–2.

[16] Snowden J, Simonsen KA. Rocky mountain spotted fever (Rickettsia rickettsii). 2023. In: StatPearls [Internet]. Treasure Island (FL): StatPearls Publishing; 2025.

[17] Hammadi SA, Al-Anbari AJK, Al-Alosi BM. Toxoplasma lymphadenopathy: a comparative diagnostic assessment of clinical, serological and histopathological findings. Iran J Otorhinolaryngol 2023;35(128):157–63.

[18] Faye A. Kawasaki disease: a new understanding of the clinical spectrum. Lancet Child Adolesc Health 2023;7(10):672–3.

[19] Metterle L, Hatch L, Seminario-Vidal L. Pediatric drug reaction with eosinophilia and systemic symptoms: a systematic review of the literature. Pediatr Dermatol 2020;37(1):124–9.

[20] Bewtra M, Lewis JD. Update on the risk of lymphoma following immunosuppressive therapy for inflammatory bowel disease. Expert Rev Clin Immunol 2010;6(4):621–31.

[21] Johnson DR, Kurlan R, Leckman J, et al. The human immune response to streptococcal extracellular antigens: clinical, diagnostic, and potential pathogenetic implications. Clin Infect Dis 2010;50(4):481–90.

[22] Harris JE, Patel NN, Wai K, et al. Management of pediatric persistent asymptomatic cervical lymphadenopathy. Otolaryngol Head Neck Surg 2024;170(1):69–75.

[23] Raja Lakshmi C, Sudhakara Rao M, Ravikiran A, et al. Evaluation of reliability of ultrasonographic parameters in differentiating benign and metastatic cervical group of lymph nodes. ISRN Otolaryngol 2014;2014:238740.

[24] Steinkamp HJ, Cornehl M, Hosten N, et al. Cervical lymphadenopathy: ratio of long- to short-axis diameter as a predictor of malignancy. Br J Radiol 1995;68(807):266–70.

[25] van de Maat JS, Garcia Perez D, Driessen GJA, et al. The influence of chest X-ray results on antibiotic prescription for childhood pneumonia in the emergency department. Eur J Pediatr 2021;180(9):2765–72.

[26] Shamberger RC. Preanesthetic evaluation of children with anterior mediastinal masses. Semin Pediatr Surg 1999;8(2):61–8.

[27] McLeod M, Dobbie M. Anterior mediastinal masses in children. BJA Educ 2019;19(1): 21–6.

[28] Bayhan Z, Ozdemir K, Gonullu E, et al. Analysis of diagnostic excisional lymph node biopsy results: 12-year experience of a single center. Acta Clin Croat 2023;62(1):58–64.

[29] Ha HJ, Lee J, Kim DY, et al. Utility and limitations of fine-needle aspiration cytology in the diagnosis of lymphadenopathy. Diagnostics (Basel) 2023;13(4):728.

[30] Cho J. Basic immunohistochemistry for lymphoma diagnosis. Blood Res 2022;57(S1): 55–61.

Advances in Pediatrics 72 (2025) 103–113

ADVANCES IN PEDIATRICS

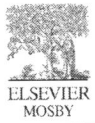

Quality Improvement in Pediatrics

Ashley Perry, MD[a],*, Shaila Siraj, MD[b]

[a]Department of Graduate Medical Education, University of South Florida, 17 Davis Boulevard, #308, Tampa, FL 33606, USA; [b]Department of Pediatrics, Johns Hopkins All Children's Hospital, 601 5th Street South, St Petersburg, FL 33701, USA

Keywords

- Quality improvement • Pediatrics • High value care • Health equity • Patient safety

Key points

- Prior initiatives demonstrated the impact that quality improvement has on patients, continued provider involvement is essential to ensuring the benefits to patients continue.
- Robust project design and utilization of quality improvement tools are crucial to a successful quality improvement project.
- Many additional resources exist to enhance understanding of quality improvement.

INTRODUCTION

Many are familiar with the landmark publication by the Institute of Medicine in 1999, *To Err is Human: Building a Safer Healthcare System*. This publication estimated that 98,000 people die yearly from hospital-associated medical errors, more than in automobile accidents or from breast cancer [1]. This shed light on the magnitude of the problem of patient safety and the need to work toward a safer system to deliver health care. Today, more than 25 years after this publication, significant gains have been achieved in improving the value of care provided to our patients. However, more work remains to be done to build a safer system and provide high quality care to all patients. This goal cannot be achieved without the engagement of providers and multidisciplinary clinical staff in identifying areas for improvement and implementing change. As you engage in clinical practice, we encourage you to continuously think about how all aspects of health care delivery can be improved. Think about the

*Corresponding author. E-mail address: Aperry2@usf.edu

https://doi.org/10.1016/j.yapd.2025.01.003
0065-3101/25/

pebble in your shoe, the one small thing that bothers you every day. With this article, we aim to provide you with the basic tools to remove the pebble and take action to make improvements.

What is quality improvement?

Quality improvement differs significantly from research in many ways, however, differentiating these methodologies can be challenging. Research typically involves rigorous testing of a single hypothesis to generate new, generalizable knowledge, whereas quality improvement aims to improve local clinical practice in real time [2]. A research project has a precise protocol that does not change over time. A subset of the population is eligible to participate in research based on strict, predefined criteria, and subjects typically consent to participation. A quality improvement project has an adaptive design using iterative cycles that may change over time based on results gathered in real-time. The entire population participates, and consent is implied. Research methods involve a hypothesis and use the scientific methods to determine an answer to the question at hand. Quality improvement involves working toward a global aim and adhering to already established best practices. Quality improvement directly impacts institutional practices and, therefore, is expected to directly improve care for patients involved in the work [3]. The Institute of Medicine has set 6 specific aims for quality improvement: health care should be safe, effective, patient-centered, timely, efficient, and equitable [4]. Achievement of these aims is monitored across health care institutions in standardized ways.

Successes in quality improvement

To date, there have been numerous successes in quality improvement, particularly surrounding reductions in adverse drug events, catheter-associated blood stream infections, ventilator-associated pneumonia, and patient handoff errors [2]. These achievements have led to a variety of benefits including improved patient outcomes with the reduction in morbidity and mortality, decreased health care costs, and enhancement of the patient provider experience. These advances have a direct impact on patients, families, and the community.

In 1993, Jerry Sternin was asked to complete what seemed like an impossible task—end childhood malnutrition in Vietnam. To achieve this, he started with a narrow scope, selecting just one small village where he would focus his efforts. He began by talking to locals to ensure he had a deep understanding of the problem before proposing any interventions. Through his work, he was able to eliminate malnutrition in 80% of children within 2 years using resources available in the community [5]. This impact was sustained, families who participated in the program had better-nourished children than controls, even when those children were too young to have participated in the initial program [6]. Ultimately, this program was spread to 20 Vietnamese provinces impacting more than 2 million children [5]. This initiative had an enormous, clinically relevant impact on the pediatric population. This improvement started with a small group of people with very limited resources who saw a problem and were motivated to make a change.

Although Sternin's initiative occurred in the community, the same principles can and have been applied in the clinic and hospital setting. One initiative across 21 primarily community hospitals aimed at reducing the use of bronchodilators, steroids, and chest X rays among pediatric patients with bronchiolitis. Avoiding the use of these evaluation and treatment modalities in bronchiolitis is the best practice. Through quality improvement methodologies, investigators were able to reduce the use of bronchodilators by 29%, the use of steroids by 68%, and the use of X ray by 44%, thereby significantly reducing unnecessary care for patients with bronchiolitis without increasing length of stay or readmission rates [7]. Eliminating one dose of medication or one imaging study may not seem like a massive shift in clinical care, but over time this reduces the risk of medication side effects, radiation exposure, costs of patients and families, and unnecessary use of hospital resources. It also increases adherence to evidence-based guidelines, which is something all health care systems strive for.

Another initiative across 29 pediatric intensive care units aimed at reducing catheter-associated blood stream infections. Through implementation of an insertion and maintenance bundle, they were able to decrease their infection rates by 43%. This work was based on prior initiatives that were successful in adult patients, some of which proved to be as successful in pediatric populations and some of which were not as successful [8]. Collaboration and sharing of quality improvement interventions between institutions, departments, and individual groups is fundamental to the continued improvement in care for our patients.

Prior successes have demonstrated that significant improvements can be made even with limited resources and simple interventions. A robust project plan using quality improvement tools and a desire to make life better are the crucial components to improving care for patients. In the next section, we review methodologies and recommendations for developing and implementing quality improvement work within your own practice.

DISCUSSION

How to complete a quality improvement project

Implementing a quality improvement project can be a daunting task. There are many different, but equally effective, strategies to develop and execute this type of work. This includes Lean, Six Sigma, and the Model for Improvement [9].

Lean focuses on maximizing value and eliminating waste, working to create more efficient processes to generate more products with fewer deficits in a shorter amount of time [10]. Six Sigma focuses on reducing variability to decrease nonconformance to the standard using the framework of define, measure, analyze, improve, and control (DMAIC) [11]. The Model for Improvement begins with 3 essential questions: what are we trying to accomplish, how will we know the change is an improvement, and what changes can be made to result in improvement? This is followed by multiple plan, do, study, act (PDSA) cycles where changes are implemented and assessed [12]. This process is often best understood through examples, so we will use a hypothetical project of improving flu vaccination rates in a pediatric clinic to demonstrate each phase. This overall process is outlined in Fig. 1, although the process may look slightly different based on which methodology is utilized. Regardless of which methodology is utilized, building a strong foundation is crucial for any successful quality improvement project.

The initial step in creating a quality improvement project is identifying the problem to be solved and outlining the problem statement. It is imperative to focus on one, solvable problem that ideally addresses one of the 6 Institute of Medicine domains for improvement. To understand the problem, completing a Gemba walk or conducting a gap analysis can clarify the current state and explore the differences between the ideal state and current state. Gemba is a Japanese word which means "the place where things happen," and taking a Gemba walk means going to the place where the process occurs and following it from start to finish. During this time, ask the people who do the work about the process, the people involved, barriers to completing the process, why those barriers occur, any workarounds, and who they contact when there are problems. Try to support the problem with data if available. Generate a clear and concise problem statement which is 1 to 2 sentences in length, devoid of assumptions and bias, and without any proposed solutions. It is important to highlight the burning platform. The burning platform outlines the consequences of not addressing the problem and highlights why people should care. Depending on the audience, this may include things like patient morbidity and mortality, financial loss, overutilization of resources, and nonadherence to widely accepted guidelines.

Problem statement: Approximately 200 children die annually from influenza, however, according to well-established data, influenza vaccination can decrease hospitalization rates by over 50%. The CDC recommends that all children over 6 months of age receive influenza vaccination and yet currently in Advances Pediatric Clinic, only 50% of patients are vaccinated against influenza annually.

After identifying the problem, the project goal should be outlined in an aim statement. The aim is the specific, measurable, attainable, relevant, and time-bound goal of your project, often referred to as an SMART aim [12]. The aim should include a specific goal to be achieved by a certain date, although this goal may change over time depending on the success of the project. In general, a 20% improvement from baseline is an appropriate starting point.

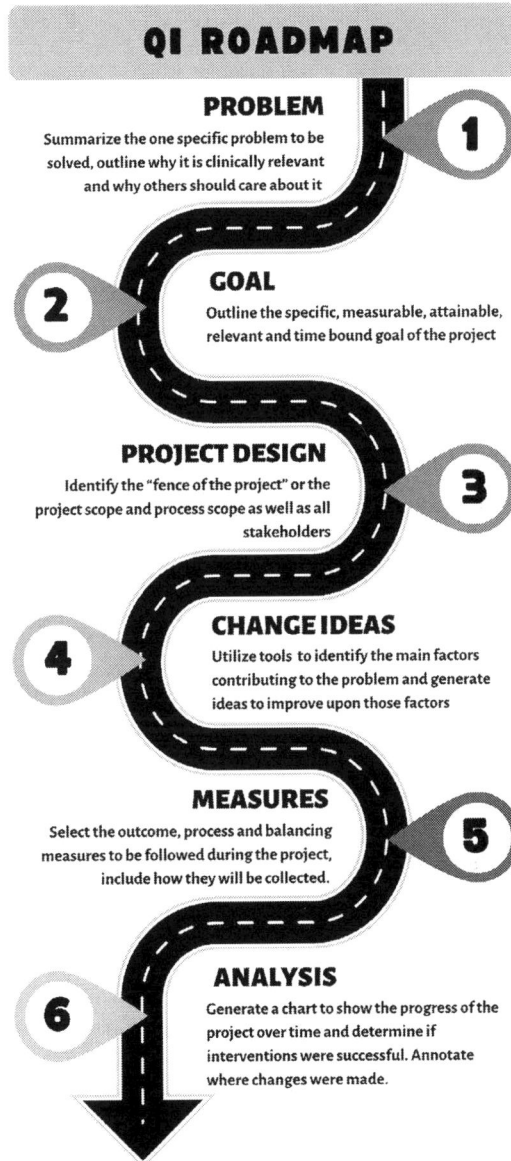

Fig. 1. An overview of the process of developing and implementing a quality improvement project.

Aim: Increase the percentage of pediatric patients (age >6 month to <18 years) seen in Advances Pediatric Clinic who receive the influenza vaccine from a baseline of 50% to a goal of 75% by April 2025.

Then, outline the scope—this is the boundary of what will be included in the project. It is typically best to start with a narrow scope and then expand successful interventions to other areas over time. The process scope includes the start and end of the process to be improved upon. Creating a map of the process or flowchart including each step and decision point within the process can clarify the current process. There are many ways to accomplish this, depending on the complexity of the process and the number of individuals involved. Some examples include basic flowcharts, swim lane diagrams, and SIPOC (suppliers, inputs, process, outputs, and customers) diagrams. The project scope identifies which population will be included in the project, similar to inclusion and exclusion criteria [13]. Quality improvement work should apply to the entire population selected, so the population should be clearly defined but should not have a significant number of exclusions.

Process scope: Patient presents to Advances Pediatric Clinic for a visit -> Patient checks out of the Advances Pediatric Clinic from that visit.

Project scope: All pediatric patients, age greater than 6 mo and less than 18 years, who have not been previously vaccinated against influenza this season and do not have medical contraindications[a] to receiving the influenza vaccine who present to the Advances Pediatric Clinic during the study period.

Now identify your stakeholders. A stakeholder is anyone involved in the process or impacted by the process. These individuals can effect change or may be affected by the change [9]. Stakeholder groups should have representation when major project decisions are made. Some stakeholders are referred to as key stakeholders–these individuals have more impact on, or authority over, the process.

Stakeholders: physicians, advanced practice providers, nurses, medical assistants, families, patients.

Next, use tools such as a cause-and-effect diagram (Ishikawa or fishbone diagrams) or key driver diagram to better understand the factors contributing to the problem and help brainstorm ideas that can bring about change. The goal of this part of the process is to fully understand all the factors that contribute to the problem being solved. A cause-and-effect diagram looks like the skeleton of the fish. This type of diagram places the problem at the head of the fish on the right side of the page and then adds likely causes as the bones under major headings. This is a structured approach to identifying the root cause of a problem. A key driver diagram also helps guide improvement efforts by outlining changes that can be made to result in improvement. Teams identify the key factors that drive the process and brainstorm change ideas in each of these categories [8]. Some of the key categories of change concepts are eliminating waste, improving workflow, optimizing inventory, changing the work environment, managing variation, managing time, and designing systems to avoid mistakes [12].

Key driver diagram: See Fig. 2.

Before implementing any changes, measures should be set forth which will determine if a change is an improvement. Each project should have an outcome measure, process measure, and a balancing measure. The outcome measure is

---

[a]Medical contraindications: severe allergic reaction (anaphylaxis) to a component of the vaccine.

Key Drivers **Change Ideas**

Smart Aim

Increase the percentage of pediatric patients who receive the influenza vaccine from a baseline of 50% to a goal of 75% by April 2025.

Patient and family medical literacy and knowledge of influenza vaccine

Provide handouts to patients and families on the benefits of influenza vaccination

Clinical staff knowledge of benefits of influenza vaccine

Educate clinical staff on benefits of influenza vaccination

Clinical staff time and competing priorities

Standardize the process of offering influenza vaccination to all patients in the clinic

Patient/family time and competing priorities / access

Create an option for walk-in influenza vaccination

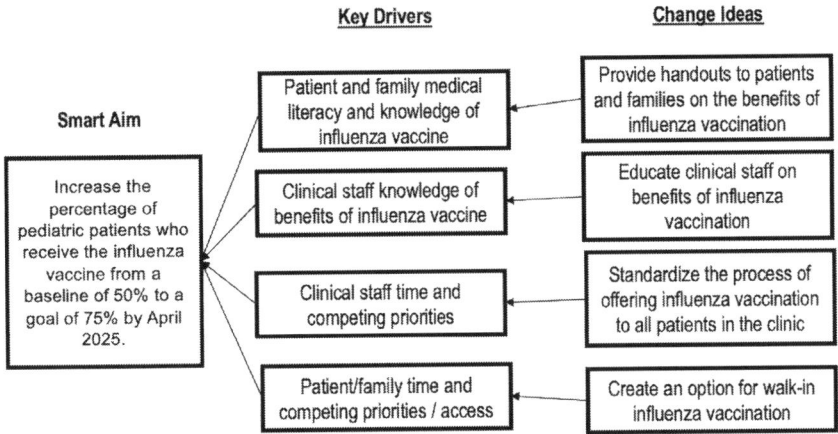

Fig. 2. Key driver diagram for the theoretic quality improvement project aimed increasing influenza vaccination rates in a pediatric clinic.

directly related to the aim of the project and determines if the goal is achieved. The outcome measure should be tracked before starting the project and throughout the duration of the project. A process measure is selected for each change idea and determines if that change occurs. A process measure may be tracked for the duration of the study or just during the PDSA cycle associated with that change. A balancing measure assesses for any unintended consequences that occur because of the changes made to achieve the project goal [12]. This measure should also be tracked prior to and for the duration of the study. For each measure, the operational definition of how that measure is defined (numerator and denominator, scoring system, etc), where the data will be obtained, and how often it will be collected should be outlined. Selected measures should reflect the change you are making; however, they do not need to be perfect. Additionally, obtaining data from a representative subset of patients is typically sufficient to determine if a change is occurring.

Measures: Outcome measure—percentage of pediatric patients seen in Advances Pediatric Clinic who are vaccinated against influenza. Process measure—percentage of patients/families provided with the influenza handout, percentage of clinical staff who attend or view influenza vaccine education sessions, percentage of patients who are offered influenza vaccine, volume of patients who attend the walk-in clinic. Balancing measure—visit wait times.

Finally, it is time to put the first change into action. Typically, change ideas that have high impact and low effort should be completed first. Creating a priority matrix with ranking criteria including the value of the change, resources needed, alignment with other strategic initiatives, etc, can help determine which change to prioritize. Viewing baseline data in a Pareto chart with causes/defects on the x-axis and incidence on the y-axis can also help determine where to focus efforts, as the Pareto principle states most of the variation (80%) of any condition comes from a small number of variables (20%) [9]. Testing a change on a small scale and then applying that change to other areas if successful can be the most manageable way to effect change. Explicitly outlining what people should do, making it easy and straightforward for people to do it, and inspiring people to appreciate the benefits of doing it are the crucial components to change [14].

Lastly, measuring data in real-time and providing feedback to those involved in the work allows for continued adaptation of the project and generation of further PDSA cycles. Collecting data should not be time-consuming–looking at a small, representative portion of the population is acceptable. Celebrate any wins and obtain more information about any challenges or obstacles to keep people engaged. Data can be presented in an annotated run chart or control chart showing the change over time and where the interventions were made. This allows for the visualization of whether a change is an improvement and if that improvement is sustainable. It can also help identify any trends that highlight the significance of the data. The definition of each trend varies depending on the type of chart used to display the data. The use of predefined trends helps differentiate inherent variation from true change [9]. Once the project is underway, share the work with others within your institution or from other institutions.

Effecting change

Changing human behavior is one of the most challenging parts of quality improvement; to be successful, it requires a strong foundation in people management. Change may be viewed as uncertain, or as a request for people to do more work without any guarantee of benefit. So how do you get people to change? Many have heard of the adage of the carrot or the stick–entice people with reward or threaten them with punishment to get them to adhere to what you want. This falls short, however, when the carrot or stick wielder is not around or if the person leading the change does not have the authority to use the carrot or stick. There are many theories on how to get people to change, which is beyond the scope of this article, but one theory comes from Chip and Dan Heath. They suggest that change requires 3 components: stating why the change is needed in a way that speaks to the individual's inner desires and motivations, clearly laying out the steps of the change, and making it as easy as possible for the change to occur [14].

Barriers to engaging in quality improvement

While the importance of quality improvement has been emphasized, engagement in this type of work is not without barriers. Studies have reported that the most common barriers were the culture of the institution, conflicting priorities, time, and resources. In some cases, physicians also perceived quality improvement as extra work and did not see the value in this work to improve patient care [15]. Additional reasons for project failure include having too large of a scope, not involving the necessary key stakeholders, having poorly defined aims, having poorly constructed measures, and ending the project rather than adapting when cycles do not go as intended [9].

FUTURE CONSIDERATIONS
Education in pediatric residency
Currently, the Accreditation Council for Graduate Medical Education (ACGME) allows pediatric residents to meet their educational requirements for quality improvement in a variety of ways. ACGME requires participation in real or simulated interprofessional quality improvement activity, such as root cause analysis, that includes formulation and implementation of actions. They also require residents to demonstrate knowledge of central principles that drive continuous quality improvement and systematically analyze practice using quality improvement methods [16]. Despite these requirements, a national survey of pediatric residency programs demonstrated that there is significant variability in the education received by trainees. Although 84% of respondents planned to use quality improvement methods to improve their clinical area after graduation, 28% did not feel confident in applying quality improvement methods and 39% felt they would be unable to lead a quality improvement project on their own. Development of a strong understanding of quality improvement during residency training can lay the foundation for continued participation in quality improvement throughout a physician's career. Key components of this education include faculty support, structured curriculum, hands-on projects, and dedicated project time [17].

Quality improvement to address health disparities
On the surface, quality improvement appears to be an excellent tool to address health disparities and improve the quality of care that is provided to vulnerable populations. However, challenges remain in implementing quality improvement initiatives in low resource settings that may serve these populations. Unfortunately, it is possible that quality improvement initiatives could worsen health disparities if there is greater success of interventions among patient populations who have better outcomes at baseline [18]. Moving forward, the inclusion of interventions focused on social determinants of health and subanalysis of intervention success in minority populations could identify and reduce these disparities. Additionally, the use of quality improvement to reduce health care costs and increase accessibility could lessen health disparities.

Additional resources for quality improvement education
This article provides an overview of quality improvement methodologies. There are many more resources that provide an in-depth understanding of the topics discussed here, and more! Discuss with your employer or institution about any training opportunities or resources available to you.

For self-directed education on quality improvement, the Institute for Healthcare Improvement Open School offers multiple courses. Some of these courses are available at no cost to qualified students and trainees. The Institute for Healthcare Improvement also offers a fellowship program for continued training in quality improvement. The American Medical Association EdHub offers a course in Foundations of Quality Improvement and Patient Safety.

There are also many books available on quality improvement, including Pediatric Patient Safety and Quality Improvement.

For publication of improvement initiatives, the Standards for Quality Improvement Reporting Excellence (SQUIRE) guidelines provide a framework for reporting system-level work to improve the quality, safety, and value of health care. Although every aspect of the framework may not be applicable to every initiative, it provides a thorough foundation for disseminating this work [19]. Sharing both successes and failures moves us toward the most efficient and safest system for health care delivery [1].

SUMMARY AND RECOMMENDATIONS

Quality improvement has been successful in improving patient safety and the value of care that is provided to patients. Continued involvement in quality improvement activities is necessary to continue to advance patient care. This article provides clinicians with basic tools to start to build a foundation in quality improvement methodologies.

For those who hope to initiate quality improvement initiatives, additional resources are available to further outline the tools discussed here and discuss additional tools. Overall, a quality improvement initiative should outline the problem, aim, scope, change ideas, and measures. Quality improvement methodologies are more flexible than traditional research, but a successful project has a well-defined outline prior to initiation of any interventions.

Further work remains to address barriers to implementation of quality improvement, improve education on quality improvement during training, and use quality improvement to promote health equity.

CLINICS CARE POINTS

- Prior initiatives have demonstrated the impact that quality improvement can have on patients, and that continued provider involvement is essential to ensuring the benefits to patients continue.
- Robust project design and utilizing the tools discussed above are crucial to a successful quality improvement project.
- Many additional resources exist to enhance understanding of quality improvement.

Disclosure

The authors have nothing to disclose.

References

[1] Institute of Medicine (US) Committee on Quality of Health Care in America. In: Kohn LT, Corrigan JM, Donaldson MS, editors. To Err is human: building a safer health system. Washington, DC: National Academies Press (US); 2000.

[2] Schwartz SP, Rehder KJ. Quality improvement in pediatrics: past, present, and future. Pediatr Res 2017;81(1–2):156–61.

[3] Bass PF 3rd, Maloy JW. How to determine if a project is human subjects research, a quality improvement project, or both. Ochsner J 2020;20(1):56–61.

[4] Committee on Quality Health Care in America, Institute of Medicine. Crossing the quality chasm: a new health system for the 21st century. Washington, DC: National Academy Press; 2011.

[5] Pascale RT, Sternin J, Sternin M. The power of positive deviance: how unlikely innovators solve the world's toughest problems. Boston: Harvard University Press; 2010.

[6] Mackintosh UA, Marsh DR, Schroeder DG. Sustained positive deviant child care practices and their effects on child growth in Viet Nam. Food Nutr Bull 2002;23(4 Suppl):18–27.

[7] Ralston SL, Garber MD, Rice-Conboy E, et al. A multicenter collaborative to reduce unnecessary care in inpatient bronchiolitis. Pediatrics 2016;137(1); https://doi.org/10.1542/peds.2015-0851.

[8] Miller MR, Griswold M, Harris JM 2nd, et al. Decreasing PICU catheter-associated bloodstream infections: NACHRI's quality transformation efforts. Pediatrics 2010;125(2): 206–13.

[9] Frush KS, Krug SE. Pediatric patient safety and quality improvement. China: McGraw Hill; 2015. p. 1–48.

[10] Womack JP, Jones DT. Lean thinking. New York: Free Press, Simon & Schuster; 2003.

[11] Arthur J. Lean six Sigma for hospitals. New York: McGraw-Hill; 2011.

[12] Langley GL, Moen R, Nolan KM, et al. The improvement guide: a practical approach to enhancing organizational performance. 2nd edition. San Francisco (CA): Jossey-Bass Publishers; 2009.

[13] Step 1: define the goals, scope, and institutional home of your stakeholder engagement process. Rockville (MD): Agency for Healthcare Research and Quality; 2019. Available at: https://www.ahrq.gov/policymakers/chipra/demoeval/what-we-learned/implementation-guides/implementation-guide1/impguide1step1.html.

[14] Heath C, Heath D. Switch: how to change things when change is hard. United States: Crown; 2010.

[15] Kiran T, Rozmovits L, O'Brien P. Factors influencing family physician engagement in practice-based quality improvement: qualitative study. Can Fam Physician 2023;69(5): e113–9.

[16] Pediatrics Accreditation Council for Graduate Medical Education (ACGME) Program Requirements. 2024.

[17] Craig MS, Garfunkel LC, Baldwin CD, et al. Pediatric resident education in quality improvement (QI): a national survey. Acad Pediatr 2014;14(1):54–61.

[18] Lion KC, Raphael JL. Partnering health disparities research with quality improvement science in pediatrics. Pediatrics 2015;135(2):354–61.

[19] Ogrinc G, Davies L, Goodman D, et al. SQUIRE 2.0 (Standards for QUality Improvement Reporting Excellence): revised publication guidelines from a detailed consensus process. BMJ Qual Saf 2016;25(12):986–92.

Advances in Pediatrics 72 (2025) 115–129

ADVANCES IN PEDIATRICS

ELSEVIER
MOSBY

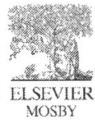

Helping Support Our Families Reach Their Breastfeeding Goals

Check for updates

Innovative Skill-Based Breastfeeding Education for Pediatric Residents

Jennifer Markwood, DO, MPH[a,1],
Karen Fugate, MSN RNC-NIC, CPHQ, LSSBB-C[b,2],
Alyssa Woodard, MD, CLC[a,3],
Cheryl Godcharles, MD, NABBLM-C, IBCLC[c,4],
Karyn Gerstle, MD, MPH, IBCLC[a,*]

[a]Department of Pediatrics, University of South Florida, Tampa, FL, USA; [b]Department of Performance Improvement, Tampa General Hospital, Tampa, FL, USA; [c]Department of Obstetrics and Gynecology, University of South Florida, Tampa, FL, USA

Keywords

• Breastfeeding • Pediatrics • Resident • Curriculum • Interprofessional

Key points

• Breastfeeding education for pediatric trainees is lacking despite program requirements for direct care of the infant–maternal dyads in both the hospital and outpatient settings.

• A novel skill-based breastfeeding curriculum can be utilized to increase breastfeeding comfort and knowledge within the pediatric trainee population.

• Supporting a family's feeding goals should be a collaborative effort that includes advanced practice providers, trainees, residents, attending physicians, and nursing team members.

[1]Present address: 7705 Willow Park Drive, Temple Terrace, FL 33637.
[2]Present address: 2806 Fairway Drive, Valrico, FL 33596.
[3]Present address: 408 N Willow Avenue, Tampa, FL 33606.
[4]Present address: 19405 Wingrove Lane, Lutz, FL33558.

*Corresponding author. Department of Pediatrics, Univeristy of South Florida, IBCLC17 Davis Island, Floor 1, Tampa, FL 33606. E-mail address: karyngerstle@usf.edu

https://doi.org/10.1016/j.yapd.2025.02.002

Abbreviations

AAP	American Academy of Pediatrics
OB/GYN	obstetrician–gynecologists
TGH	Tampa General Hospital
UNICEF	United Nations Children's Fund
WHO	World Health Organization

INTRODUCTION

It is well established that providing breast milk to infants yields health benefits to both mother and baby. In 2022, the American Academy of Pediatrics (AAP) updated its guidelines to recommend exclusive breastfeeding for the first 6 months of life, and continued breastfeeding for 2 years or beyond, if desired by both mother and infant [1]. This change from the 2012 stance meant the AAP recommendations now align with the World Health Organization (WHO) [2], United Nations Children's Fund (UNICEF) [3], American Academy of Family Physicians [4], and American College of Obstetricians and Gynecologists [5]. Despite the recommendations from these organizations, little has changed to update resident and medical school curricula to include breastfeeding medicine.

While all pediatric, family medicine, and obstetrician–gynecologists (OB/GYN) residency trainees have the opportunity to work with families and their newborns during labor and delivery, nursery, and neonatal intensive care unit rotations, most residents and early career physicians report a lack of confidence in discussing breastfeeding with these families [6]. Moreover, this discomfort extends outside of the initial newborn hospitalization and impacts clinic conversations. A 2008 study that surveyed pediatric providers found that clinicians were less likely to encourage breastfeeding than those who took the same survey in 1995, with study authors noting a lack of breastfeeding-specific training and personal experience with breastfeeding as 2 main contributors to this decline [7]. Other studies validate this notion that a lack of resident and medical student training contributes to reduced provider likelihood of supporting breastfeeding. A 2017 review with the keywords "breastfeeding + medical education" noted a lack of standardization in education opportunities, differing modes of delivery (lecture vs didactics vs rounding lectures) and a deficiency in general research evaluating breastfeeding education [8]. Furthermore, Osband and colleagues [9] reported that program directors believed the average number of hours devoted to breastfeeding training was low—just 3 hours per year of training. Most of this training is virtual material that residents review on their own time without any formal in-person reinforcement or competency assessment. Of pediatricians who graduated from residency in the past 5 years, only 1 in 4 endorsed adequate exposure and training to support lactating caregivers [10].

This problem is not unique to the United States. According to the 2018 Breastfeeding Resident Education Study, which surveyed 201 pediatric residents and 14 program directors in Canada, the majority of both directors and trainees reported a lack of breastfeeding education at their respective programs. Of the trainees surveyed, only 28% had observed a patient breastfeeding during their residency rotations [11]. Inadequacy in breastfeeding training is also reported by trainees in other specialties that manage birthing parents and their newborns. For example, a comprehensive survey of family medicine residency programs showed a similar deficiency, with trainees receiving on average 8 hours of informal education over the course of 3 years [9]. To put this in perspective, most residency programs require a minimum of 144 hours (or 36 half-day sessions) every year as part of their continuity clinic/longitudinal outpatient experience hours [12], which regularly includes newborn well visits and weight checks. In addition, pediatric residency programs require at least 4 additional weeks of newborn nursery exposure. If we do not devote more time to breastfeeding education despite our trainees' roles in newborn care, we are missing a valuable opportunity to optimize early nutrition, maternal mental health, and trust in the health care team.

Although time constraints to providing continuing medical education can be a limiting factor, many studies show that even minimal effort to provide in-person skills training can have a large impact. For example, a 2020 quality improvement project by Busler and colleagues [13], surveyed 24 pediatric residents who completed a 1 hour in-person skills training, and all reported improvement in their self-efficacy in breastfeeding counseling in clinic. Additionally, the American Board of Pediatrics has published their list of "Entrustable Professional Activities 3," which affirms that all general pediatricians should be able to apply "key evidence-based guidelines for care of the newborn," which includes addressing common problems that develop in the first 28 days of life. The AAP Breastfeeding Curriculum, which is available to pediatricians—both trainees and practicing physicians—provides education on many of these common problems such as perceived breastmilk insufficiency, nipple soreness, and low milk supply. Furthermore, a 2010 prospective study published in the journal *Pediatrics* [14] surveyed 417 pediatric, family medicine, and obstetrics residents and found that trainees who completed the AAP Breastfeeding curriculum felt they had significant improvements in "knowledge, practice patterns, and confidence in breastfeeding management." This training also provides a competency component—those completing the curriculum are given the opportunity to evaluate their learning with pretest and posttest assessments [15].

Despite suboptimal efforts to improve pediatrician knowledge of breastfeeding medicine, the need to support breastfeeding parents has been widely recognized. This recognition started with the Baby Friendly Hospital Initiative in 1991 led by the WHO and UNICEF to "assist hospitals in giving mothers the information, confidence, and skill necessary to successfully initiate and continue breastfeeding their babies." [16] Currently, 25% of babies born in the United States are born in a hospital with a Baby Friendly designation, and there is at least 1 hospital with a Baby Friendly designation in all 50 states, Washington D.C, and Puerto Rico. Furthermore, Healthy People 2030, a 10 year plan that outlines various public health objectives to improve the well-being of people living in the United States, has proposed an objective to improve the proportion of infants who are breastfed at 1 year of life [17].

While hospital policies and nationwide initiatives have made great impacts on supporting the feeding goals of parents, the majority of families still does not reach its breastfeeding goals by the time their child is 6 months old [18]. Although the first "golden" hour that the mother/baby dyad shares and the subsequent 24 to 48 hour newborn nursery stay is a crucial time for establishing breastfeeding, it is in the weeks thereafter that many common breastfeeding concerns (eg, engorgement, clogged ducts, painful latch, jaundice due to breastfeeding insufficiency, and mastitis) tend to arise. To this end, it is the outpatient pediatrician who will be seeing families regularly for the first year of children's lives and providing continued breastfeeding support. Here, we describe an innovative approach to improve general pediatric competency in providing bedside breastfeeding counseling in both the inpatient and outpatient settings. This training is an in-person skills session that aims to reinforce a pediatrician's knowledge of breastfeeding medicine. Specifically, we adapted a national nursing curriculum known as EMPower Best Practice Initiative into a condensed training experience delivered to pediatric residents and combined medicine-pediatric residents at a large academic medical center in the southeast United States during resident Academic Half Day. We describe the development of this curriculum to include counseling that is appropriate for a general pediatrician, and we present the data regarding changes to trainee confidence in providing breastfeeding support to families. We also discuss a model for expanding this curriculum to pediatricians already in practice, along with OB/GYN and family medicine residents and practicing providers. To our knowledge, this is the first adaptation of the EMPower curriculum that has added content relevant to physicians practicing in the ambulatory setting who will be managing patients after the initial nursery hospitalization.

GENERAL CONTENT
Curriculum development

EMPower Breastfeeding is a national quality improvement initiative, funded by the Centers for Disease Control, aimed at improving hospital-based maternity care practices [19]. The initiative began in 2014, and as of September 2024, the EMPower curriculum is in use by 125 hospitals, and the skill-based training has been completed by more than 10,000 nurses [20]. The overarching goal is to improve equitable care to support optimal infant nutrition and lactation health. The initiative is designed to be interactive, as practical skill-based training that includes an emphasis on communication and cultural competency has consistently proven to enhance breastfeeding success.

Tampa General Hospital (TGH) was accepted to participate in the EMPower Best Practices Initiative 2022 cohort, and was successfully redesignated as a Baby Friendly hospital in 2023, an accreditation process that occurs every 5 years. As part of participation in the EMPower Initiative, the hospital was given comprehensive training materials and resources, along with eLearning modules and a suggested curriculum covering all Baby-Friendly staff competency performance indicators. TGH, which received the initial Baby Friendly designation in 2015, selected a group of registered nurses with subject matter expertise to develop 12 skill stations covering all baby-friendly performance indicators. These stations required EMPower participants to show competency in each of the indicated skills. The skill stations were developed using relatable, common scenarios experienced by labor and delivery and nursery staff. Staff were required to complete eLearning modules prior to attending a scheduled skills assessment. Groups of 4 nurses rotated through 20 minute skills stations giving ample time for each to demonstrate competency. Over 200 registered nurses from the labor and delivery, postpartum, and newborn wards successfully completed the prerequisite eLearning modules and skills checkoffs.

Program evaluation occurred regularly after implementation and data collected during the 2 years since initiation of EMPower with nursing staff showed overall improvements in breastfeeding rates at the time of hospital discharge. In addition, patients from backgrounds traditionally impacted by health inequity saw the largest improvements in breastfeeding rates (Figs. 1–3).

Curriculum adaptation

Prior to the initiation of EMPower in 2022, nurses (along with nurse practitioners, residents, and attending physicians) with privileges to round on families in the TGH nursery were required to complete 3 hours of breastfeeding management content. The curriculum used is called Bella Breastfeeding, a peer-reviewed virtual course offered through a web-based continuing medical education platform called OPENPediatrics [21]. Although this online course offers many benefits, including free access around the world, it does not offer a skill-based competency component. In addition, hospital staff take this course on their own time without a follow-up discussion with other members of the hospital team to discuss hospital-specific breastfeeding policies or review barriers to breastfeeding for a hospital system's unique patient population.

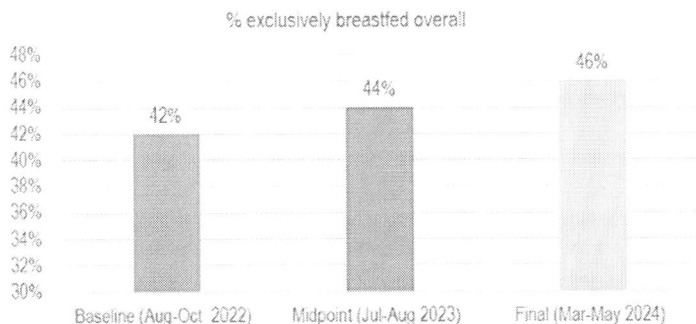

% exclusively breastfed overall

Fig. 1. Rates of exclusive breastfeeding for infants who were older than 36 weeks' gestational age at the time of hospital discharge. Rates were recorded at baseline, and at the midpoint and final time points following implementation of the EMPower Breastfeeding Training program.

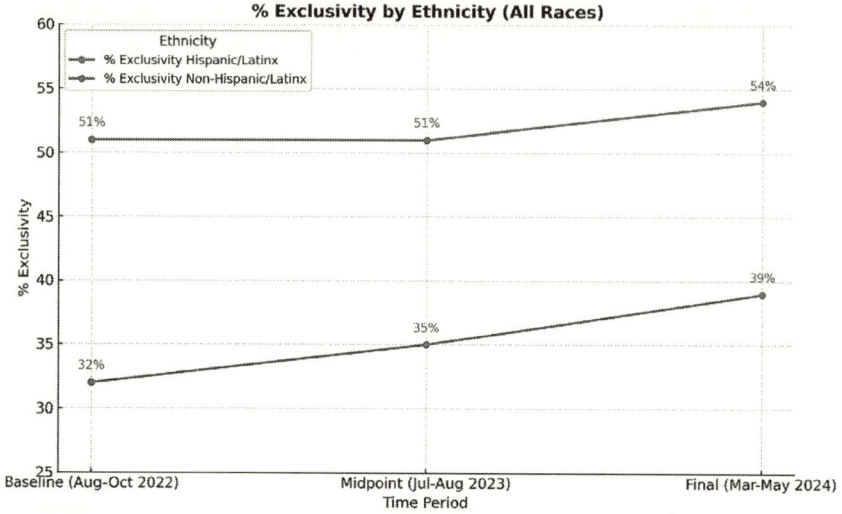

Fig. 2. Rates of exclusive breastfeeding for infants who were older than 36 weeks' gestational age among Hispanic/LatinX and non-Hispanic/LatinX families. Rates were recorded at baseline, and at the midpoint and final time points following implementation of the EMPower Breastfeeding Training program.

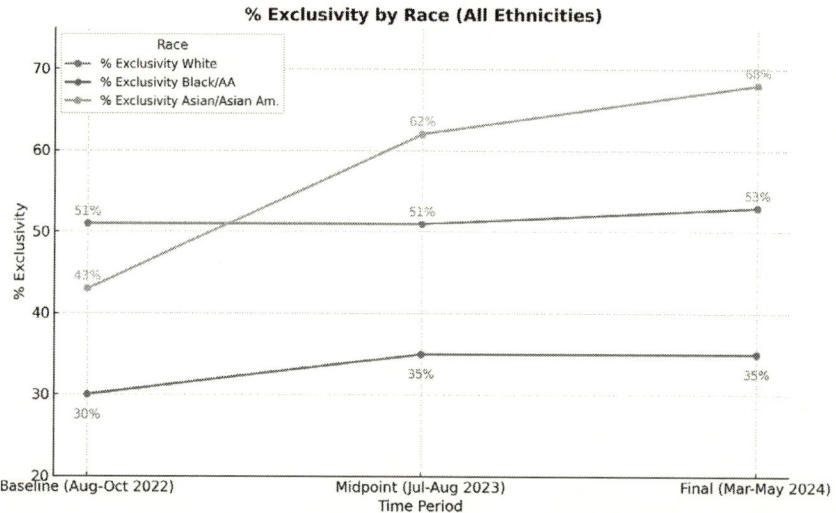

Fig. 3. Rates of exclusive breastfeeding for infants who were older than 36 weeks' gestational age among Black/AA and Asian/Asian Am Families compared to White families. Rates were recorded at baseline, and at the midpoint and final time points following implementation of the EMPower Breastfeeding Training program.

Although a self-paced learning format has benefits to allow for flexibility in schedules and access, it may not encourage collaboration among a multidisciplinary team given the solitary nature of an online prerecorded curriculum. Currently, pediatric providers, including residents who see patients at TGH, complete the Bella Breastfeeding curriculum prior to seeing their first patient in the mother/baby nursery.

As previously reviewed, self-directed learning that is followed by competency assessment is a validated method of improving provider confidence [22]. Thus, this group of authors decided to adapt the already established EMPower skill-based curriculum to include new content relevant for the outpatient setting and include a competency component. As far as we know, this is the first adaptation of the EMPower curriculum to add curriculum relevant to the ambulatory provider.

We adapted the curriculum to add content appropriate for pediatricians at different levels of training, as some providers attending the session had minimal to no baseline education in breastfeeding medicine. This adapted curriculum added content to include skills related to fourth trimester breastfeeding challenges that arise after discharge from the hospital. For example, one added station explored conversations about the transition from colostrum to mature milk, engorgement, cluster feeding, and expected weight loss at a newborn well check during days of life 3 to 5. A second station was added to discuss the 2 week well visit and to review how to assess maternal milk supply, manage oversupply or low supply, and how to evaluate newborn milk transfer by performing a prebreastfeeding and postbreastfeeding weight check. A final station was added for the 2 month well visit with emphasis on pumping education for breastfeeding parents who may be returning to work (see Fig. 5, pediatric resident trainee stations).

Pediatric resident trainee stations
- Station 1: Position, latch, and hand expression: Demonstrate how to help a mother achieve a comfortable position for breastfeeding and to achieve an effective and comfortable latch.
- Station 2: Evaluation of breastfeeding session, infant feeding patterns, and milk transfer: Observe a breastfeeding session and identify key points; demonstrate hand expression, describe signs of adequate milk transfer and engage in a conversation regarding normal feeding patterns in the first 36 hours of life.
- Station 3: Management of common breastfeeding conditions: Review management of common concerns such as sore nipples, engorgement, low milk supply, and infant not sucking well.
- Station 4: Artificial feeding methods: Demonstrate cup feeding. Describe at least 4 ways to supplement breastfeeding in a safe manner. Engage in a conversation with parents who request feeding bottles, pacifiers, and soothers.
- Station 5: Support after discharge: Engage in a conversation with parent noting at least 4 ways to facilitate breastfeeding in order to prevent or resolve most common conditions; review community resources.
- Station 6: Newborn visit: Review newborn weight gain expectations, engage in a conversation about jaundice management and medical indications for

supplementation, engage in a conversation regarding family support of breastfeeding parents' goals.

- Station 7: The 2 week weight check: Describe at least 4 reasons why a breastfed baby may not be back at birthweight, review steps to performing predirect and postdirect breastfeed weight assessments.
- Station 8: Planning for return to work: Review the different types of pumps (bring examples). Describe how to schedule pumping sessions at work. Discuss the difference between clogged ducts and mastitis and review management of both conditions.

Participants

Trainees were sent eLearning modules along with the AAP Breastfeeding Curriculum prior to the in-person skills checkoff and were encouraged to review the content. Completion of the modules was not required. The curriculum was offered to all pediatric trainees (36 residents) and combined medicine-pediatric trainees (16 residents) during their regularly scheduled Academic Half Day. Twenty-two residents participated in the adapted EMPower curriculum. The residents rotated through 8 stations in groups of 4 during a 2 hour session. Each group included a mix of senior residents and interns to enable collaboration among residents at different stages of training who had different levels of exposure to breastfeeding and newborn care prior to this skills session.

Survey results

The pediatric residents were provided a presurvey and a postsurvey on the breastfeeding curriculum that queried clinical knowledge and comfort in breastfeeding skills. After the session, residents reported that they were more confident in the skills needed to address common breastfeeding concerns (57% said they were very confident; 43% said moderately confident) as compared to before the training (Fig. 4). More than 90% of respondents said they were likely to use at least one skill from the training session in their outpatient clinic. Respondents were also asked to rank the stations that they found most valuable to their practice. Stations with the most votes were those that reviewed infant attachment at the breast, common breastfeeding concerns at day of life 3 to 5, and community resources that support breastfeeding (Fig. 5, stations ranked highest were stations 1, 5, and 6).

Curriculum expansion

While this adapted curriculum was piloted with pediatric residents, this structured and tested lactation curriculum also fulfills learning objectives for continuing medical education for practicing pediatricians, along with providers in other specialties including OB/GYN and family medicine. For example, the Council on Resident Education in Obstetrics and Gynecology objectives include counsel patients on breastfeeding and chestfeeding, describe the effects of medical and surgical conditions on breastfeeding and chestfeeding, understand drug transfer or effect of medication on breastfeeding and chestfeeding, describe the approach to successful lactation and troubleshooting difficulty. Previous studies have demonstrated improvement in lactation knowledge and counseling by OB/GYN residents after formal lactation training [23]. Implementation of a targeted breastfeeding curriculum within an OB/GYN division has also been associated

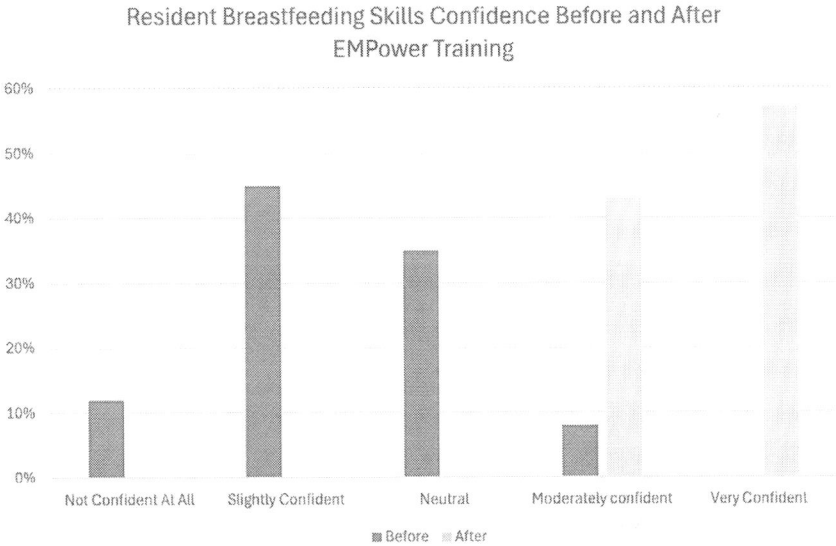

Resident Breastfeeding Skills Confidence Before and After EMPower Training

Fig. 4. Resident confidence in providing breastfeeding support before and after the EMPower training. Before the training, no one reported being "very confident" while after, a significant number (57%) reported being "very confident." After the training, no one reported being "Not confident at all."

with improved breastfeeding rates at 6 weeks postpartum [24]. Expanding this curriculum to other specialties increases the opportunity for interdisciplinary learning, ensures required Baby Friendly USA knowledge and skills are being taught, and increases evidence-based support for patients at institutions who adopt initiatives to support the mother/infant dyad.

Although this current education model using the expanded EMpower curriculum was developed for residents, this same training can be offered to providers already practicing in the community with support from hospital leadership, accrediting boards and professional organizations such as the AAP and the American College of Obstetrics and Gynecology. There are already systems in place to allow for consistent recertification for other valued training programs such as the Neonatal Resuscitation Program and Advanced Cardiac Life Support, which both require renewal every 2 years and offer in person skills training by accredited instructors. In addition, many hospitals require providers to perform a certain number of procedures per year to maintain privileges. If this same value was applied to breastfeeding skills, providers could complete the required training on a regular basis to stay up to date on current breastfeeding guidelines and maintain lactation support skills.

Other pathways for general pediatricians to support feeding goals

While this article focuses on using a specific curriculum to improve physician skill-based knowledge of breastfeeding medicine, there are several other ways

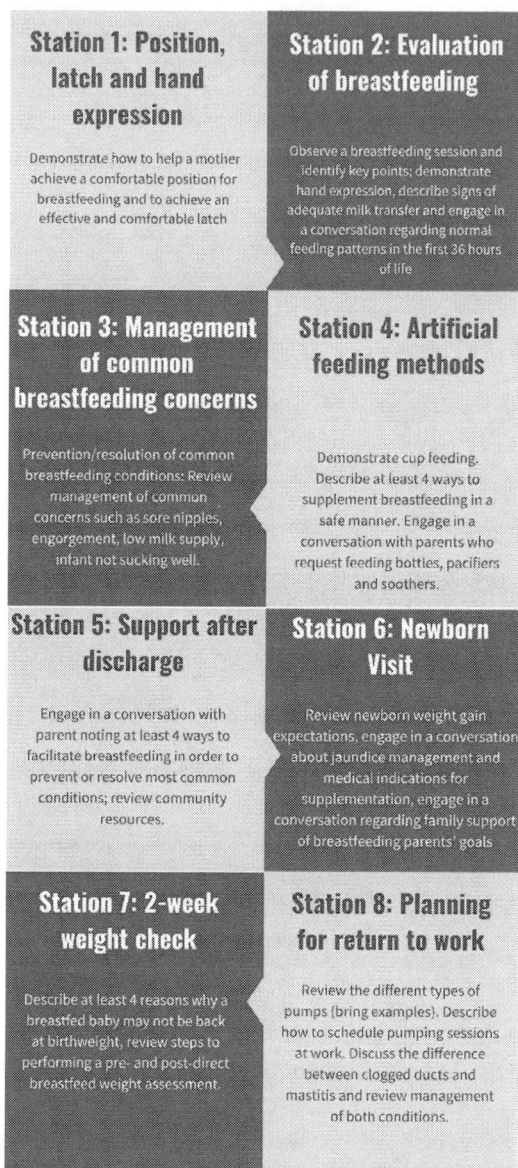

Station 1: Position, latch and hand expression

Demonstrate how to help a mother achieve a comfortable position for breastfeeding and to achieve an effective and comfortable latch

Station 2: Evaluation of breastfeeding

Observe a breastfeeding session and identify key points; demonstrate hand expression, describe signs of adequate milk transfer and engage in a conversation regarding normal feeding patterns in the first 36 hours of life

Station 3: Management of common breastfeeding concerns

Prevention/resolution of common breastfeeding conditions: Review management of common concerns such as sore nipples, engorgement, low milk supply, infant not sucking well.

Station 4: Artificial feeding methods

Demonstrate cup feeding. Describe at least 4 ways to supplement breastfeeding in a safe manner. Engage in a conversation with parents who request feeding bottles, pacifiers and soothers.

Station 5: Support after discharge

Engage in a conversation with parent noting at least 4 ways to facilitate breastfeeding in order to prevent or resolve most common conditions; review community resources.

Station 6: Newborn Visit

Review newborn weight gain expectations, engage in a conversation about jaundice management and medical indications for supplementation, engage in a conversation regarding family support of breastfeeding parents' goals

Station 7: 2-week weight check

Describe at least 4 reasons why a breastfed baby may not be back at birthweight, review steps to performing a pre- and post-direct breastfeed weight assessment.

Station 8: Planning for return to work

Review the different types of pumps (bring examples). Describe how to schedule pumping sessions at work. Discuss the difference between clogged ducts and mastitis and review management of both conditions.

Fig. 5. EMPower stations. Stations 6 to 8 are part of the adapted curriculum and not included in the standard nursing curriculum. Stations 1, 5, and 6 were ranked highest when residents were asked which content they found most practical for patient management.

that general pediatricians can support families who desire to breastfeed. For example, hiring ancillary support staff who specialize in lactation counseling would provide families additional opportunities to work on breastfeeding skills while at their already scheduled well baby visits. Additionally, pediatricians can attain specialized training in breastfeeding medicine and be a provider who offers both well child visits coupled with lactation counseling during the first 2 weeks of a child's life (Fig. 6, list of pathways for lactation training). Prioritizing convenience for families who are sleep deprived and adjusting to the early postpartum period sends a strong message of support to families. Physicians can also partner with local breastfeeding coalitions and community organizations to create a workflow to get families established with a lactation specialist during a child's first well visit. Families who desire breastfeeding may also need support in attaining their breast pump, which can be attained for free for individuals with both public and private insurance. Adding a checklist in the electronic medical record or note template to establish a standardized system among providers would also offer additional support to families and allow providers to track feeding goals.

DISCUSSION

EMPower Breastfeeding is a well-established national quality improvement initiative with comprehensive training materials and resources. We successfully adapted this innovative nursing-targeted training into a more expansive breastfeeding curriculum designed for pediatricians. To our knowledge, this is the first adaptation for graduate medical education. Not only is this skill-based curriculum practical for daily practice in both the outpatient clinic and newborn nursery setting, but it is essential as part of their residency training if pediatricians are to play an impactful role in improving breastfeeding success rates.

Although the residents who attended the skills training reported an improvement in their breastfeeding knowledge and comfort, the initial cohort was small and it will be challenging to offer this education to all residents regularly due to scheduling conflicts (eg, residents on overnight rotations who do not attend daytime education activities or residents on vacation). To offer the EMPower curriculum at different time points to accommodate common resident scheduling conflicts, residency program leadership will need to support these efforts so that residents have protected time to participate.

Furthermore, the EMPower curriculum was provided to just one resident program cohort, but to have broader impact, the curriculum would need to be expanded. This expansion could include physicians who have already completed their training but do not feel confident in their breastfeeding knowledge. This curriculum would also be appropriate for other providers who work with pregnant persons and newborns, such as OB/GYN and family medicine specialists. As the EMPower curriculum is already used at more than 100 hospital systems for training nursery and labor and delivery nurses [19], expanding the curriculum to physicians at these sites first would be feasible once this concept is spread to reach other audiences through efforts such as conference workshops or publications. Expansion of this curriculum to other EMPower sites and additional residency specialties will broaden the impact. With widespread uptake of this education, the United States is more likely to reach the Healthy People 2030 breastfeeding goals.

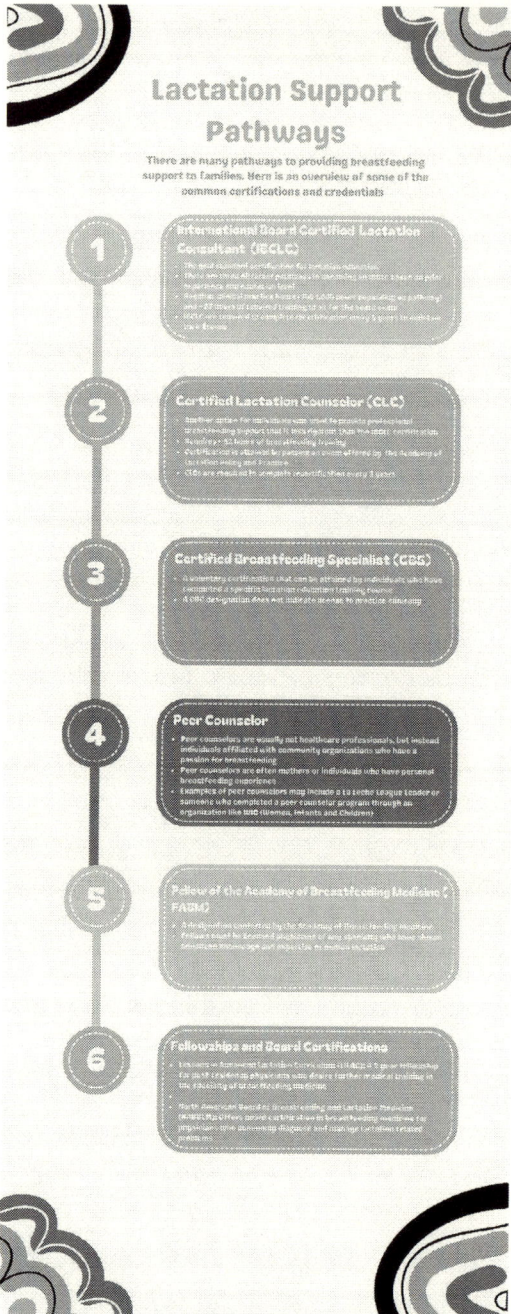

Fig. 6. An overview of different certification and education pathways for individuals who desire increased knowledge in the field of breastfeeding medicine.

While the primary goal of this curriculum was aimed at improving resident breastfeeding competency through skills training, there was an important side effect. The nurses and lactation specialists involved in the resident skills training session reported immense fulfillment from this collaborative effort and reported that working on interprofessional education allowed for the cultivation of teamwork. Learning from different professionals across different roles fosters a culture of respect and encourages appreciation for each individual's unique contribution to the team. The residents also provided positive feedback on this interprofessional collaboration and noted that they were meeting many members of the mother/baby nursery team for the first time. We hope that collaborative skills training like this can encourage an inclusive approach to breastfeeding support that leverages the strengths of each team member in the inpatient and outpatient settings.

SUMMARY

The Centers for Disease Control and Prevention-funded EMPower curriculum can be adapted to provide a standardized skill-based breastfeeding curriculum to general pediatricians. Increasing physician breastfeeding education is an easy and effective way to support families during children's first months of life. Creating a supportive breastfeeding environment in the primary care setting is ideal as children see their pediatrician regularly for well-child and weight check visits. Formal skills training in addition to self-directed learning is critical for reinforcing principles that improve learners' comfort level and their practice in the real world. Apart from using the EMPower Breastfeeding curriculum to improve the general pediatrician's role in providing breastfeeding support, the curriculum has the opportunity to provide a broader impact by improving interdisciplinary collaboration. Next steps include expanding this curriculum to other residency programs and early career physicians, and adapting the training to be appropriate for medical students as part of their third-year pediatric clerkship.

CLINICS CARE POINTS

- Support breastfeeding goals at early well care visits by routinely providing lactation counseling during newborn encounters.
- Observe a breastfeed when possible to assess latch and positioning, offer real-time guidance and address nipple and breast pain.
- Be prepared to counsel on pain, low milk supply, oversupply, difficulty with latch, and maternal mental health.
- Encourage breastfeeding-friendly supplementation strategies when needed, such as hand expression, paced bottle feeding, or syringe feeds at the breast.
- Know when to refer to breastfeeding specialists and what resources are available in your community.

Disclosure

The authors have nothing to disclose.

References

[1] Sulaski Wyckoff A. Updated AAP guidance recommends longer breastfeeding due to benefits. In: AAP news. 2022. Available at: https://publications.aap.org/aapnews/news/20528/Updated-AAP-guidance-recommends-longer?autologincheck=redirected. Accessed September 10, 2024 2022.

[2] World Health Organization. Breastfeeding. In: WHO health topics. Available at: https://www.who.int/health-topics/breastfeeding#tab=tab_1. Accessed July 12, 2024.

[3] UNICEF. Breastfeeding: a Mother's Gift for every child. In: UNICEF resources. 2018. Available at: https://data.unicef.org/resources/breastfeeding-a-mothers-gift-for-every-child/. Accessed September 18, 2024 2018.

[4] Breastfeeding AAFP. Family physicians supporting (position paper). In: AAFP policies. 2019. Available at: https://www.aafp.org/about/policies/all/breastfeeding-position-paper.html. Accessed July 12, 2024 2019.

[5] Louis-Jacques AF, Joyner AB, Crowe SD. In: Breastfeeding challenges. ACOG; 2021. Available at: https://www.acog.org/clinical/clinical-guidance/committee-opinion/articles/2021/02/breastfeeding-challenges#: ~ :text=The%20American%20College%20of%20Obstetricians%20and%20Gynecologists%20recommends%20exclusive%20breastfeeding,the%20woman%20and%20her%20infant.

[6] Rodriguez Lien E, Shattuck K. Breastfeeding education and support services provided to family medicine and obstetrics–gynecology residents. Breastfeed Med 2017;12(9):548–53.

[7] Feldman-Winter LB, Schanler RJ, O'Connor KG, et al. Pediatricians and the promotion and support of breastfeeding. Arch Pediatr Adolesc Med 2008;162(12):1142.

[8] Kim YJ. Important role of medical training curriculum to promote the rate of human milk feeding. Pediatr Gastroenterol Hepatol Nutr 2017;20(3):147–52.

[9] Osband YB, Altman RL, Patrick PA, et al. Breastfeeding education and support services offered to pediatric residents in the US. Acad Pediatr 2011;11(1):75–9.

[10] Meek JY. Pediatrician competency in breastfeeding support has room for improvement. Pediatrics 2017;140(4):e20172509.

[11] Esselmont E, Moreau K, Aglipay M, et al. Residents' breastfeeding knowledge, comfort, practices, and perceptions: results of the breastfeeding resident education study (BRESt). BMC Pediatr 2018;18(1):1150.

[12] Accreditation Council for Graduate Medical Education (ACGME). Pediatric program requirements. 2025. Available at: https://www.acgme.org/globalassets/pfassets/programrequirements/2025-prs/320_pediatrics_2025.pdf. Accessed November 20, 2024.

[13] Busler CR, Datta I, Newsome M, et al. Revamping breastfeeding education for pediatric residents: a quality improvement initiative towards breastfeeding-friendly practices in an inner-city hospital. Pediatrics 2020;146(1_MeetingAbstract):134–5.

[14] Feldman-Winter L, Barone L, Milcarek B, et al. Residency curriculum improves breastfeeding care. Pediatrics 2010;126(2):289–97.

[15] American Academy of Pediatrics. Breastfeeding curriculum. 2024. Available at: https://www.aap.org/en/pedialink/breastfeeding-curriculum/?srsltid=AfmBOor9Wd-nE-neA2_I8vsnCOm8ayzM-lOi9M3JthWwoNvno2iYgtCej. Accessed November 20, 2024.

[16] Baby-Friendly USA. About the baby-friendly hospital initiative. 2024. Available at: https://www.babyfriendlyusa.org/about/. Accessed November 20, 2024.

[17] Noiman A, Kim C, Chen J, et al. Gains needed to achieve Healthy People 2030 breastfeeding targets. Pediatrics 2024;154(3).

[18] Centers for Disease Control and Prevention. Breastfeeding report card: United States. 2022. Available at: https://www.cdc.gov. Accessed November 20, 2024.

[19] EMPower best practices. 2024. Available at: https://www.empowerbestpractices.org/best-practices/. Accessed November 20, 2024.

[20] Mulcahy H, Philpott LF, O'Driscoll M, et al. Breastfeeding skills training for healthcare professionals: a systematic review. Heliyon 2022;8(11); https://doi.org/10.1016/j.heliyon.2022.e11747.

[21] OPENPediatrics. Bella breastfeeding Curriculum.OPENPediatrics. Available at: https://learn.openpediatrics.org/learn/courses/3696/bella-breastfeeding-provider-training/lessons. Accessed June 21, 2022.

[22] Douangchak KE. Breastfeeding education of medical students and resident physicians. Intellectus 2023;1(1); https://doi.org/10.61442/2994-4384.1005.

[23] DiGirolamo AM, Grummer-Strawn LM, Fein SB. Effect of maternit-care practices on breastfeeding. Pediatrics 2008;122(Supple 2):S43–9.

[24] McGuire S. Centers for Disease Control and Prevention. 2013. Strategies to prevent obesity and other chronic diseases: the CDC guide to strategies to support breastfeeding mothers and babies. Atlanta, GA: U.S. Department of Health and Human Services, 2013. Adv Nutr 2014;5(3):291–2.

Advances in Pediatrics 72 (2025) 131–141

ADVANCES IN PEDIATRICS

Neonatal Resuscitation Program
Then and Now

Devin McKissic, MD, Ivana Brajkovic, MD, MPH*

Division of Neonatology, Department of Pediatrics, Seattle Children's Hospital and University of Washington, 4800 Sand Point Way Northeast Mail Stop: FA.2.113, Seattle, WA 98105, USA

Keywords
- Neonatal Resuscitation Program • Neonatal resuscitation • History • Technology

Key points
- The Neonatal Resuscitation Program (NRP) has provided education on quality neonatal resuscitation over the last 4 decades.
- Emerging research has informed changes to NRP recommendations over time.
- Various technologies have utility in augmenting neonatal resuscitation education and delivery.

HISTORY OF NEONATAL RESUSCITATION PROGRAM

In the overall scheme of medicine, neonatology is a relatively new field. It was not until the 1960s that neonatology began to emerge as a distinct field, rather than part of general pediatric practice. The death of President John F. Kennedy and Jacqueline Kennedy's son, Patrick Bouvier Kennedy, in 1964 due to respiratory failure at 34 weeks' gestation brought neonatology into the public eye and helped to accelerate the development of significant advances in neonatal research [1]. But even as focus shifted to specific care of the neonate, guidance regarding neonatal resuscitation remained sparse [2].

In 1952, Virginia Apgar, an obstetric anesthesiologist, presented her system for the evaluation of the newborn at the Annual Congress of Anesthetists and International College of Anesthetists, and went on to publish it in Anesthesia and Analgesia in 1953 [2,3]. She described 5 areas of clinical presentation to score in the immediate period after birth: color, pulse, reflex activity, activity, and respiration. Each area could receive a 0, 1, or 2, with the total score ranging from 0 to 10. This scoring system provided a standardized method to assess the need for resuscitation of the infant; however, standardized

---

*Corresponding author. E-mail address: ivana.brajkovic@seattlechildrens.org

https://doi.org/10.1016/j.yapd.2025.03.003

Abbreviations

AAP	American Academy of Pediatrics
AHA	American Heart Association
CoSTR	Consensus on Science with Treatment Recommendations
DCC	delayed cord clamping
ECG	electrocardiographic
HBB	Helping Babies Breathe
ILCOR	International Liaison Committee on Resuscitation
IVH	intraventricular hemorrhage
MSAF	meconium-stained fluid
NEP	Neonatal Educational Program
NIH	National Institutes of Health
NRP	Neonatal Resuscitation Program
NRVR	neonatal resuscitation video review
PPV	positive pressure ventilation
SBE	simulation-based education
SGA	supraglottic airway
UCM	umbilical cord milking

recommendations for neonatal resuscitation, based on suboptimal Apgar score, were still lacking.

Guidelines for adult resuscitation were developed in 1966 by the National Academy of Sciences. Subsequently, in the 1970s, the American Heart Association (AHA) and the American Academy of Pediatrics (AAP) acknowledged the need for improvement in neonatal resuscitation practices [4]. Although the number of neonatologists in the United States was increasing at the time, many infants were born at a hospital without a neonatal intensive care unit and thus, if needed, were resuscitated by individuals without specific neonatal training [5]. The National Institutes of Health (NIH) funded 5 projects aimed to educate providers in Level 1 nurseries (nurseries focused on caring for well term infants) about neonatal resuscitation. Ronald Bloom, MD, and Catherine Cropley, RN, MSN, received one of these grants [4] and used the money to create a 6-module educational series on newborn resuscitation, which they called the Neonatal Educational Program (NEP) [2].

In the early 1980s, Dr George Peckham became the chair of the AAP's Section on Perinatal Pediatrics and advocated for a standardized approach to neonatal resuscitation education. In 1986, the AAP Executive Committee approved the Section on Perinatal Pediatrics' proposal to further develop NEP. Representatives from the AAP and AHA collaborated to further explore this idea and found a strong ally in pediatric cardiologist, Dr Leon Chameides, as they established the Neonatal Resuscitation Program (NRP). Subsequently, the first edition of the *Textbook of Neonatal Resuscitation* was published in 1986, and the first NRP national faculty training session was held at the AAP Annual Meeting in New Orleans in 1987 [4,6].

Five key principles guided the development of NRP. These included: (1) using the best available evidence to develop recommendations, and when this was lacking, expert consensus; (2) recognizing the variety of skills required for a successful resuscitation; (3) emphasizing the importance of self-education, (4) adequate trainer preparation; and (5) regionalizing training (eg, national instructors teach regional instructors, who teach hospital-based instructors) [5]. These tenets remain central to NRP today. The uptake of NRP was swift and by the end of 1988, national faculty and hospital-based instructors were present in 48 states and Canada.

In 2000, the AAP and AHA partnered with the International Liaison Committee on Resuscitation (ILCOR). This committee is composed of experts from around the world who review the current evidence on resuscitation for newborns, children, and adults. When consensus opinions are achieved or relevant updates become available, a Consensus on Science with Treatment Recommendations (CoSTR) document is released. The AAP and AHA use these recommendations to update specific resuscitation guidelines for the United States and Canada, and the NRP Steering Committee, in turn, uses these to update NRP educational materials. Currently, new editions of NRP are published every 5 years, unless there is compelling evidence requiring an earlier update [2,4,5,7]. The most recent edition—the eighth—was released in June 2021.

Although the initial intent of the AAP and the AHA was to develop NRP for use in the United States and Canada, it has been gradually introduced outside of North America; to date, it has been introduced in 130 countries and translated into 24 languages [8]. However, awareness of the ongoing global burden of neonatal mortality—particularly with the focus on reducing under-5 child mortality with United Nations' Millennium Development Goal 4 created in 2000—highlighted the need for a different approach to neonatal resuscitation education in resource-limited settings [9]. Thus, Helping Babies Breathe (HBB), a curriculum created to support the education of basic skills in neonatal resuscitation in low-income and middle-income countries, was released in 2010. While using the same scientific approach as NRP, it deliberately focused on incorporating universally understood pictograms (use of pictorial image in place of words) and limiting text to a simple few words that could be consistently translated into multiple languages and understood by providers with low literacy [10]. Since its inception, HBB has been introduced in over 80 countries [11]. Its implementation has had substantial impacts; one study in Tanzania found that HBB implementation was associated with a reduction in early neonatal mortality by up to 47% [12]. An HBB second edition was published in 2016, which incorporated updates from the 2015 ILCOR CoSTR and 2012 World Health Organization Guidelines on Basic Newborn Resuscitation, as well as updated guidance on quality improvement and program implementation [13].

Basic tenets of Neonatal Resuscitation Program

It is difficult to succinctly summarize NRP, but there are some key guiding principles that are important to highlight. The first of these is the importance of ventilation of the newborn's lungs. To successfully transition from intrauterine to extrauterine life (sometimes referred to simply as "transition"), a newly born infant must replace the fluid in their alveoli with air—either by breathing spontaneously or, if needed, with the assistance of positive pressure ventilation (PPV). In utero, the placenta provides oxygen for the fetus; most blood bypasses the lungs because of high pulmonary vascular resistance and then flows to the systemic circulation via the patent ductus arteriosus. As the newly born infant's lungs fill with air, pulmonary vascular resistance drops, allowing blood to flow from the right ventricle to the lungs. Blood flowing to the lungs where appropriate oxygenation and ventilation can occur is required for tissue perfusion and optimal end-organ function. This physiology underlies the primary focus on ventilation prior to addressing issues with circulation and perfusion in NRP [14]. The process of transition (as described earlier) is seamless for most newborns, but there are several points at which things can go wrong, leading to an infant in distress.

Another major focus of NRP is teamwork and communication. The successful resuscitation of an infant who is not transitioning well relies on many components and a variety of skills that require effective collaboration among team members. NRP recognizes that interprofessional teams that communicate clearly and effectively are best positioned to provide the care to infants' requiring resuscitation. Some key strategies include clearly defining roles, designating a team leader, and recognizing when to call for additional assistance. Important communication behaviors include closed-loop communication and calling out safety concerns (eg, inappropriate respiratory rate with PPV) [14]. Closed-loop communication is defined as a method of exchanging information that ensures understanding from both the giver and receiver of the instruction. The person initiating the communication (or sender) provides information, the receiver repeats the information back, and the sender confirms that the receiver has properly understood the information.

Finally, NRP emphasizes the importance of adequate preparation and planning. Staff involved in newborn resuscitations should be knowledgeable on equipment location in their hospital and its proper use [14]. Resuscitation equipment that works and is ready for immediate use is critical for an effective resuscitation, as is having the appropriate personnel ready for specific prenatal and perinatal risk factors.

Changes in Neonatal Resuscitation Program over time

As previously mentioned, NRP uses the latest evidence, and when necessary, expert consensus, to develop and update their curriculum and recommendations. Since its inception, there have been several major changes in NRP. One of these changes was a revision to the learning format of NRP. Instructors have become facilitators, rather than teachers, and material is now taught through simulations, rather than lectures. Simulations are opportunities for health care providers to practice how they would behave in and respond to a scenario with a simulated patient. Simulations are followed by debriefings, which allow facilitators to provide feedback and reinforce NRP behaviors

[15]. Research to support the value and efficacy of simulation in health care education continues to grow, and simulation remains a key component to NRP instruction to this day [14]. The eighth edition of NRP also introduced resuscitation quality improvement, in which learners complete quarterly cognitive and skills activities as an alternative learning method to the traditional sequential practice and evaluation method (ie, a class with an instructor who facilitates skills stations and simulated scenarios). Additionally, the eighth edition introduced distinctions between curriculums called NRP essentials and NRP advanced provider status. This allows providers to identify which category most closely matches their clinical responsibilities when reviewing and maintaining NRP education [14].

A second change in NRP was the removal of the recommendation for tracheal intubation and suctioning for infants born through meconium-stained amniotic fluid (MSAF). In earlier NRP iterations, tracheal suctioning was recommended for infants with MSAF, with the intent to prevent meconium aspiration syndrome. However, studies throughout the 1990s and early 2000s failed to show any benefit of tracheal suctioning in reducing the incidence of meconium aspiration syndrome [16–21]. The sixth edition of NRP recommended that infants with MSAF who were vigorous at birth need not be intubated, and the seventh edition went farther, removing the recommendation for tracheal suctioning for all, including nonvigorous, infants born through MSAF [22,23].

A third change involves recognition of the deleterious effect of hyperoxia (excessive oxygen levels in body tissues) on infants, particularly in those infants who are born preterm. The sixth edition addressed the negative impacts of excessive oxygen administration, and recommended initiating resuscitation with fraction of inspired oxygen (FiO_2) at 21% for term infants but did not address a specific FiO_2 for initial resuscitation of preterm infants [21]. Ongoing research has failed to show a benefit of initiating resuscitation with higher oxygen concentrations for preterm infants, and thus the seventh edition formally recommended an initial FiO_2 of 21% to 30% during resuscitation for infants born at less than 35 weeks gestation [22]. This recommendation remains in the current eighth edition [14].

A fourth change focuses on accurate measurement of the infant's heart rate as a critical component of NRP; underestimating the heart rate can lead to unnecessary interventions, while overestimation of the heart rate may lead to inadequate resuscitation. Recommendations for how to best monitor heart rate in resuscitations have changed over time. Reliance on palpating cord pulsations to assess heart rate was replaced with recommendations for pulse oximetry use for infants requiring resuscitation. However, pulse oximetry, which is meant to measure oxygen saturation (but also provides a heart rate) may not always give an accurate heart rate measurement, particularly in the first few minutes of an infant's life. The 2015 ILCOR CoSTR identified that cardiac monitoring with placement of electrocardiographic (ECG) leads is a reasonable option for measurement of an infant's heart rate, and the seventh edition of

NRP recommends considering use of cardiac monitoring with the initiation of PPV and recommends use of cardiac monitoring during chest compressions [20,22]. The eighth edition recommends cardiac monitoring if the heart rate remains below 100 bpm with PPV [14].

A fifth change has centered on umbilical cord management after birth. Umbilical cord management refers to what is done with the umbilical cord after delivery, with options including clamping, delayed cord clamping (DCC, where the cord is not clamped for some time after delivery, allowing passive blood flow from the placenta to the baby), and milking (where the blood in the cord is actively "milked" toward the baby). DCC was first recommended for vigorous infants in the seventh edition of NRP after research demonstrated its association with multiple beneficial clinical outcomes; for preterm infants, these include higher blood pressure and blood volume, less need for blood transfusions, lower rates of intraventricular hemorrhage (IVH), and decreased risk for necrotizing enterocolitis, and in term infants, potentially less anemia and better neurodevelopmental outcomes [22]. The eighth edition continues to recommend DCC for vigorous infants and does not make a recommendation on cord clamping for nonvigorous infants [14].

In contrast to DCC, NRP does not make any recommendations regarding umbilical cord milking (UCM). A recent ILCOR clinical update summarized recent systematic reviews of umbilical cord practices after birth and presented different recommendations depending on gestational age and clinical status of the infant [24]. UCM is not recommended in any patients born at gestational ages less than 28 weeks, as it has been shown to be associated with higher rates of severe IVH as compared with DCC [25]; because this association did not persist for infants of higher gestational ages in this particular study, UCM can be considered an appropriate alternative for preterm infants ≥ 28 weeks who do not require resuscitation and for whom DCC cannot be performed. There are no data to support UCM as superior to DCC in infants born at ≥ 34 weeks who do not require resuscitation at birth. For those late preterm and term infants that do require some resuscitation, UCM may be reasonable as compared with early cord clamping—one randomized crossover trial of infants ≥ 35 weeks found that infants who received UCM had increased hemoglobin levels and reduced need for cardiorespiratory support [26]. Further studies are needed to better understand the benefits and limitations of UCM in both preterm and term neonates and to help inform appropriate use of these interventions in the setting of neonatal resuscitation. Given the fact that UCM has the advantage of potentially improving stability in some infants with hemodynamic instability by providing volume resuscitation in a very short amount of time, it may have utility in avoiding increased interventions in this select subset of patients [27].

Lastly, another addition to the seventh edition of NRP is guidance on the use of supraglottic airways (eg, laryngeal mask airways) as an alternative method for administration of PPV if face mask ventilation is not effective and if the placement of an endotracheal tube is not feasible [28]. Updates to the eighth edition of NRP include simplified recommendations for the placement of an alternative airway, in which both supraglottic airway (SGA) and endotracheal tube are now both listed as initial options [29]. Future iterations of NRP may consider introducing SGA use as an intermediary step between PPV and endotracheal intubation in some clinical scenarios. A recent systematic review comparing the administration of initial PPV immediately after birth via SGAs versus facemasks showed that infants that received PPV via SGA were more likely to improve and to do so more quickly than those receiving PPV via face mask [30]. Use of an SGA for PPV when ventilation via face mask is unsuccessful may help to avoid traumatic endotracheal intubation in select cases; in fact, recent updates from the AHA and AAP highlight consideration for SGA use as the primary interface for administration of PPV as opposed to face mask for infants ≥34 weeks' gestation [24]. SGA use may be of particular benefit as a corrective ventilatory measure in situations where the skill of bag-mask ventilation has not yet been mastered [31]; this is of particular interest in low-resource settings, where randomized clinical trials comparing use of SGAs versus face mask during newborn resuscitation have shown decreased time to spontaneous breathing with SGAs [32].

New frontiers in Neonatal Resuscitation Program: use of technology to optimize education and quality

Ongoing education and practice are crucial to maintain skill retention and prevent deterioration of knowledge surrounding neonatal resuscitation [33,34]. Currently, recommendations emphasize simulation-based education (SBE) if possible. Simulation-based teaching, however, may not be readily available for a variety of reasons (eg, cost, time, and/or other resource limitations). Serious games (board, computer, and virtual reality games that are played for a reason other than entertainment) are alternative approaches to SBE that have the potential to not only be useful but also less expensive and less labor-intensive and time-intensive than SBE [35]. Digital game-based learning has been shown to be efficacious in improving pediatric trainees' neonatal resuscitation skills [36]. Similarly, neonatal resuscitation gamification (which refers to the use of game-based elements as learning tools) using virtual reality has been studied as an alternative to SBE for nursing students [37]. Virtual reality training has even been shown to be effective in maintaining NRP skills in resource-limited settings, where constraints for SBE may be most evident [38].

Neonatal resuscitation video review (NRVR) is another adjunctive technological tool that is increasingly utilized by neonatal clinicians. It involves recording real or simulated resuscitations and then reviewing them with the clinical team; providers can learn from watching their own performance in a resuscitation or from reviewing the performance of other individuals. NRVR can also be used as a quality assurance tool to study compliance with NRP guidelines [39]. NRVR has been shown to improve teamwork and skill retention, as well as increase exposure to resuscitations and improve situational awareness [39–41]. Regular NRVR sessions present an opportunity for all members of a team to learn from one another and empower providers to address areas for improvement [42]. Video debriefing has even been shown to improve skill attainment and competency retention for birth attendants receiving training through HBB [43].

Mobile phone applications ("apps") provide an important tool in resource-limited settings where standard equipment for neonatal resuscitations, such as pulse oximetry and ECG, are not universally available. One example is Neo-TapLifeSupport, an app used to generate a number that estimates heart rate based on screen-tapping of at least 3 auscultated heart sounds [44,45]. Such apps can also be useful in providing opportunities for education and simulation; the HBB Prompt app which utilizes training videos, simulation of resuscitation scenarios, and quizzes to test knowledge retention is one example which has been demonstrated to help mitigate skill decay in practitioners in Uganda [46].

Lastly, novel advances in technology have the potential to provide real-time feedback to optimize life-saving measures. Sensors inside infant mannequins have been shown to help perform adequate compressions during high-quality CPR simulations [47]. Interventions that can be worn on the body of individuals providing chest compressions, such as smartwatch-based feedback devices that measure variables like chest compression depth and rates, have been explored as potential adjuncts to optimizing infant CPR [48]. Object detection (using machine or deep learning to identify and classify images of objects such as bag mask) during videos of infant resuscitations may also one day be useful for debriefing after resuscitations and possibly for real-time feedback and corrective measures during actual resuscitations [48]. As technologic advances improve, and access to such resources broadens, future iterations of NRP may find utility in including these options as adjuncts to education and clinical practice.

SUMMARY

For the past 4 decades, NRP has focused on training providers in the delivery of quality neonatal resuscitation. Emerging research in neonatology, resuscitation medicine, education, and simulation has informed changes to recommendations over time, which, in turn, have improved outcomes. Use of technology in NRP is a current area of clinical and scholarly interest that may shape changes to NRP in the future.

CLINICS CARE POINTS

- Resuscitation with oxygen should start at an initial range of 21-30% for infants less than 35 weeks gestation and at 21% for infants at older gestational ages.
- Cardiac monitoring via ECG leads is recommended for all infants receiving chest compressions as well as those that remain bradycardic with positive pressure ventilation.

- Delayed cord clamping is recommended for infants who are vigorous at birth.
- Use of supraglottic airways can be useful for administration of positive pressure ventilation if placement of endotracheal tube is not feasible.

Disclosure

The authors have nothing to disclose.

References

[1] Zaichkin J, Wiswell TE. The history of neonatal resuscitation. Neonatal Network 2002;21(5):21–8.

[2] Apgar V. A proposal for a new method of evaluation of the newborn infant. Anesth Analg 1953;32(4):1056–9.

[3] NRP history. American Academy of Pediatrics; 2024. Available at: https://www.aap.org/en/pedialink/neonatal-resuscitation-program/nrp-history/?srsltid=AfmBOopwKQLOjDJ-wLUPqG_v9-CEENRfbW-iRQXd6Dspz2HSXjus67Ewf. Accessed November 1, 2024.

[4] Halamek LP. Educational perspectives: the genesis, adaptation, and evolution of the neonatal resuscitation program. NeoReviews 2008;9(4):e142–9.

[5] Bloom R, Cropley C. Textbook of neonatal resuscitation. Dallas (TX): American Academy of Pediatrics and American Heart Association; 1987.

[6] Zaichkin J, Kamath-Rayne BD, Weiner G. The NRP 8th edition: innovation in education. Adv Neonatal Care 2021;21(4):322–32.

[7] American Academy of Pediatrics. NRP global overview. 2022. Available at: https://www.aap.org/en/pedialink/neonatal-resuscitation-program/nrp-global-overview/?srsltid=AfmBOooOMeC9a_Bz2wP-Rka92W44kvMuGN4jP614vpHofwl_1QF4Tg5Y. Accessed November 1, 2024.

[8] Niermeyer S. From the neonatal resuscitation program to helping babies breathe: global impact of educational programs in neonatal resuscitation. Semin Fetal Neonatal Med 2015;20(5):300–8.

[9] Niermeyer S, Little GA, Singhal N, et al. A short history of helping babies breathe: why and how, then and now. Pediatrics 2020;146(Supplement_2):S101–11.

[10] Helping Babies Breathe. American Academy of Pediatrics; 2023. Available at: https://www.aap.org/en/aap-global/helping-babies-survive/our-programs/helping-babies-breathe/?srsltid=AfmBOorzROW__Jrbiblt-hxkWl94llWolCob1Th9eiw3XHshdKKMptlB. Accessed November 1, 2024.

[11] Msemo G, Massawe A, Mmbando D, et al. Newborn mortality and fresh stillbirth rates in Tanzania after helping babies breathe training. Pediatrics 2013;131(2):e353–60.

[12] Helping Babies Breathe. 2nd Edition. American Academy of Pediatrics; 2021. Available at: https://www.aap.org/en/aap-global/helping-babies-survive/our-programs/helping-ba-bies-breathe/helping-babies-breathe-2nd-edition/. Accessed November 1, 2024.

[13] Weiner GM, Zaichkin J, editors. Textbook of neonatal resuscitation. 8th edition. Elk Grove Village, IL: American Academy of Pediatrics and American Heart Association; 2021.

[14] Sawyer T, Ades A, Ernst K, et al. Simulation and the neonatal resuscitation program 7th edition curriculum. NeoReviews 2016;17(8):e447–53.

[15] Linder N, Aranda JV, Tsur M, et al. Need for endotracheal intubation and suction in meconium-stained neonates. J Pediatr 1988;112(4):613–5.

[16] Peng TC, Gutcher GR, Van Dorsten JP. A selective aggressive approach to the neonate exposed to meconium-stained amniotic fluid. Am J Obstet Gynecol 1996;175(2):296–303.

[17] Wiswell TE, Gannon CM, Jacob J, et al. Delivery room management of the apparently vigorous meconium-stained neonate: results of the multicenter, international collaborative trial. Pediatrics 2000;105(1):1–7.

[18] Myers P, Gupta AG. Impact of the revised NRP meconium aspiration guidelines on term infant outcomes. Hosp Pediatr 2020;10(3):295–9.

[19] Kattwinkel J, Perlman JM, Aziz K, et al. Part 15: neonatal Resuscitation: 2010 American Heart Association guidelines for cardiopulmonary resuscitation and emergency cardiovascular care. Circulation 2010;122(18_suppl_3):S909–19.

[20] Wyckoff MH, Aziz K, Escobedo MB, et al. Part 13: neonatal Resuscitation: 2015 American Heart Association guidelines update for cardiopulmonary resuscitation and emergency cardiovascular care. Circulation 2015;132(18_suppl_2):S543–60.

[21] Kattwinkel J, McGowan JE, Zaichkin J, editors. Textbook of neonatal resuscitation. 6th edition. Elk Grove Village, IL: American Academy of Pediatrics and American Heart Association; 2011.

[22] Weiner GM, Zaichkin J, editors. Textbook of neonatal resuscitation. 7th edition. Elk Grove Village, IL: American Academy of Pediatrics and American Heart Association; 2016.

[23] Yamada NK, Szyld E, Strand ML, et al. 2023 American Heart Association and American Academy of Pediatrics focused update on neonatal resuscitation: an update to the American Heart Association guidelines for cardiopulmonary resuscitation and emergency cardiovascular care. Pediatrics 2024;153(2):e2023065030.

[24] Katheria A, Reister F, Essers J, et al. Association of umbilical cord milking vs delayed umbilical cord clamping with death or severe intraventricular hemorrhage among preterm infants. JAMA 2019;322(19):1877–86.

[25] Katheria AC, Clark E, Yoder B, et al. Umbilical cord milking in nonvigorous infants: a cluster-randomized crossover trial. Am J Obstet Gynecol 2023;228(2):217.e1.

[26] Katheria A, Blank D, Rich W, et al. Umbilical cord milking improves transition in premature infants at birth. PLoS One 2014;9(4):e94085.

[27] Perlman JM, Wyllie J, Kattwinkel J, et al. Part 7: neonatal resuscitation: 2015 international consensus on cardiopulmonary resuscitation and emergency cardiovascular care science with treatment recommendations. Circulation 2015;132(16_suppl_1):S204–41.

[28] Weiner GM, Zaichkin J. Textbook of neonatal resuscitation. 8th edition. Itasca (IL): American Academy of Pediatrics; 2021. p. 84–9.

[29] Yamada NK, McKinlay CJD, Quek BH, et al. Supraglottic airways compared with face masks for neonatal resuscitation. Pediatrics 2022;150(3):e2022056568.

[30] Zhu XY, Lin BC, Zhang QS, et al. A prospective evaluation of the efficacy of the laryngeal mask airway during neonatal resuscitation. Resuscitation 2011;82(11):1405–9.

[31] Pejovic NJ, Trevisanuto D, Lubulwa C, et al. Neonatal resuscitation using a laryngeal mask airway: a randomised trial in Uganda. Arch Dis Child 2018;103(3):255–60.

[32] Patel J, Posencheg M, Ades A. Proficiency and retention of neonatal resuscitation skills by pediatric residents. Pediatrics 2012;130(3):515–21.

[33] McCaw JM, Yelton SE, Tackett SA, et al. Effect of repeat refresher courses on neonatal resuscitation skill decay: an experimental comparative study of in-person and video-based simulation training. Adv Simul 2023;8(1):7.

[34] Ghoman SK, Patel SD, Cutumisu M, et al. Serious games, a game changer in teaching neonatal resuscitation? A review. Arch Dis Child Fetal Neonatal Ed 2020;105(1):98–107.

[35] Bardelli S, Del Corso G, Ciantelli M, et al. Improving pediatric/neonatology residents' newborn resuscitation skills with a digital serious game: diana. Front Pediatr 2022;10:842302.

[36] Yang SY, Oh YH. The effects of neonatal resuscitation gamification program using immersive virtual reality: a quasi-experimental study. Nurse Educ Today 2022;117:105464.

[37] Umoren R, Bucher S, Hippe DS, et al. eHBB: a randomised controlled trial of virtual reality or video for neonatal resuscitation refresher training in healthcare workers in resource-scarce settings. BMJ Open 2021;11(8):e048506.

[38] Carbine DN, Finer NN, Knodel E, et al. Video recording as a means of evaluating neonatal resuscitation performance. Pediatrics 2000;106(4):654–8.

[39] Nadler I, Sanderson PM, Van Dyken CR, et al. Presenting video recordings of newborn resuscitations in debriefings for teamwork training. BMJ Qual Saf 2011;20(2):163–9.

[40] Weimar Z, Nestel D, Battista A, et al. Impact of the Neonatal Resuscitation Video Review program for neonatal staff: a qualitative analysis. Pediatr Res 2024;1–10. https://doi.org/10. 1038/s41390-024-03602-9.

[41] Heesters V, van Zanten HA, Heijstek V, et al. Record, reflect and refine: using video review as an initiative to improve neonatal care. Pediatr Res 2024;96:299–308.

[42] Odongkara B, Tylleskär T, Pejovic N, et al. Adding video-debriefing to helping-babies-breathe training enhanced retention of neonatal resuscitation knowledge and skills among health workers in Uganda: a cluster randomized trial. Glob Health Action 2020;13(1):1743496.

[43] Myrnerts Höök S, Pejovic NJ, Marrone G, et al. Accurate and fast neonatal heart rate assessment with a smartphone-based application - a manikin study. Acta Paediatr 2018;107(9): 1548–54.

[44] Myrnerts Höök S, Pejovic NJ, Cavallin F, et al. Smartphone app for neonatal heart rate assessment: an observational study. BMJ Paediatrics Open 2020;4(1):e000688.

[45] Chan NH, Merali HS, Mistry N, et al. Utilization of a novel mobile application,"HBB Prompt", to reduce Helping Babies Breathe skills decay. PLOS Global Public Health 2023;3(5):e0000705.

[46] Martin P, Theobald P, Kemp A, et al. Real-time feedback can improve infant manikin cardiopulmonary resuscitation by up to 79%—a randomised controlled trial. Resuscitation 2013;84(8):1125–30.

[47] Lee J, Song Y, Oh J, et al. Smartwatch feedback device for high-quality chest compressions by a single rescuer during infant cardiac arrest: a randomized, controlled simulation study. Eur J Emerg Med 2019;26(4):266–71.

[48] Meinich-Bache Ø, Engan K, Austvoll I, et al. Object detection during newborn resuscitation activities. IEEE Journal of Biomedical Health and Informatics 2020;24(3):796–803.

Advances in Pediatrics 72 (2025) 143–156

ADVANCES IN PEDIATRICS

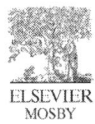

Renal Physiology
From Fetus to Newborn and Beyond

Benjamin Holland, BS[a], Cara L. Slagle, MD[b],
Michelle C. Starr, MD, MPH[c,d],*

[a]Department of Pediatrics, Indiana University School of Medicine, Indianapolis, IN, USA; [b]Division of Neonatology, Department of Pediatrics, Indiana University School of Medicine, Indianapolis, IN, USA; [c]Division of Nephrology, Department of Pediatrics, Indiana University School of Medicine, Indianapolis, IN, USA; [d]Division of Child Health Service Research, Department of Pediatrics, Indiana University School of Medicine, Indianapolis, IN, USA

Keywords

- Kidney • Renal physiology • Neonate • Preterm • Glomerular filtration rate
- Urine output

Key points

- Nephron number is determined by the time of birth or soon after. Low nephron number increases the risk of hypertension, proteinuria, and renal insufficiency.
- Renal blood flow (RBF) and renal function are low before birth but increase after birth as vascular resistance decreases, resulting in a progressive increase in function.
- Urine output (UOP) for the first 24 h is low; oliguria or anuria after 24 h and during the first week can indicate abnormal renal function.
- Due to relative physiologic immaturity, newborns are uniquely susceptible to kidney injury, commonly indicated by high serum creatinine and low UOP.

INTRODUCTION

Renal physiology in the neonate is a complex and highly regulated process. This process begins with embryologic development, followed by dramatic changes in function during the perinatal and early neonatal period. This period is one of high-risk for additional kidney injuries and insults, and ultimately progressing to maturation, typically by 2 y of age. In this review, we seek to provide an overview of developmental renal physiology in the context

*Corresponding author. Division of Child Health Service Research, Department of Pediatrics, Indiana University School of Medicine, 410 West 10th Street, Suite 200A, Indianapolis, IN 46202. E-mail address: mcstarr@iu.edu

https://doi.org/10.1016/j.yapd.2025.03.004
0065-3101/25/

Abbreviations

AKI	acute kidney injury
CAKUT	congenital abnormalities of the kidney and urinary tract
CKD	chronic kidney disease
ECF	extracellular fluid
GFR	glomerular filtration rate
NSAID	non-steroidal anti-inflammatory drug
RBF	renal blood flow
UOP	urine output

of clinical implications using patient cases and examples. A nuanced understanding of this process will inform the counseling of families on anticipated kidney changes in the perinatal period, what to anticipate in terms of kidney function during the immediate postnatal period, and ongoing kidney function and maturation after discharge.

Case 1: You are covering the neonatal service at a delivery unit and are called to counsel parents on the implications of preterm birth at 31 w gestational age. A 20-w prenatal ultrasound showed bilateral kidneys and normal amniotic fluid. The expectant mother is an adult nephrologist and remembers "just a little" about prenatal kidney development and function. After hearing about possible complications of prematurity affecting other body systems, she has specific questions about how early delivery affects future renal health in her soon-to-be newborn.

PRENATAL KIDNEY DEVELOPMENT

Kidney development begins with the appearance of the Wolffian duct during the third week of gestation [1]. This duct then forms the pronephros, mesonephros, and metanephros—the first 2 of these embryonic structures ultimately regress. The pronephros develops first and then regresses around 5 w of gestation. Second, the mesonephros forms around weeks 3 to 4 of gestation, but degenerates from weeks 5 to 12 of gestation [2]. The mesonephros serves no function in females, but in males forms the efferent ductules of the gonad, the epididymis, and the ductus deferens. The metanephros develops into the future kidney, developing caudally to the mesonephros, starting in weeks 4 to 5 of gestation. The ureteric bud—an outgrowth of the metanephros—interacts with the metanephric mesenchyme via tightly regulated, complex signaling [3]. Ureteric induction and branching is controlled by multiple highly regulated genes [4]. Nephrogenesis only occurs at the tips of the ureteric tree, and thus, the process of branching morphogenesis is essential for the development of nephrons.

NEPHROGENESIS, NEPHRON NUMBER, AND RESPONSE TO NEPHRON LOSS

As branching morphogenesis occurs, the potential maximum number of nephrons increases. There is variability in nephron number in healthy individuals, with normal nephron number ranged from approximately 200,000 to almost 2 million per kidney [5,6]. Branching morphogenesis occurs during the second trimester until 36 w gestation. Based on our current understanding of nephrogenesis, it appears that no new nephrons are made after 36 w of gestation.

Premature infants delivered before 36 w have fewer nephrons relative to infants born at term. One study estimated an increase of approximately 250,000 nephrons for each additional kilogram of birth-weight [7]. In preterm infants, nephrogenesis can potentially continue for up to 40 d following birth (Fig. 1), although postnatal nephrogenesis can result in nephrons with abnormal morphology, including larger glomeruli that may be more at risk for progression to abnormal kidney function during childhood [8,9]. As such, an infant born at 24 w gestation will have, after 40 d of postnatal nephron development, a potential maximum number of nephrons equivalent to an infant born at 31 w. Furthermore, prenatal stressors, such as ischemia, fetal malnutrition, growth restriction, or exposure to maternal medications, such as Angiotensin-Converting Enzyme (ACE) inhibitors, non-steroidal anti-inflammatory drugs (NSAIDs), and aminoglycosides can further reduce nephron number in utero [1,10,11].

Infants born prematurely have increased susceptibility to acute kidney injury (AKI) during periods of clinical instability due to their fewer nephrons. Following AKI and subsequent recovery, accelerated postnatal compensatory maturation results in remaining nephrons undergoing hypertrophy leading to hyperfiltration necessary to maintain adequate kidney function, and then to progressive glomerular injury [12,13]. Long-term consequences of fewer nephrons and AKI include increased risk of hypertension, proteinuria, and chronic kidney disease (CKD) in childhood and adulthood [14,15]. Despite this well-

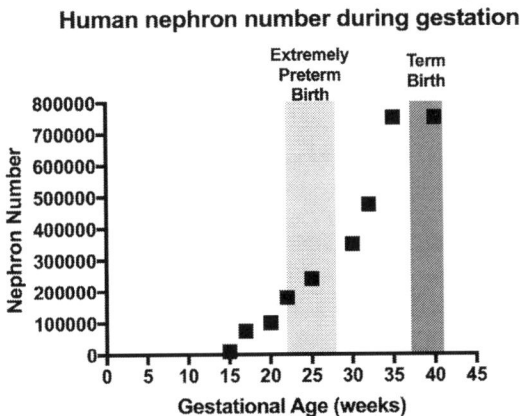

Fig. 1. Figure demonstrating nephron number during gestation, as several studies have demonstrated the cessation of human nephrogenesis at ~32 to 36 w. (*From* Harer MW, Charlton JR, Tipple TE, et al. Preterm birth and neonatal acute kidney injury: implications on adolescent and adult outcomes. J Perinatol 2020;40(9):1286–95. Epub 2020/04/12. https://doi.org/10.1038/s41372-020-0656-7. PubMed PMID: 32277164.)

described association, neither we know little about risk of future CKD nor about predicting the timeline of CKD progression in neonates with lower nephron number [1].

Disruptions in nephron signaling during in utero nephrogenesis lead to developmental abnormalities, often referred to as congenital abnormalities of the kidney and urinary tract (CAKUT). There are many genes that are closely linked with CAKUT, including but not limited to PAX2, RET, and GFRα1. Some of these genes (such as PAX2) are associated with other abnormalities, such as eye or ear findings, which may be identifiable at birth by physical examination. For example, PAX2 and RET ear findings include ear pits or tags, which can be identified as part of a routine newborn examination and should raise suspicion for genetic etiology of CAKUT in infants with known kidney abnormality. CAKUT represents 20% to 30% of all anomalies identified during the prenatal period and is responsible for 50% of childhood kidney failure worldwide [3]. Most second trimester ultrasounds identify severe cases of CAKUT, with severity determined by the amount of amniotic fluid [1].

AMNIOTIC FLUID

A critical role of the kidneys during gestation is amniotic fluid production. Amniotic fluid is fetal urine, which serves to both protect the fetus and support fetal lung development. Urine production begins around the 10th week of gestation and is hypotonic [1,9,16]. At 10 w of gestation, there are ~25 mL of amniotic fluid with the volume gradually increasing to a peak of ~800 mL at 28 w. This amount remains relatively stable for the remainder of pregnancy, decreasing slightly each week until near term [1,17]. Oligohydramnios, defined as too little amniotic fluid, or polyhydramnios, excessive amniotic fluid, has a large differential diagnosis and should prompt further urgent investigation. While oligohydramnios first seen close to term is relatively common, oligohydramnios or anhydramnios (no amniotic fluid) identified earlier in gestation is concerning for diminished or absent kidney development or other structural abnormality and may result in pulmonary hypoplasia.

Clinical application of case 1

For this case, it is important to highlight that the neonate reassuringly has both kidneys, which appear to have normal function, as demonstrated by appropriate amniotic fluid volumes. Postnatally, her baby will have fewer nephrons present than if delivered at term. Even with subsequent nephron development over the next 40 d, the number of nephrons is reduced, placing this infant at an increased risk for AKI, as well as an increased risk of CKD in the future compared to a term infant.

Case 2

As the overnight covering provider for the newborn nursery, you are called at 2 AM by the bedside nurse of a 16-h old newborn. The nurse notes that the infant has not yet voided, and she is concerned that this is abnormal. She also reports that she received a "critical value" serum creatinine level of 0.9 mg/dL. She asks when you expect the infant to make urine and whether further imaging, testing or evaluation is needed.

RENAL BLOOD FLOW AND GLOMERULAR FILTRATION RATE

As birth nears, dramatic changes occur in kidney function and blood flow occurs. At delivery, the kidneys take over many of the roles previously performed by the placenta. Glomerular filtration rate (GFR), the rate at which plasma is filtered across the glomerular membrane, and renal blood flow (RBF), the rate at which blood flows through the glomerulus, are tightly connected and highly regulated as RBF in part determines GFR and the maturation of neonatal GFR depends on RBF development [18].

RBF in newborn infants is initially low, primarily due to small blood vessel size, decreased glomeruli number, and high renal vascular resistance [1]. Following delivery, RBF begins to increase due to a drop in renal vascular resistance, which occurs at around 24 h of life. In the fetus, RBF is 3% to 7% of cardiac output, increasing to 10% within the first week of life, and then to the adult level of 25% by 2 y of age [2]. RBF increase is mediated by vasoactive factors, with Angiotensin II being the primary vasoconstrictor and smaller roles played by arginine vasopressin, endothelin, and the sympathetic nervous system. Nitric oxide is primary vasodilator and smaller contributions are made by atrial natriuretic peptide, bradykinin, and prostaglandins [19–21].

In addition to their vasodilatory role, prostaglandins also provide critical protection against pathologic hypoperfusion and related injury [1]. NSAIDs, such as indomethacin and ibuprofen, inhibit synthesis of prostaglandins. These medications are commonly administered to premature infants for a variety of reasons, most commonly to induce closure of a patent ductus arteriosus. Neonatal kidneys are particularly sensitive to NSAID's effects on the kidney due to the inhibition of protective vasodilation [22]. Indomethacin has long been associated with an increased risk of kidney injury in premature infants [22,23]. The relative adverse kidney injury potential of ibuprofen versus indomethacin remains unclear [24,25].

Similar to RBF, newborns have low GFR that progressively increases after birth due to changes in vascular resistance, blood pressure, and oncotic pressure. GFR is established during intrauterine life but is insignificant compared to the role of the placenta [2]. At birth, GFR increases from ~5 mL/min/1.73 m^2 to 40 mL/min/1.73 m^2 within the first week of life, which is still significantly lower than adult GFR (100 – 125 mL/min/1.73 m^2). This low GFR in young infants contributes to a decreased ability to handle fluid and solute loads [2]. A number of factors can interfere with establishment of appropriate GFR after birth—both specific to the infant and as a consequence of treatment for critical illness; these include hypoxemia, asphyxia, mechanical ventilation, and medications (eg, ACE inhibitors and NSAIDs). Neonates are particularly susceptible to the detrimental impact of such insults on their GFR [26].

Clinically, kidney function or GFR is assessed by serum creatinine. Creatinine is an endogenous compound, which is freely filtered across the glomerulus and not reabsorbed or metabolized by the kidney, making it the best clinical marker for GFR. At birth, newborn serum creatinine reflect maternal creatinine levels as creatinine readily crosses the placenta, making interpretation of neonatal kidney function more challenging in the first few post-natal days [27]. By postnatal day 2 or 3, serum creatinine increasingly reflects neonatal kidney function [28]. Serum creatinine levels over the first several days may further be impacted by fluid status, as creatinine concentration is affected by fluid levels in the vascular space [1,16].

FURTHER MATURATION OF KIDNEY FUNCTIONS

Even after the dramatic initial changes in renal function that occur around delivery, the kidneys continue to develop and mature in the postnatal period. Within the first week of life, GFR increases from 5 to 40 mL/min/1.73 m^2. Depending on the infant (including their birth weight, gestational age, and complications during the perinatal period), it can take 6 mo to 2 y to reach "normal" adult GFR range [20,21,29]. Prematurity delays this increase and maturation of GFR, as well as other renal functions. For example, in very low birth weight infants, GFR is lower and reaches adult levels around 8 y of age [2].

Prematurely born infants have lower GFR, which increases more slowly than in term infants [30]. In preterm infants, one study estimated median GFRs of 13.4, 16.2, 19.1, 21.9, and 24.8 mL/min/1.73 m^2 in neonates born at 27, 28, 29, 30, and 31 w' gestation, respectively. These lower GFR values make preterm infants more susceptible to kidney injury after delivery. Premature birth also delays the stabilization of creatinine levels. In term infants, serum creatinine stabilizes around 5 to 10 d of life, but in VLBW infants, it stabilizes somewhat later, around 1 to 3 mo of age [16]. While an elevation of serum creatinine may indicate slow to mature GFR, it also can represent an acute change in function, that is, AKI (Table 1) [31].

Table 1
Neonatal acute kidney disorder KDIGO classification

Stage	SCr	Urine output
0	No change in SCr or rise <0.3 mg/dL	≥0.5 mL/kg/h
1	Increase in SCr of ≥0.3 mg/dL within 48 h or SCr rise ≥1.5–1.9 X reference SCr[a] within 7 d	<0.5 mL/kg/h for 6–12 h
2	SCr rise ≥2–2.9 X reference SCr[a] within 7 d	<0.5 mL/kg/hour for ≥12 h
3	SCr ≥3 X reference SCr[a] or SCr >2.5 mg/dL[b] or receipt of RRT	<0.3 mL/kg/hour for ≥24 h or anuria for ≥12 h

Differences between the neonatal AKI definition and KDIGO include the following:
[a]Reference SCr defined as the lowest previous SCr value.
[b]SCr value of 2.5 mg/dL represents <10 mL/min/1.73m2.

FLUID REGULATION AND URINE OUTPUT

At the time of delivery, the fetus transitions from an "aquatic" intrauterine environment to a "terrestrial" extrauterine environment and kidney function replace placental function. Shortly after birth, the kidneys facilitate a loss of body water [1,32]. At birth, extracellular fluid (ECF) comprises 44% of total body water, which decreases to ~30% at 6 mo, reflecting ECF contraction that parallels an increased urine output (UOP) [2].

For ease of understanding, postnatal fluid shifts can be broken into 3 phases based on water and sodium homeostasis [33,34]. The pre-diuretic phase begins at birth and lasts up to 36 h of life. This phase is characterized by low UOP with minimal water and sodium excretion regardless of intake [16]. Weight loss during this period is attributable to insensible losses. The diuretic phase follows, beginning approximately 24 to 96 h of life, and marks the beginning of diuresis and natriuresis. As urine output increases, ECF contraction begins, resulting in an average decrease of 5% to 10% of body weight during the first week of life [2]. The diuretic phase lasts 2 to 4 d. This decrease in weight is normal and in the first few days of life does not represent dehydration or inadequate intake. The post-diuretic phase follows and is characterized by an appropriate UOP response and sodium excretion based on intake. Clinically, postnatal diuresis is a physiologic process that results in weight loss. This physiologic process is often challenging to interpret and sometimes is interpreted as pathologic.

Most healthy, full-term babies will urinate at least once in the first 36 h of life followed by an increase in frequency of urination over the next few days. Although no or low urine output on the first 1 to 2 d of life is often concerning to parents and providers, it can be normal in full-term healthy newborns [35]. In infants with no urine output after 36 to 48 h of life, a prenatal ultrasound showing normal kidneys, ureters, and bladder is reassuring against other more concerning causes of low UOP, including structural kidney abnormalities or obstructive processes, such as posterior urethral valves in males.

Further complicating the interpretation of UOP in the first few days of life is the immaturity of urine concentration and dilution mechanisms in the neonate, especially in preterm infants [36]. The clinical implications are that neonates and infants are less able to handle fluid loads and may not be able to appropriately concentrate their urine in the setting of volume depletion [37,38]. Specifically, newborns may continue to have what appears to be adequate UOP even in the setting of evolving volume depletion. Therefore, in the first few weeks of life, acute weight loss rather than UOP may be a better indicator of hydration status. Contributors to a lower concentrating capacity in the newborn period include poor ADH responsiveness, shorter loops of Henle, decreased urinary urea solute content, and delayed establishment of the corticomedullary gradient [39,40]. During the first week, the maximum concentrating capacity is 600 mOsm/kg H2O, which increases to 1300 to 1400 mOsm/kg H2O by 9 to 12 m [41].

Pathologic causes of oliguria or anuria beyond the first several days include CAKUT, perinatal hypoxia or asphyxia resulting in AKI, syndrome of inappropriate antidiuretic hormone, or kidney dysfunction (either AKI or congenital kidney failure) [35,42]. Preterm infants are more likely to have oliguria or anuria in the first few days of life; however, administration of antenatal steroids can facilitate earlier diuresis and natriuresis, increased GFR and UOP. [43,44]. In very preterm infants, a UOP <2 mL/kg/h over 24 h between days 1 and 7 strongly predicts neonatal mortality or severe morbidities [45]. For this reason, careful UOP monitoring is important in the Neonatal Intensive Care Unit setting.

TUBULAR IMMATURITY AND MATURATION
During the several weeks after birth, the renal tubules remain relatively immature in their ability to maintain ion and acid-base homeostasis. This immaturity is in addition to immaturity in fluid balance described earlier. The fetus has high urinary sodium losses, indicating tubular immaturity. High urinary sodium losses are inversely correlated with gestational age (eg, losses are higher in a 26 w infant than a 34 w infant) as Na/K ATPase activity increases, ENaC expression upregulate, and ANP decreases [1]. Preterm infants are at risk for negative sodium balance that can precipitate hyponatremia [2,46]. This can be prevented or managed by supplementing with sodium. However, sodium provision must be balanced with fluid status changes that will occur. Positive sodium balance, which is typically present in term infants, is essential for growth.

Kidney specific acid-base regulation does not reach adult-level function until after the first year of life. In term and near term infants net acid excretion in the urine is adequate to maintain homeostasis [1]. However in preterm infants, a reduction in net acid excretion and decreased urinary acidification can have clinical consequences [47]. Low bicarbonate reabsorption, as well as higher acid load due to rapid growth, osteogenesis, and other processes [1] leads to a relative predilection for metabolic acidosis, the most common acid-base abnormality observed during the early neonatal period, especially in premature or sick neonates. This is due to a transient renal tubular acidosis that resolves as neonatal tubular function matures. Bicarbonate reabsorption increases in the early postnatal period and reaches adult levels at around 1 y of age, driven mostly by increased cytosolic carbonic anhydrase activity [48]. Additionally, the mature kidney has a greater ability to generate new bicarbonate. Urinary acidification matures around 1 y of age as well, with a greater capacity to secrete organic and inorganic acids [1].

Clinical application of case 2
For this case, an astute clinician will pay attention to whether there was normal prenatal kidney imaging and/or any perinatal event (such as a traumatic delivery, prolonged resuscitation, or maternal medications) that warrants closer observation for adequate UOP. In the setting of a normal pregnancy, prenatal anatomy scan, and birth history, the nurse and family can be reassured that the first urination is likely forthcoming (if it was not missed earlier, for example,

occurring in the delivery room but not documented). No additional intervention or evaluation is necessary at this time, but the newborn should be observed in the hospital until urination occurs.

Case 3

You are discharging home a 10-d old term infant from the nursery. While she is now doing well, she had a difficult delivery with neonatal asphyxia and was treated for hypoxic ischemic encephalopathy with therapeutic cooling in the neonatal intensive care unit. She had no urine output for the first 72 h of life. The family wants to know what they should expect from a kidney standpoint for her life and if she is at increased risk of kidney problems after she goes home.

Interpreting serum creatinine and acute kidney injury
Broadly speaking, incidence of AKI in NICU patients is approximately 30% [49]. High-risk groups for developing AKI in the neonatal period include those with low birth-weight or premature birth, perinatal asphyxia, congenital heart disease, or requiring cardiopulmonary bypass/extracorporeal membrane oxygenation [50].

AKI has 3 major classifications of etiologies: prerenal, renal, and postrenal (Table 2). Prerenal AKI (sometimes referred to as "functional AKI") represents around 85% of neonatal AKI cases and is defined as elevated serum creatinine and/or low UOP and is generally due to decreased RBF [51]. This can be because of decreased intravascular volume, perceived poor renal blood flow (due to maldistribution of fluid or poor cardiac output), or medications (NSAIDs, ACE inhibitors, AT1-R antagonists). Intrinsic AKI represents ~ 10% of neonatal AKI cases and is commonly due to acute tubular necrosis, which could be caused by either prolonged hypoperfusion or nephrotoxic medications, such as aminoglycosides, vancomycin, or acyclovir [51]. Postrenal AKI represents <5% of neonatal AKI cases and is due to anatomic obstructions, with the most common cause being posterior urethral valves in males.

Even after resolution of AKI, neonates with a history of AKI are at increased risk of childhood CKD and hypertension [52–54]. This risk appears to be the highest in those with AKI requiring dialysis, prolonged episodes of AKI, or

Table 2
Epidemiology, risk factors, and associated findings with neonatal acute kidney disorder

Prenatal	Perinatal	Postnatal
Factors that increase risk of preterm or LBW neonate	Exposure to nephrotoxic medications	Prematurity
Placental insufficiency	(ACE inhibitors, NSAIDs)	Low birth weight
	Delivery complications,	Congenital Heart Disease
	resulting in hypoxia	Inborn errors of metabolism
	and/or asphyxia	Sepsis
	Hypoxic ischemic	Nephrotoxin exposure
	encephalopathy	PDA
		Extracorporeal therapies

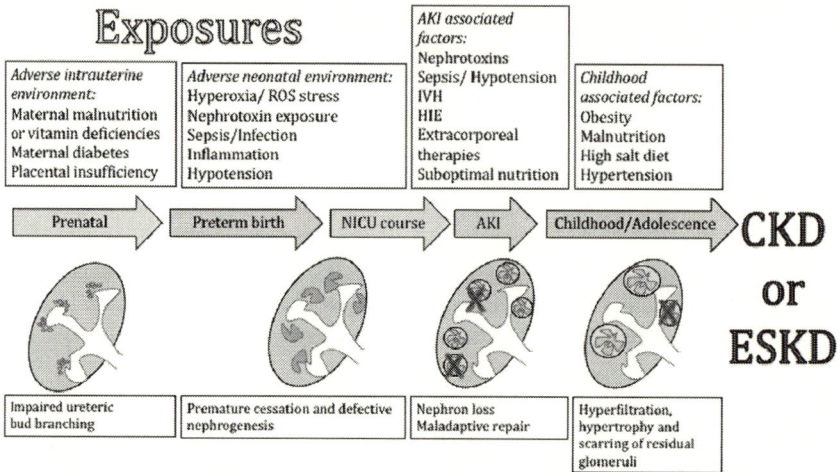

Fig. 2. Summary of incurred by neonate that may lead to an enhanced risk of acute kidney injury, as well as chronic kidney disease. (*From* Harer MW, Charlton JR, Tipple TE, et al. Preterm birth and neonatal acute kidney injury: implications on adolescent and adult outcomes. J Perinatol 2020;40(9):1286–95. Epub 2020/04/12. https://doi.org/10.1038/s41372-020-0656-7. PubMed PMID: 32277164.)

those with recurrent episodes of AKI [53]. One major challenge is that neonates with AKI are often not identified or recognized as having kidney dysfunction, either due to lack of laboratory monitoring, awareness, or recognition of AKI risk in the neonatal period [55–57]. Recent work has focused on standardizing the approach to the diagnosis and recognition of AKI in neonates to improve their care both during their initial hospitalization but also to facilitate long-term management and screening [55,58]. While no current evidence-based guidelines exist for neonates with AKI, recent expert consensus recommends risk stratification at the time of neonatal discharge and then follow-up for at least the first 2 y of life, to include monitoring for hypertension and/or evidence of CKD [59] (Fig. 2).

Clinical application of case 3. This infant had severe AKI (Stage 3) based on urine output. The family and their infant's primary care provider should be aware of diagnosis of AKI, its stage and severity, as well as potential implications for future health. Surveillance for kidney health include monitoring of blood pressure at all clinical visits, avoidance of nephrotoxic medications when possible, and assessment of kidney function at 2 y, or sooner if concerns arise, with measurement of serum creatinine and urine protein.

SUMMARY

Development and maturation of the kidney involve complex, regulated processes that are essential for long-term homeostasis and health. Kidney development begins in utero and maturation continues after birth. While kidney development is essentially completed by 2 y of age, maturation may be delayed in preterm or critically-ill neonates. Assessment of kidney function (often by measurement of serum creatinine and UOP) is critical to identify neonates with kidney dysfunction, specifically AKI. Furthermore, there is growing recognition that neonatal kidney dysfunction may have long-term implications, which requires ongoing surveillance for hypertension and/or CKD.

CLINICS CARE POINTS

- While kidney development occurs mostly during the prenatal period, with the bulk of nephrons formed during the second trimester, perinatal and early postnatal kidney development continues for about 40 d in neonates born prior to 36 w' gestation.
- Kidney function in the early days to weeks of neonatal life is immature, only approximately 10% of adult levels. While this is adequate for a healthy term neonate, a premature or critically-ill neonate may have challenges with fluid, sodium, and/or acid-base homeostasis due to immature kidney function.
- Urine output can be a helpful marker of kidney function in the neonate. However, the interpretation can be made challenging by immature tubular function and natriuresis in the early postnatal period.
- Premature neonates, as well as critically-ill term neonates, are at high-risk of AKI. This risk is highest in extremely premature infants, those born low birthweight, and those with perinatal events, such as asphyxia.
- Infants who experience AKI are at increased risk of CKD and hypertension. Infants with AKI should have their diagnosis communicated to their primary care provider and should be carefully monitored during childhood for evidence of hypertension and/or CKD, so appropriate treatment can mitigate their long-term consequences.

Disclosures

All authors report no real or perceived conflicts of interest that could affect the study design, collection, analysis, and interpretation of data, the writing of the report, or the decision to submit the article for publication. For full disclosure, we provide an additional list of authors' other funding not directly related to this article. M. Starr is supported in part by the Indiana University School of Medicine Physician Scientist Initiative and K23HL168362. B. Holland was supported by the IMPRS program and the Indiana Clinical and Translational Sciences Institute, United States funded, through an award made by the National Center for Advancing Translational Sciences of the National Institutes of Health, under the award number UL1TR00252. The authors have nothing to disclose.

References

[1] Polin RA. Fetal and neonatal physiology. 6th edition. Philadelphia: Elsevier; 2021.
[2] Sulemanji M, Vakili K. Neonatal renal physiology. Semin Pediatr Surg 2013;22(4):195–8.
[3] Walker KA, Bertram JF. Kidney development: core curriculum 2011. Am J Kidney Dis 2011;57(6):948–58.

[4] Wickremsinhe E, Fantana A, Berthier E, et al. Standard venipuncture vs a capillary blood collection device for the prospective determination of abnormal liver chemistry. J Appl Lab Med 2023;8(3):535–50.

[5] Sampogna RV, Schneider L, Al-Awqati Q. Developmental programming of branching morphogenesis in the kidney. J Am Soc Nephrol 2015;26(10):2414–22.

[6] Hoy WE, Douglas-Denton RN, Hughson MD, et al. A stereological study of glomerular number and volume: preliminary findings in a multiracial study of kidneys at autopsy. Kidney Int Suppl 2003;83:S31–7.

[7] Hughson M, Farris AB, Douglas-Denton R, et al. Glomerular number and size in autopsy kidneys: the relationship to birth weight. Kidney Int 2003;63(6):2113–22.

[8] Akalay S, Rayyan M, Fidlers T, et al. Impact of preterm birth on kidney health and development. Front Med (Lausanne) 2024;11:1363097.

[9] Baum M. Neonatal nephrology. Curr Opin Pediatr 2016;28(2):170–2.

[10] Wanner N, Vornweg J, Combes A, et al. DNA methyltransferase 1 controls nephron progenitor cell renewal and differentiation. J Am Soc Nephrol 2019;30(1):63–78.

[11] Liu J, Edgington-Giordano F, Dugas C, et al. Regulation of nephron progenitor cell self-renewal by intermediary metabolism. J Am Soc Nephrol 2017;28(11):3323–35.

[12] Sutherland MR, Gubhaju L, Moore L, et al. Accelerated maturation and abnormal morphology in the preterm neonatal kidney. J Am Soc Nephrol 2011;22(7):1365–74.

[13] Hostetter TH, Olson JL, Rennke HG, et al. Hyperfiltration in remnant nephrons: a potentially adverse response to renal ablation. Am J Physiol 1981;241(1):F85–93.

[14] Abitbol CL, Bauer CR, Montané B, et al. Long-term follow-up of extremely low birth weight infants with neonatal renal failure. Pediatr Nephrol 2003;18(9):887–93.

[15] Luyckx VA, Brenner BM. Clinical consequences of developmental programming of low nephron number. Anat Rec (Hoboken) 2020;303(10):2613–31.

[16] Botwinski CA, Falco GA. Transition to postnatal renal function. J Perinat Neonatal Nurs 2014;28(2):150–4.e3–4.

[17] Underwood MA, Gilbert WM, Sherman MP. Amniotic fluid: not just fetal urine anymore. J Perinatol 2005;25(5):341–8.

[18] Su SW, Stonestreet BS. Core concepts: neonatal glomerular filtration rate. NeoReviews 2010;11(12):e714–21.

[19] Solhaug MJ, Wallace MR, Granger JP. Nitric oxide and angiotensin II regulation of renal hemodynamics in the developing piglet. Pediatr Res 1996;39(3):527–33.

[20] Suessenbach FK, Burckhardt BB. Levels of angiotensin peptides in healthy and cardiovascular/renal-diseased paediatric population-an investigative review. Heart Fail Rev 2019;24(5):709–23.

[21] Wolf G. Angiotensin II and tubular development. Nephrol Dial Transplant 2002;17(suppl_9):48–51.

[22] van Bel F, Guit GL, Schipper J, et al. Indomethacin-induced changes in renal blood flow velocity waveform in premature infants investigated with color Doppler imaging. J Pediatr 1991;118(4 Pt 1):621–6.

[23] Akima S, Kent A, Reynolds GJ, et al. Indomethacin and renal impairment in neonates. Pediatr Nephrol 2004;19(5):490–3.

[24] Overmeire BV, Smets K, Lecoutere D, et al. A comparison of ibuprofen and indomethacin for closure of patent ductus arteriosus. N Engl J Med 2000;343(10):674–81.

[25] Hammerman C, Shchors I, Jacobson S, et al. Ibuprofen versus continuous indomethacin in premature neonates with patent ductus arteriosus: is the difference in the mode of administration? Pediatr Res 2008;64(3):291–7.

[26] Nada A, Bonachea EM, Askenazi DJ. Acute kidney injury in the fetus and neonate. Semin Fetal Neonatal Med 2017;22(2):90–7.

[27] Rodríguez MM, Gómez AH, Abitbol CL, et al. Histomorphometric analysis of postnatal glomerulogenesis in extremely preterm infants. Pediatr Dev Pathol 2004;7(1):17–25.

[28] Kiyoshige A, Osawa K, Watanabe Y, et al. Association of neonatal serum creatinine concentration with maternal serum creatinine concentration and birth weight. Clin Lab 2023;69(3); https://doi.org/10.7754/Clin.Lab.2022.220601.

[29] Kotchen TA, Strickland AL, Rice TW, et al. A study of the renin-angiotensin system in newborn infants. J Pediatr 1972;80(6):938–46.

[30] Coulthard MG, Hey EN, Ruddock V. Creatinine and urea clearances compared to inulin clearance in preterm and mature babies. Early Hum Dev 1985;11(1):11–9.

[31] Jetton JG, Askenazi DJ. Update on acute kidney injury in the neonate. Curr Opin Pediatr 2012;24(2):191–6.

[32] Friis-Hansen B. Body water compartments in children: changes during growth and related changes in body composition : kenneth D. Blackfan Memorial Lecture. Pediatrics 1961;28(2):169–81.

[33] Lorenz JM, Kleinman LI, Ahmed G, et al. Phases of fluid and electrolyte homeostasis in the extremely low birth weight infant. Pediatrics 1995;96(3 Pt 1):484–9.

[34] Jose PA, Fildes RD, Gomez RA, et al. Neonatal renal function and physiology. Curr Opin Pediatr 1994;6(2):172–7.

[35] Gomella TL, Eyal FG, Bany-Mohammed F. No urine output in 24 hours. Gomella's neonatology: management, procedures, on-call problems, diseases, and drugs. 8th edition. New York: McGraw-Hill Education; 2020.

[36] Calcagno PL, Rubin MI, Weintraub DH. Studies on the renal concentrating and diluting mechanisms in the premature infant. J Clin Investig 1954;33(1):91–6.

[37] Arant BS Jr. Postnatal development of renal function during the first year of life. Pediatr Nephrol 1987;1(3):308–13.

[38] Ames RG. Urinary water excretion and neurohypophysial function in full term and premature infants shortly after birth. Pediatrics 1953;12(3:1):272–82.

[39] Vieux R, Hascoet JM, Merdariu D, et al. Glomerular filtration rate reference values in very preterm infants. Pediatrics 2010;125(5):e1186–92.

[40] Osathanondh V, Potter EL. Development of human kidney as shown by microdissection. IV. Development of tubular portions of nephrons. Arch Pathol 1966;82(5):391–402.

[41] Torrey TW. The Kidney: developmental Nephrology. Wallace W. McCrory. Harvard University Press, Cambridge, Mass., 1973. xiv, 216 pp. + plates. $12. A Commonwealth Fund Book. Science 1973;182(4107):48.

[42] Leipälä JA, Boldt T, Turpeinen U, et al. Cardiac hypertrophy and altered hemodynamic adaptation in growth-restricted preterm infants. Pediatr Res 2003;53(6):989–93.

[43] Omar SA, DeCristofaro JD, Agarwal BI, et al. Effects of Prenatal Steroids on Water and Sodium Homeostasis in Extremely Low Birth Weight Neonates. Pediatrics 1999;104(3): 482–8.

[44] Dimitriou G, Kavvadia V, Marcou M, et al. Antenatal steroids and fluid balance in very low birthweight infants. Arch Dis Child Fetal Neonatal Ed 2005;90(6):F509–13.

[45] De Mul A, Heneau A, Biran V, et al. Early urine output monitoring in very preterm infants to predict in-hospital neonatal outcomes: a bicentric retrospective cohort study. BMJ Open 2023;13(1):e068300.

[46] Siegel SR, Oh W. Renal function as a marker of human fetal maturation. Acta Paediatr Scand 1976;65(4):481–5.

[47] Sulyok E, Heim T. Assessment of maximal urinary acidification in premature infants. Biol Neonat 2009;19(1–3):200–10.

[48] Edelmann CM, Soriano JR, Boichis H, et al. Renal bicarbonate reabsorption and hydrogen ion excretion in normal infants. J Clin Investig 1967;46(8):1309–17.

[49] Jetton JG, Boohaker LJ, Sethi SK, et al. Incidence and outcomes of neonatal acute kidney injury (AWAKEN): a multicentre, multinational, observational cohort study. Lancet Child Adolesc Health 2017;1(3):184–94.

[50] Charlton JR, Boohaker L, Askenazi D, et al. Incidence and risk factors of early onset neonatal AKI. Clin J Am Soc Nephrol 2019;14(2):184–95.

[51] Starr MC, Charlton JR, Guillet R, et al. Advances in neonatal acute kidney injury. Pediatrics 2021;148(5); https://doi.org/10.1542/peds.2021-051220.

[52] Starr MC, Hingorani SR. Prematurity and future kidney health: the growing risk of chronic kidney disease. Curr Opin Pediatr 2018;30(2):228–35.

[53] Selewski DT, Hyatt DM, Bennett KM, et al. Is acute kidney injury a harbinger for chronic kidney disease? Curr Opin Pediatr 2018;30(2):236–40.

[54] Harer MW, Charlton JR, Tipple TE, et al. Preterm birth and neonatal acute kidney injury: implications on adolescent and adult outcomes. J Perinatol 2020;40(9):1286–95.

[55] Starr MC, Kula A, Lieberman J, et al. Improving the recognition and reporting of acute kidney injury in the neonatal intensive care unit. J Perinatol 2020;40(9):1301–7.

[56] Sethi SK, Agrawal G, Wazir S, et al. Neonatal acute kidney injury: a survey of perceptions and management strategies amongst pediatricians and neonatologists. Front Pediatr 2019;7:553.

[57] Carmody JB, Swanson JR, Rhone ET, et al. Recognition and reporting of AKI in very low birth weight infants. Clin J Am Soc Nephrol 2014;9(12):2036–43.

[58] Vincent K, Murphy HJ, Ross JR, et al. Acute kidney injury guidelines are associated with improved recognition and follow-up for neonatal patients. Adv Neonatal Care 2020;20(4):269–75.

[59] Starr MC, Harer MW, Steflik HJ, et al. Kidney health monitoring in neonatal intensive care unit graduates: a modified Delphi Consensus Statement. JAMA Netw Open 2024;7(9):e2435043.

Advances in Pediatrics 72 (2025) 157–169

ADVANCES IN PEDIATRICS

ELSEVIER
MOSBY

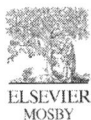

Neonatal Endocrine Emergencies

Check for
updates

Grace K. Kim, MD, Alejandro F. Siller, MD, MSCI,
Meghan Craven, MD, Nidhi Bansal, MD, MPH*

Division of Diabetes and Endocrinology, Department of Pediatrics, Baylor College of Medicine and
Texas Children's Hospital, Houston, TX, USA

Keywords

- Neonatal emergencies • Endocrine • Hypoglycemia • Hyperglycemia
- Hypocalcemia • Hyperthyroidism • Adrenal insufficiency

Key points

- Delayed diagnosis and treatment of neonatal endocrine emergencies may be associated with increased mortality and morbidity.
- Signs and symptoms of neonatal endocrine disorders may be subtle and nonspecific.
- A high degree of suspicion and thorough history and evaluation are important to screening and diagnosing endocrine emergencies in neonates.
- Initial treatment of endocrine emergencies focuses on stability of neonate, and correcting electrolyte abnormalities and dehydration.

INTRODUCTION

Neonatal endocrine emergencies are important to diagnose, as delay in recognition and treatment may be related to high morbidity and mortality. Initial symptoms may be vague or nonspecific; thus, a high degree of suspicion and thorough evaluation are needed for diagnosis. The following sections discuss the diagnosis and initial management of common neonatal emergencies related to disorders of glucose metabolism, calcium metabolism, thyroid disorders, and adrenal disorders.

HYPOGLYCEMIA

Neonatal hypoglycemia can affect up to 15% of neonates [1]. Expert consensus on glucose levels to use for identifying neonatal hypoglycemia varies owing to lack of evidence supporting a glucose threshold that will prevent morbidity

*Corresponding author. 6701 Fannin Street, Suite 1020, Houston, TX 77030. E-mail address: nidhi.bansal@bcm.edu

https://doi.org/10.1016/j.yapd.2025.03.006
0065-3101/25/© 2025 Elsevier Inc.

Abbreviations

ACTH	adrenocorticotropic hormone
AI	adrenal insufficiency
ATD	antithyroid drug
CAH	congenital adrenal hyperplasia
DOL	day of life
DKA	diabetic ketoacidosis
ELBW	extremely low birth weight
GIR	glucose infusion rate
HI	hyperinsulinemia
IV	intravenous
MMI	methimazole
17OHP	17-hydroxyprogesterone
PHA	pseudohypoaldosteronism
PTH	parathyroid hormone
TRAb	thyrotropin receptor antibodies
TSH	thyrotropin
VLBW	very low birth weight
UTI	urinary tract infection

and mortality [1–3]. Furthermore, because of the presence of the physiologic nadir of serum glucose as the neonate adapts to extrauterine life, initial lower glucose levels in the newborn period should be tolerated [2]. Recommendations focus on treatment goals, with minimal glucose levels of 50 mg/dL in the first 48 hours where congenital hyperinsulinemia (HI) is not suspected, 60 mg/dL after the first 48 hours of life when HI is not suspected, and 70 mg/dL when HI is suspected or confirmed [2,4]. However, variations exist on recommendations for timing and glucose thresholds for screening [1]. Independent of the exact values, diagnosis of hypoglycemia in neonates is challenging, as neonates are unable to report symptoms, and signs of hypoglycemia are nonspecific [2–4]. However, it is critical that hypoglycemia is recognized promptly and treated immediately to prevent irreversible neurologic damage and/or death [3]. Screening should be limited to at-risk and symptomatic neonates to avoid capturing and overtreating healthy neonates who may transiently dip below these thresholds [1,3]. Risk factors for development of neonatal hypoglycemia and symptoms that should prompt screening in any neonate are listed in Table 1.

Initial treatment of hypoglycemia should focus on immediately raising the blood glucose. This may include feeding, especially in the first 48 hours of life, and if glucose is not too far below threshold [3]. Initial intravenous (IV) boluses of 2 mL/kg with 10% dextrose can be used for immediate treatment in severe hypoglycemia [2]. In severe hypoglycemia, while cause is being established, the neonate should be placed on continuous dextrose-containing IV fluids, initially at maintenance rate for weight [2]. Glucose infusion rate (GIR) should be titrated to maintain a glucose level between 70 mg/dL and 90 mg/dL [4]. Need for prolonged supraphysiologic GIR should significantly increase suspicion for HI as the cause of hypoglycemia in the neonate.

Table 1
A list of maternal, fetal, and perinatal risk factors for transient neonatal hypoglycemia, and a list of the nonspecific symptoms of neonatal hypoglycemia to prompt immediate measurement of blood or plasma glucose

Risk factors for development of neonatal hypoglycemia	• Large for gestational age (LGA) • Small for gestational age (SGA) • Intrauterine growth restriction (IUGR) • Maternal diabetes mellitus • Perinatal stress, birth asphyxia • Preterm or postterm delivery • Maternal use of beta-blockers • Antenatal corticosteroids • Family history of congenital hypoglycemia syndrome • Diagnosis of syndrome associated with hypoglycemia (such as Beckwith-Wiedemann syndrome)
Symptoms of neonatal hypoglycemia	• Jitteriness • Tachycardia • Hypothermia • Cyanosis • Seizure • Apnea • Tachypnea • Weak or high-pitched cry • Lethargy • Irritability • Poor tone • Difficulty feeding • Abnormal eye movements • Lip smacking

Adapted from Refs. [3,4].

Diagnosis of specific causes (Table 2) should be a priority once the infant is stabilized, and pediatric endocrinology should be consulted. Critical laboratory tests should be obtained at the time of hypoglycemia, which include confirmatory serum glucose, insulin, beta-hydroxybutyrate, free fatty acid, bicarbonate, lactate, cortisol, and growth hormone. Fig. 1 provides an algorithm for interpretation of critical laboratory tests.

HYPERGLYCEMIA

Hyperglycemia is common in preterm or low-birth-weight infants, in whom perinatal stress, iatrogenic factors such as administration of IV dextrose or treatment with steroids, or physiologic factors, such as increased insulin resistance, can result in transient hyperglycemia [5]. Such hyperglycemia tends to be transient, resolving within the first week. Symptoms may include polyuria, polydipsia, and failure to thrive. However, symptoms can be insidious and nonspecific, and hyperglycemia is often detected incidentally or once the infant has progressed to diabetic ketoacidosis (DKA) [5].

There are differing recommendations for thresholds to treat hyperglycemia with insulin owing to insulin resistance in neonates and the potential risk of

Table 2
Neonatal hypoglycemia causes

Broad category for neonatal hypoglycemia	Specific cause for neonatal hypoglycemia
Poor glucose production	• Prematurity • Small for gestational age • Impaired gluconeogenesis • Galactosemia
Increased glucose demand	• Sepsis • Hypothermia • Hypoxia • Cyanotic heart disease • Polycythemia
Hyperinsulinism	• Perinatal stress-induced transient hyperinsulinism • Infant of diabetic mother • Maternal drugs (anti–diabetic drugs, beta-blockers, antiarrhythmic drugs, and so forth) • Congenital hyperinsulinism (*ABCC8, KCNJ11* mutation) • Beckwith-Wiedemann syndrome • Insulinoma • Hyperinsulinism hyperammonemia syndrome
Endocrine abnormalities	• Cortisol deficiency • Growth hormone deficiency • Pan-hypopituitarism

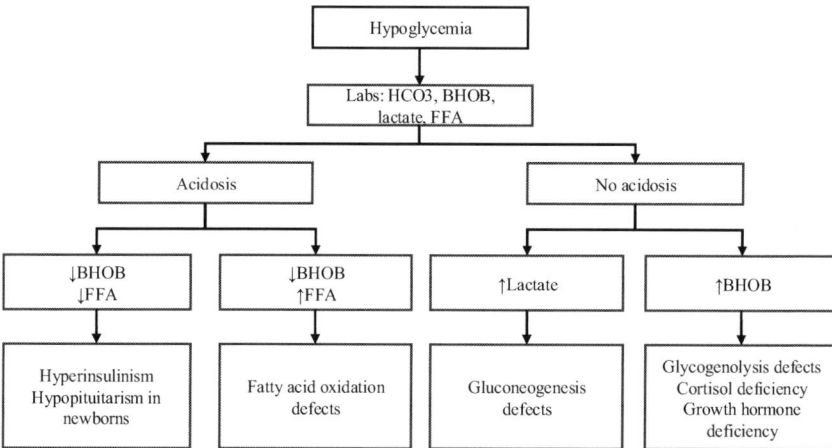

Fig. 1. Algorithm for interpretation of hypoglycemia critical laboratory tests. BHOB, beta-hydroxybutyrate; FFA, free fatty acid; HCO$_3$, bicarbonate. (*Adapted from* Thornton PS, Stanley CA, De Leon DD, et al. Recommendations from the Pediatric Endocrine Society for Evaluation and Management of Persistent Hypoglycemia in Neonates, Infants, and Children. J Pediatr 2015;167(2):238–45. https://doi.org/10.1016/j.jpeds.2015.03.057.)

hypoglycemia [5,6]. Adjusting GIR or transitioning to enteral nutrition when possible, or adjusting doses of medications that may be provoking hyperglycemia, should be considered first [5]. Aggressive control of mild hyperglycemia is controversial, as despite association with numerous adverse outcomes, there is no consensus that it plays a causal role. Moreover, treatment does not improve outcomes of mortality, retinopathy of prematurity, or sepsis [6]. In severe hyperglycemia, or where clinical factors are suggestive of possible neonatal diabetes mellitus, treatment with insulin is necessary to avoid progression to DKA [5].

Persistent hyperglycemia beyond the first week of life above 250 mg/dL should prompt concern for neonatal diabetes [5]. In the acute phase, continuous insulin infusion at 0.02 to 0.05 units/kg per hour can be started. IV dextrose infusion can be administered in tandem to prevent hypoglycemia [5]. Once stabilized, transition to subcutaneous insulin can be considered.

HYPOCALCEMIA

Neonatal hypocalcemia is relatively common and is classified by timing of onset and birth weight. It is typically defined by serum calcium levels, with thresholds varying based on birth weight and gestational age. For term infants and preterm infants with a birth weight of $\geq$1500 g, hypocalcemia is defined as a serum calcium level of less than 8 mg/dL (<2 mmol/L). In contrast, for very-low-birth-weight (VLBW) and extremely low-birth-weight (ELBW) preterm infants (<1500 g), hypocalcemia is defined as a total serum calcium level of less than 7 mg/dL (<1.75 mmol/L) [7].

Although many neonates with hypocalcemia are asymptomatic, clinical manifestations can include irritability, jitteriness, tremors, facial spasms, and tetany. Symptoms are often triggered by external stimuli. Seizures are a serious manifestation, and rarely, neonates may present with laryngospasm, vomiting, or apnea [8]. Table 3 provides common causes of neonatal hypocalcemia.

Early-onset neonatal hypocalcemia is an inappropriate physiologic response to the calcium nadir. It is often asymptomatic owing to preservation of ionized calcium levels, although the exact mechanism is unclear, likely related to

Table 3 Causes of neonatal hypocalcemia	
Early neonatal hypocalcemia 48–72 h after birth	Late neonatal hypocalcemia 3–7 d after birth
• Prematurity • Birth asphyxia • Infant of diabetic mother • Intrauterine growth retardation • Maternal hyperparathyroidism • Maternal anticonvulsant exposure	• Phosphate-rich cow's milk or formula • Transient hypoparathyroidism of newborn • Hypomagnesemia • Hypoparathyroidism • Vitamin D deficiency • Hyperbilirubinemia and phototherapy • Intestinal malabsorption • Parathyroid hormone resistance

relative acidosis and hypoproteinemia [7]. Late-onset neonatal hypocalcemia is more likely to be symptomatic and is often related to nutritional factors [9]. Routine monitoring is recommended in VLBW and ELBW infants for at least the first 48 hours, as well as in neonates who are critically ill, neonates with congenital heart disease, and neonates with symptoms of hypocalcemia. It is not necessary to screen asymptomatic healthy preterm infants or infants of diabetic mothers who are feeding on the first day [9].

Before initiating treatment, a laboratory evaluation to determine the underlying cause of hypocalcemia is recommended. This workup should include measurements of total calcium, ionized calcium, phosphate, magnesium, alkaline phosphatase, albumin, intact parathyroid hormone (PTH), creatinine, 25-hydroxyvitamin D, and the urine calcium-creatinine ratio. Treatment should address any underlying conditions, such as hypomagnesemia or hyperphosphatemia [10].

The recommended treatment for neonates with acute symptomatic hypocalcemia is IV calcium gluconate, preferably administered via a central line. The initial dose is 10% (100 mg/mL) solution at 100 mg/kg, infused over 10 minutes, with heart rate monitoring owing to the risk of bradyarrhythmia from rapid serum calcium elevation. The infusion site should also be carefully monitored to prevent extravasation, which could lead to subcutaneous necrosis. It is important to note that hepatic necrosis can occur if the infusion is given through an umbilical venous catheter with the tip located in a branch of the portal vein. In addition, calcium should not be infused through an umbilical artery catheter, as this may cause arterial spasm, potentially compromising intestinal blood flow [11]. If there is no response to the initial dose, a repeat dose can be administered after 10 minutes. In life-threatening cases, calcium chloride, which is metabolized more rapidly, may be given at a dose of 20 mg/kg if available. Once asymptomatic, intermittent doses of IV calcium gluconate can be infused slowly for over an hour until target calcium levels are achieved. After, maintenance therapy should be initiated through an oral dose of 50 mg/kg of elemental calcium (rather than the total calcium salt) per day divided in 4 to 6 doses or via a continuous infusion. Maintenance therapy may be gradually weaned over approximately a week if serum calcium remains stable, and cause is resolved [7,12,13].

In asymptomatic infants, especially with early-onset hypocalcemia, most will recover with nutritional support alone. Oral calcium supplementation can be considered as needed, or for infants not yet on full enteral feeds, calcium can be given through IV fluids, providing 10% calcium gluconate at 500 mg/kg per day (equivalent to 50 mg/kg of elemental calcium) as a continuous infusion. If parenteral calcium infusion continues for more than 48 hours, phosphate supplementation is required based on serum phosphate levels [12].

For late-onset hypocalcemia, it is additionally recommended to administer 400 IU of vitamin D3 per day. Calcitriol, at a dose of 0.08 to 0.1 µg/kg, may also be used as an adjunct therapy to support calcium metabolism and maintain adequate calcium levels [14].

HYPERCALCEMIA

Neonatal hypercalcemia is uncommon and is defined as total blood calcium concentration 2 standard deviations above the mean, typically greater than 11.3 mg/dL; however, symptoms may not occur until the total serum calcium level exceeds 13 mg/dL. In a neonate, these symptoms include failure to thrive, lethargy, poor appetite, vomiting, constipation, polyuria leading to dehydration, hypotonia, irritability, seizures, as well as hypertension with a shortened S-T segment and associated heart block and death [15]. When hypercalcemia is suspected, an accurate diagnosis requires a thorough dietary history, family history, assessment for physical features, and biochemical evaluation. Biochemical evaluation should include ionized calcium, serum albumin, serum phosphate, creatinine, PTH, vitamin D metabolites, and urinary calcium, phosphate, creatinine [15,16].

After obtaining evaluation laboratory tests, acute treatment should be initiated in symptomatic neonates. Treatment for hypercalcemia initially involves avoidance of excessive calcium and vitamin D intake, and hydration with IV fluids. Loop diuretics may be used to enhance calcium excretion; however, it may exacerbate dehydration. Subcutaneous calcitonin is an effective antiresorptive agent, but tachyphylaxis may occur. Use of IV bisphosphonates leads to sustained reduction of hypercalcemia. Glucocorticoids may be considered if hypercalcemia is mediated by granulomatous inflammatory cells with increased 1-alpha-hydroxylase activity, such as in subcutaneous fat necrosis of the newborn [15,16].

HYPERTHYROIDISM

Neonatal thyrotoxicosis occurs frequently because of neonatal Graves disease caused by placental transfer of thyrotropin (TSH) receptor antibodies (TRAb) from mother to fetus [17]. Neonatal Graves occurs in approximately 1:25,000 to 1:50,000 neonates and affects male and female neonates equally. Rarer causes of neonatal thyrotoxicosis include McCune-Albright syndrome, genetic defect of the TSH receptor, and fetal iodine exposure [18–21].

Neonatal Graves typically presents in the first 2 weeks of life but may be delayed because of interplay between TSH receptor simulating and blocking antibodies [17]. Clinical manifestations of neonatal hyperthyroidism include tachycardia, irritability, tremors, poor feeding, poor weight gain, sweating, and difficulty sleeping. Newborns may have proptosis with stare, and a goiter. Goiter may be a result of maternal antithyroid drug (ATD) treatment or owing to neonatal Graves disease. Infants with neonatal Graves disease may rarely present with thrombocytopenia, jaundice, and hepatomegaly and may be confused with congenital infections or sepsis. Other rare presentations of neonatal Graves disease include fulminant liver failure, pulmonary hypertension, and persistent hypoglycemia [22–24]. Short-term complications include arrhythmias and cardiac failure and may even result in death if treatment is delayed or inadequate. Although most children with neonatal hyperthyroidism do not develop severe long-term impairments, recent studies suggest subtle neurodevelopmental variations in affected children [25].

Because a large majority of neonatal hyperthyroidism is due to placental transfer of TRAb, guidelines for management of thyroid disease during pregnancy recommend determining TRAb levels in pregnant women with a history of Graves disease at 20 to 24 weeks' gestation [26]. All neonates born from women with TRAb-positive pregnancy are at risk of developing neonatal hyperthyroidism. The risk is markedly increased if maternal TRAb level is greater than 2 to 3 times the upper limit of normal [27]. Nomograms for fetal thyroid gland are available and can be used to make early diagnosis of fetal hyperthyroidism [28]. Fetal ultrasound is recommended at 20 weeks' gestation and then repeated every 4 to 6 weeks [29]. A screening algorithm for newborns at risk for neonatal hyperthyroidism has been proposed. The recommendations include testing TRAb in the cord blood or day of life (DOL) 1 and again during DOL 10 to 14 and thyroid function studies on DOL 3 to 5 and DOL 10 to 14 [17].

Fetal hyperthyroidism can be prevented with adequate management of maternal hyperthyroidism with ATDs. Normalization of fetal heart rate is the goal of maternal therapy. A management algorithm for neonatal hyperthyroidism has been proposed. Methimazole (MMI), starting dose of 0.2 to 0.5 mg/kg per day, divided twice daily is recommended for neonates with biochemical hyperthyroidism. Propranolol should be added at a dose of 2 mg/kg per day divided twice daily for tachycardia and hypertension. In severe cases with hemodynamic instability, Lugol solution or potassium iodide at a dose of 1 drop 3 times daily should be considered. The first dose of iodine should be given at least 1 hour after the first dose of MMI. In addition, glucocorticoid therapy with hydrocortisone 2.5 to 10 mg/kg per day divided 3 times daily or prednisolone 1 to 2 mg/kg per day divided twice daily may be considered [17].

HYPOTHYROIDISM

Congenital hypothyroidism should be managed urgently owing to long-term implications on growth and cognitive development; however, congenital hypothyroidism rarely presents as a neonatal emergency. Respiratory distress caused by compressive hypothyroid goiter is a rare neonatal emergency. Treatment frequently includes surgical decompression along with levothyroxine replacement [30].

ADRENAL INSUFFICIENCY

Symptoms of neonatal adrenal insufficiency (AI) may be nonspecific and can be confused with sepsis, metabolic conditions, or cardiovascular disease. Primary AI occurs when there is either primary adrenal failure (primary AI) or disruption of the hypothalamic pituitary axis (central AI) leading to inadequate cortisol production. In preterm, low-birth-weight, and critically ill neonates, relative AI may also be present [31,32].

Primary adrenal insufficiency

Primary AI is associated with insufficiency of both glucocorticoids and mineralocorticoids. Patients present with hyponatremia, hyperkalemia, hypoglycemia, poor feeding, dehydration, failure to thrive, and cholestatic jaundice. Adrenal crisis is a life-threatening complication owing to the body's inability to respond to physiologic stress. This occurs more often in primary AI. Symptoms include hypotension, dehydration, vomiting, shock, coma, and death [33].

The most common cause of primary AI in neonates is congenital adrenal hyperplasia (CAH) [31]. The prevalence of CAH is 1:14,000 to 1:18,000. Approximately 95% of CAH is due to mutations in *CYP21A1* gene, which encodes the 21-hydroxylase enzyme, which converts 17-hydroxyprogesterone (17OHP) into precursors for cortisol and aldosterone. Deficiency of this enzyme leads to accumulation of cortisol precursors that are diverted to androgen biosynthesis, which leads to variable degrees of virilization in girls. Neonates with atypical genitalia and nonpalpable gonads should be highly suspicious for CAH. Newborn screening, now universal in the United States and many developed countries, detects elevated levels of 17OHP to diagnose promptly. Delayed diagnosis of classic CAH is associated with salt-wasting crisis, leading to neonatal morbidity and mortality [34].

There are other rare forms of CAH that affect adrenal steroidogenesis, and many are associated with atypical genitalia because of the impact on androgens. Other causes of primary AI in neonates include adrenal hypoplasia, adrenocorticotropic hormone (ACTH) resistance, other genetic conditions, bilateral adrenal injury, hemorrhage, or infiltration [31]. Diagnosis of primary AI involves laboratory tests that show low cortisol, high ACTH, also hypoglycemia, hyponatremia, hyperkalemia, metabolic acidosis, and hyperreninemia. Cosyntropin stimulation test may be done if clinically stable [31,33].

Treatment of neonatal primary AI and salt-wasting crisis involves fluid resuscitation with IV normal saline fluid boluses, dextrose-containing fluid boluses for hypoglycemia, and IV stress dose of hydrocortisone 25 mg or 50 to 100 mg/m^2 per day, and then divided every 6 hours over 24 hours [31,34]. Recommendations for stress doses of hydrocortisone are empiric and not based on randomized controlled trials. Hydrocortisone at these stress doses also activates mineralocorticoid receptors; thus, fludrocortisone is not needed acutely. As AI resolves, hydrocortisone can be weaned to daily maintenance doses of 10 to 15 mg/m^2 day for primary AI, divided 3 times daily. Fludrocortisone and sodium chloride supplementation should also be added for mineralocorticoid deficiency. Education is needed for the family, that any time patient is acutely ill, the patient will need immediate stress doses of hydrocortisone (oral or intramuscular or IV if unable to tolerate oral) to prevent adrenal crisis (3–10 times higher than physiologic replacement, 30–100 mg/m^2 per day) divided 3 to 4 times per day [13,31,34].

Secondary adrenal insufficiency

Secondary or central AI may be due to disease or injury to the hypothalamic-pituitary area, or prolonged exogenous glucocorticoid administration and subsequent negative feedback inhibition on the pituitary. In secondary AI, mineralocorticoid function is generally spared, as it is primarily regulated by the renin-angiotensin system [35]. Isolated ACTH deficiency is rare, most frequently owing to recessive mutations in *TBX19* gene (or previously known as *TPIT*), or also mutations in *POMC* or *PC1*. However, ACTH deficiency is more commonly associated with combined pituitary hormone deficiencies, panhypopituitarism, involving mutations in transcription factors, and signaling pathways of the hypothalamic pituitary axis (*PROP1, LHX1, LHX4, HESX1,* and so forth) [35].

Signs and symptoms of central AI are due to glucocorticoid deficiency. Neonates present with severe hypoglycemia, seizures, failure to thrive, prolonged cholestatic jaundice, even coma. Cholestasis may be due to physiologic delay of maturation of bile acid synthesis and transport related to cortisol deficiency. Because aldosterone production is spared, typically sodium and potassium levels may be normal. However, cortisol contributes to regulating free water clearance and excretion, so patients may have mild dilutional hyponatremia from water retention, with normal serum potassium levels. Neonates with other pituitary deficiencies may have symptoms of other hormone deficiencies and midline defects [35].

Diagnosis of secondary AI, especially in critically ill neonates, requires a high degree of clinical suspicion, as exact testing and interpretation are variable. Random basal cortisol level may be low or normal. Generally, a cosyntropin stimulation test is the preferred method for diagnosis if patient is stable [32]. However, if a patient is critically ill and there is a high degree of clinical suspicion, one should consider starting empiric treatment and monitor clinically.

Treatment is the same as primary AI in the acute period for glucocorticoid deficiency, with rapid restoration of intravascular volume with IV fluid boluses, dextrose-containing fluid boluses for hypoglycemia, and stress doses of hydrocortisone. As the patient stabilizes, they can wean physiologic doses of hydrocortisone. Doses tend to be lower than primary AI, around 6 to 9 mg/m^2 per day divided 2 to 3 times daily with education on an outpatient basis on how to give stress dose hydrocortisone for illness to prevent adrenal crisis [31,35,36].

ALDOSTERONE RESISTANCE DISORDERS

Pseudohypoaldosteronism (PHA) type 1 is characterized by renal resistance to aldosterone. It can cause severe salt wasting, hyponatremia, life-threatening hyperkalemia (arrythmia, cardiac arrest), metabolic acidosis, and failure to thrive. PHA type 1A, autosomal dominant form, is due to mutation in the mineralocorticoid receptor (*NR3C2*), limited to kidneys, and is transient. PHA type 1B, autosomal recessive form, or systemic form, results from defects in the epithelial sodium channel (*SCNN1A, SCNN1B, SCNN1G*) and affects multiple organs, including salivary glands, colon, respiratory tract, and sweat glands, and requires lifelong management. To diagnose, CAH needs to be ruled out, and laboratory tests show high renin and aldosterone, hyponatremia, and hyperkalemia. It is also important to rule out secondary PHA (see later discussion). Treatment involves initial IV hydration with normal saline for dehydration, and high doses of sodium chloride supplement. If presenting with severe hyperkalemia and metabolic acidosis, patients may also need bicarbonate, kayexalate, and dialysis [37].

PHA type 2, or Gordon syndrome, is a heterogenous syndrome, involving defects in the sodium chloride cotransporter in the distal convoluted tubules, causing a rare familial hypertension syndrome. Clinical symptoms include volume overload, hypertension, hyperkalemia, and metabolic acidosis. Renin is normal or low, and aldosterone is low or low-normal. Treatment involves dietary salt restriction or thiazide diuretics [38].

Secondary PHA is unique in infancy and is transient. It is often associated with urinary tract infections (UTIs) or congenital malformations of the kidney and/or urinary tract, is more common in boys, and presents within the first few months of life. Patients may present with nonspecific symptoms of weight loss, decreased oral intake, vomiting, and dehydration. Laboratory tests show hyponatremia, metabolic acidosis, and hyperkalemia, along with elevated serum aldosterone and renin. Renal ultrasound and evaluation for UTI should be performed. Once the underlying cause is treated, PHA typically resolves [39].

SUMMARY

Neonatal endocrine emergencies may present insidiously, and thus, a high degree of suspicion is needed for further evaluation, for prompt diagnosis, and for acute stabilization of symptoms to prevent mortality and morbidity.

CLINICS CARE POINTS

- Hypoglycemia is common in neonates and may present insidiously; thus, it is important to screen for it in high-risk patients.
- Neonatal hypocalcemia may present early, within 72 hours, or late, within a week.
- Neonatal Graves disease should be screened for if there is a history of maternal Graves.
- The most common cause of primary adrenal insufficiency in neonates is congenital adrenal hyperplasia.
- Central adrenal insufficiency may present as isolated or more commonly as panhypopituitarism, with symptoms related to other pituitary hormone defects, or midline defects.
- Pseudohypoaldosteronism can present with severe life-threatening hyperkalemia.

Disclosures
The authors have nothing to disclose.

References
[1] Roeper M, Hoermann H, Kummer S, et al. Neonatal hypoglycemia: lack of evidence for a safe management. Front Endocrinol (Lausanne) 2023;14; https://doi.org/10.3389/fendo.2023.1179102.

[2] Thornton PS, Stanley CA, De Leon DD, et al. Recommendations from the Pediatric Endocrine Society for evaluation and management of persistent hypoglycemia in neonates, infants, and children. J Pediatr 2015;167(2):238–45.

[3] Adamkin DH, Papile LA, Baley JE, et al. Clinical report - postnatal glucose homeostasis in late-preterm and term infants. Pediatrics 2011;127(3):575–9.

[4] De Leon DD, Thornton P, Stanley CA, et al. Hypoglycemia in the newborn and infant. In: Sperling MA, editor. Pediatric endocrinology. 5th edition. Philadelphia (PA): Elsevier; 2021. p. 175–201.

[5] Lemelman MB, Letourneau L, Greeley SAW. Neonatal diabetes mellitus: an update on diagnosis and management. Clin Perinatol 2018;45(1):41–59.

[6] Hay WW, Rozance PJ. Neonatal hyperglycemia—causes, treatments, and cautions. J Pediatr 2018;200:6–8.

[7] Cheng E, George AA, Bansal SK, et al. Neonatal hypocalcemia: common, uncommon, and rare etiologies. NeoReviews 2023;24(4):e217–28.

[8] Root AW, Levine MA. 20 - Disorders of mineral metabolism II. Abnormalities of mineral homeostasis in the newborn, infant, child, and adolescent. In: Sperling MA, editor. Pediatric endocrinology. 5th Edition. Philadelphia (PA): Elsevier Inc; 2021. p. 705–813.

[9] Vuralli D. Clinical approach to hypocalcemia in newborn period and infancy: who should be treated? Int J Pediatr 2019;2019; https://doi.org/10.1155/2019/4318075.

[10] Nadar R, Shaw N. Investigation and management of hypocalcaemia. Arch Dis Child 2020;105(4):399–405.

[11] Mimouni F, Tsang RC. Neonatal hypocalcemia: to treat or not to treat? (A review). J Am Coll Nutr 1994;13(5):408–15.

[12] Abrams SA. Neonatal hypocalcemia. In: Connor RD, UpToDate. Wolters Kluwer. Available at: https://www.uptodate.com/contents/neonatal-hypocalcemia?search=hypocalcemia%20 neonate&source=search_result&selectedTitle=1%7E150&usage_type=default&display_ rank=1 (Accessed 1 October 2024).

[13] Root AW, Diamond FB. Disorders of mineral homeostasis in children and adolescents. In: Sperling MA, editor. Pediatric Endocrinology. 4th edition. Philadelphia (PA: Elsevier; 2014. p. 746–9.

[14] Misra M, Pacaud D, Petryk A, et al. Vitamin D deficiency in children and its management: review of current knowledge and recommendations. Pediatrics 2008;122(2):398–417.

[15] Hsu SC, Levine MA. Perinatal calcium metabolism: physiology and pathophysiology. Semin Neonatol 2004;9(1):23–36.

[16] Stokes VJ, Nielsen MF, Hannan FM, et al. Hypercalcemic disorders in children. J Bone Miner Res 2017;32(11):2157–70.

[17] van der Kaay DC, Wasserman JD, Palmert MR. Management of neonates bto mothers with Graves' disease. Pediatrics 2016;137(4):e20151878.

[18] Lourenço R, Dias P, Gouveia R, et al. Neonatal McCune-Albright syndrome with systemic involvement: a case report. J Med Case Rep 2015;9(1); https://doi.org/10.1186/ s13256-015-0689-2.

[19] Watkins MG, Dejkhamron P, Huo J, et al. Persistent neonatal thyrotoxicosis in a neonate secondary to a rare thyroid-stimulating hormone receptor activating mutation: case report and literature review. Endocr Pract 2008;14(4):479.

[20] Chester J, Rotenstein D, Ringkananont U, et al. Congenital neonatal hyperthyroidism caused by germline mutations in the TSH receptor gene: case report and review of the literature. J Pediatr Endocrinol Metab 2008;21:479–86.

[21] Bryant W, Zimmerman D. Iodine-induced hyperthyroidism in a newborn. Pediatrics 1995;95(3):434–6.

[22] Hasosah M, Alsaleem K, Qurashi M, et al. Neonatal hyperthyroidism with fulminant liver failure: a case report. J Clin Diagn Res 2017;11(4):SD01–2.

[23] Oden J, Cheifetz IM. Neonatal thyrotoxicosis and persistent pulmonary hypertension necessitating extracorporeal life support. Pediatrics 2005;115(1):e105–8.

[24] Fine S, Gottschalk M, Marc-Aurele K. Neonatal Graves disease with persistent hypoglycemia: a case report. SAGE Open Med Case Rep 2024;12; https://doi.org/10.1177/2050313X241237433.

[25] Grob F, Brown A, Zacharin M. Neurodevelopmental follow-up of children born to mothers with Graves' disease and neonatal hyperthyroidism. Horm Res Paediatr 2024; https://doi.org/10.1159/000539268.

[26] Alexander EK, Pearce EN, Brent GA, et al. 2017 guidelines of the American Thyroid Association for the diagnosis and management of thyroid disease during pregnancy and the postpartum. Thyroid 2017;27(3):315–89.

[27] De Groot L, Abalovich M, Alexander EK, et al. Management of thyroid dysfunction during pregnancy and postpartum: an Endocrine Society Clinical Practice Guideline. J Clin Endocrinol Metab 2012;97(8):2543–65.

[28] Ranzini AC, Ananth CV, Smulian JC, et al. Ultrasonography of the fetal thyroid: nomograms based on biparietal diameter and gestational age. J Ultrasound Med 2001;20(6):613–7.

[29] Léger J. Management of fetal and neonatal Graves' disease. Horm Res Paediatr 2017;87(1):1–6.

[30] Dufort G, Larrivée-Vanier S, Eugène D, et al. Wide spectrum of DUOX2 deficiency: from life-threatening compressive goiter in infancy to lifelong euthyroidism. Thyroid 2019;29(7):1018–22.

[31] Shulman DI, Palmert MR, Kemp SF. Adrenal insufficiency: still a cause of morbidity and death in childhood. Pediatrics 2007;119(2); https://doi.org/10.1542/peds.2006-1612.

[32] Langer M, Modi BP, Agus M. Adrenal insufficiency in the critically ill neonate and child. Curr Opin Pediatr 2006;18:448–53.

[33] Rushworth RL, Torpy DJ, Falhammar H. Adrenal crisis. N Engl J Med 2019;381(9):852–61; https://doi.org/10.1056/NEJMra1807486, Ingelfinger JR, editor.

[34] Speiser PW, Arlt W, Auchus RJ, et al. Congenital adrenal hyperplasia due to steroid 21-hydroxylase deficiency: an Endocrine Society Clinical Practice Guideline. J Clin Endocrinol Metab 2018;103(11):4043–88.

[35] Patti G, Guzzeti C, Di Iorgi N, et al. Central adrenal insufficiency in children and adolescents. Best Pract Res Clin Endocrinol Metab 2018;32(4):425–44.

[36] Fleseriu M, Hashim IA, Karavitaki N, et al. Hormonal replacement in hypopituitarism in adults: an Endocrine Society Clinical Practice Guideline. J Clin Endocrinol Metab 2016;101(11):3888–921.

[37] Gao Z, Sun J, Cai C, et al. Pseudohypoaldosteronism type 1b in fraternal twins of a Chinese family: report of two cases and literature review. Arch Endocrinol Metab 2023;67(4); https://doi.org/10.20945/2359-3997000000620.

[38] O'Shaughnessy KM. Gordon syndrome: a continuing story. Pediatr Nephrol 2015;30(11):1903–8.

[39] Moreno SA, García Atarés Á, Molina Herranz D, et al. Secondary pseudohypoaldosteronism: a 15-year experience and a literature review. Pediatr Nephrol 2024;39:3233–9.

Advances in Pediatrics 72 (2025) 171–184

ADVANCES IN PEDIATRICS

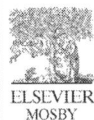

Ethical Issues in Pediatric Endocrinology
A Primer for the Practitioner

Jennifer M. Ladd, MD, MSc, Rohan K. Henry, MD, MS*

Section of Endocrinology & Diabetes, Department of Pediatrics, Nationwide Children's Hospital, The Ohio State University College of Medicine, Columbus, OH, USA

Keywords
• Beneficence • Non-maleficence • Respect for autonomy • Justice

Key points

- Consideration should be given to benefits versus unknown risks, medication coverage, and patient/family autonomy when growth hormone is used to treat idiopathic short stature.
- When providing endocrine care for neurologically devastated children, beneficence, and non-maleficence should be evaluated for this vulnerable population.
- Beyond the applicability of the 4 ethical pillars, endocrine care of transgender youth is highly influenced by political and legal landscapes.
- Although diabetes technologies fulfill the ethical principle of beneficence, access to these technologies is not just.
- With expanding use of glucagon-like peptide 1 receptor agonists, both in terms of indication and age range, principles of non-maleficence and justice must be strongly considered.

Pediatric endocrinology practitioners have witnessed an expansion of care through technological and treatment advancements and through the use of existing therapies to treat new patient populations. In managing clinical conditions with new treatments, or with older therapeutic modalities used for new indications, ethical dilemmas may arise. Another potential driver of ethical dilemmas

*Corresponding author. Section of Endocrinology, Nationwide Children's Hospital, The Ohio State University College of Medicine, 700 Children's Drive, Columbus, OH 43205. E-mail address: rohan.henry@nationwidechildrens.org

https://doi.org/10.1016/j.yapd.2024.12.002

Abbreviations

AAP	American Academy of Pediatrics
AID	automated insulin delivery
BMI	body mass index
CGM	continuous glucose monitor
FDA	Food and Drug Administration
GHD	growth hormone deficiency
GLP-1 RA	glucagon-like peptide 1 receptor agonists
GLP-1	glucagon-like peptide 1
hGH	human growth hormone
ISS	idiopathic short stature
WPATH	World Professional Association for Transgender Health

is the cost of health care, how the cost of a treatment is assigned, and who is responsible for paying this expense [1].

As many clinical situations may generate controversy, it is not feasible to present an exhaustive discourse on the myriad of ethical issues facing pediatric endocrinology practitioners. Hence, the discourse herein will focus on 5 of the more common issues, which may arise during clinical practice: use of growth hormone therapy, care of the neurologically devastated child, non-surgical care of transgender youth, access to diabetes technology, and prescription of GLP-1 receptor agonists.

These dilemmas are each placed in historical context and then approached using the influential ethical framework proposed by Beauchamp and Childress [2]. This framework is based on the 5 ethical pillars of clinical practice: *beneficence, non-maleficence, respect for autonomy,* and *justice.* Table 1 shows the pillars and their significance. Within the health care system, this last pillar also includes *distributive justice,* incorporating fair allocation in the setting of finite or scarce resources.

GROWTH HORMONE THERAPY
To gain an appreciation of the ethical issues, which occur in practice surrounding growth hormone therapy, knowledge of its therapeutic evolution

Table 1
The ethical pillars of Beauchamp and Childress and their significance

Ethical pillar	Significance
Beneficence	Therapeutic benefits should outweigh burdens in order to promote well-being
Non-maleficence	Harmful or ineffective therapies should not be knowingly prescribed
Respect for Autonomy	Freedom of voluntary decision-making, including informed consent or assent
Justice	Treatment equitability regardless of socioeconomic status or other factors

is important. A 1958 article by Dr Raben first chronicled the height gains of a 17-year-old-male with growth hormone deficiency (GHD) treated with human growth hormone (hGH) [3]. At that time, growth hormone was cadaveric in origin, and there was a relative shortage such that only 30 pediatric patients per year were eligible to receive this product [4,5].

In the early 1960s, the National Pituitary Agency and National Cooperative Growth Hormone treatment project were then established, and over a period of 10 years, more than 100 children with GHD were treated [5]. At that time, the imposition of a height cap of 5 feet in the United States ensured that the cadaveric pituitary derived hGH product would be used only to treat the shortest individuals. Subsequently, with rising commercial interest in hGH, the biochemical structure of hGH was elucidated in 1972 [4]. This event catapulted the production of growth hormone by recombinant DNA technology, and in 1981 biosynthetic recombinant hGH was produced. This synthetic production was fortuitous in that 4 adults in North America treated with the cadaveric pituitary derived hGH acquired Creutzfeldt-Jacob disease, leading to the cessation of its use [6,7].

In 1985, the United States' Food and Drug Administration (FDA) approved the use of recombinant hGH. With increasing abundance of hGH, there was an expansion of its use beyond the treatment of disease (eg, for GHD) to becoming a commodity to enhance health in pediatrics [8]. In his thesis, *Growth Hormone: A Paradigm of Expansive Biotechnologies*, the philosopher Alan Buchanan referred to growth hormone as a bio-expansive technology, which *breaks down the conceptual boundaries between treatment and health and between health and other services.* [9] Beyond medical conditions, which are associated with growth failure, hGH has now been approved for idiopathic short stature (ISS) in the United States. This diagnosis of exclusion is made when medical work-up does not yield a definitive cause for short stature, or height under the 2.3rd percentile for sex and age. Initial arguments for treating ISS were based on literature extrapolating psychosocial distress in these patients, from clinic referrals of individuals with other medical conditions coexisting with short stature [10]. However, a more recent systematic review on the impact of short stature (not ISS) on quality-of-life was inconclusive. This review again included some studies in which the presence of short stature was confounded by other diseases [11].

In the United States, an early estimate within the first 10 years after its approval for GHD was that at least a third of the pediatric patients on hGH were treated under the ISS indication [12]. Studies have also shown a male predominance of individuals receiving hGH worldwide, likely related to societal biases regarding heights of males versus females [13–15]. Since August 2021, there has also been FDA approval of long-acting hGH, although not for the ISS indication [16]. Fig. 1 shows the evolution of hGH therapy in the United States.

With the use of hGH for height augmentation in the absence of a true pathologic cause of short stature, the principles of *beneficence* and *non-maleficence* must

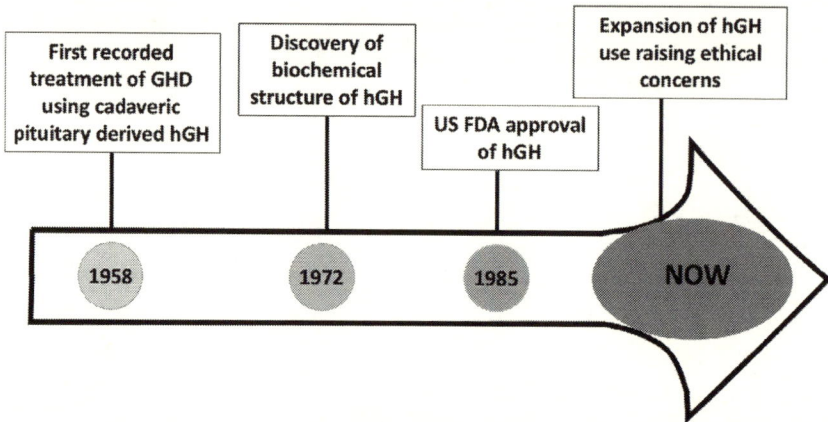

Fig. 1. Evolution of growth hormone use. FDA, Food and Drug Administration; GHD, growth hormone deficiency; hGH, human growth hormone; US, United States.

be considered. While hGH therapy has been shown to be safe overall, in the absence of true pathology, there may be uncertainty regarding supplementation benefits [17]. This uncertainty arises from the inherent weaknesses and limitations of the hGH post-marketing surveillance data acquired by the National Cooperative Growth Study [18]. Limitations of these data include the inability to capture events occurring after treatment has ended, dependence on physician reporting, and an undefined risk to patients who receive hGH without the existence of true pathology [19].

Regarding *respect for autonomy*, in the absence of pathology such as GHD, which requires supplementation to prevent metabolic sequelae, the question of whether a child should be able to provide assent for a therapy, which arguably is not a medical necessity remains unaddressed [1]. From a population statistics viewpoint, the use of hGH for height augmentation should be viewed within the context that in every normal population, some individuals will fall below the 2.3rd percentile [20]. It cannot be argued that all of these individuals should be treated. Flawed arguments in support of ISS treatment can be posited as a guide to perpetuate cosmetic endocrinology in the absence of true pathology [21]. With continued use of hGH under this sphere, there may also be a redefining of heights of the normal population with hGH use as an enhancement.

The principle of *justice* thus comes into play as access to hGH for ISS is inequitable given the differences in insurance coverage and patient/family means [22]. Those most well-off may be able to afford hGH that would not otherwise be covered, at a cost of tens of thousands of dollars per year [23]. Even with insurance coverage, the treatment cost to society needs to be considered, especially during the teenage years where there are diminishing returns from hGH as the cost of treatment per inch of height gain rises [23]. Additionally, access to hGH, including long-acting hGH, may be inequitable even for medical pathologies such as GHD, given the widely varying coverage and copays of different insurance policies.

CARING FOR THE NEUROLOGICALLY DEVASTATED CHILD

This topic was brought to international attention in the early 2000s through the Ashley *Pillow Angel* case. The parents of Ashley, a cognitively and neurologically devastated six-year-old child, voiced concerns about their ability to continue to care for her at home with progression of growth and puberty. As Ashley had a static encephalopathy, she would be dependent on caregivers lifelong. After careful consideration and discussion among the family, physicians, and hospital ethics committee, Ashley underwent a novel case of growth attenuation therapy using high-dose estrogen to fuse growth plates and halt linear growth. At the time when this therapy was proposed, the complete risks were unknown. Hence, prophylactic hysterectomy and appendectomy were performed to decrease the risk of uterine complications and appendicitis, respectively. Ashley also had breast bud removal aimed at preventing breast growth, which the medical team felt was justified, considering the risks imposed by a family history of fibrocystic breast disease and cancer [24,25].

There are arguments both for and against Ashley's treatment, and these may be extended to other pediatric patients with severe neurologic impairment. Regarding the well-being of children with limited capacities, their care should be viewed within the context of the family environment. In Ashley's case, it could be argued that if she could not be managed at home due to increasing physical size, this may cause a disruption in the family's dynamics and lead her to having to be placed outside of a loving home [26]. Therefore, treating Ashley such that she could continue to safely remain at home would fall under *beneficence*, especially given the profundity of her developmental disability and considering that she would always be dependent on her caregivers [27]. In addition, it has been suggested by some scholars that in the context of inability to consent to sexual activities, minimization of physical development of womanhood including hysterectomy could protect Ashley against those who might take advantage, and thus, *non-maleficence* was met [26].

Conversely, Ashley's treatment could be regarded as being done without medical indication, and it has been suggested by others that she was physically harmed without an indication, thus instead a violation of *non-maleficience* [28]. For example, some may argue that as compared to hysterectomy, intrauterine device placement or oral medications would be less drastic, and reversible, for menstrual suppression, and thus the tenet of *do not harm* was not recognized by Ashley's treatment.

In terms of *respect for autonomy*, some may argue that as Ashley did not have the capacity to assent, her rights were violated given that she was not able to fulfill her natural development and preserve her right to be valued and respected [28]. However, given the fact that she would not attain a developmental stage congruent with an adult member of society, and would never be able to attain capacity for decision-making, such arguments may be misinformed

[28]. Some individuals argue that children with profound disabilities lack interests, or the capacity to have those in the future, and thus are incapable of utilizing opportunities presented to them, even if they are physically the size of an adult [25]. On the other hand, it can be argued that Ashley's treatment was performed as a means to fulfill a parental agenda and not as an end herself [29].

Regarding *justice*, factors such as caregivers having the educational background and means to advocate for interventions, which they believe could ease the burden of care, insurance coverage of these interventions, and the possibility that some interventions may not be equitably accessible at all medical centers should be considered.

NON-SURGICAL CARE OF TRANSGENDER YOUTH

Discussion of treatments of pubertal development dovetails into another area of care for the pediatric endocrinology practitioner: medical management of transgender youth. Transgenders or gender diverse individuals include those who identify with a gender different than their assigned sex at birth [30]. These individuals may seek care from pediatric endocrinology practitioners for suppression of puberty (eg, with GnRH agonists), in order to prevent the body from maturing into an adult form incongruent with gender identity, and/or for gender-affirming hormones (eg, estrogen or testosterone), which will allow them to develop physical characteristics more compatible with gender identity. Beyond physical transitions, care for transgender youth often includes attention to psychological and social well-being, with transgender adolescents having increased risks of suicidality and depression [30]. Transgender care has been formally available since the mid-1900s [31], with specialized clinics for adolescents first available in the 1980s [30]. International guidelines for care (eg, through the World Professional Association for Transgender Health [WPATH]) have been available since the late 1990s, with more recent updates [30,32].

Ethical arguments both for and against medical care for transgender youth exist in the literature. Some scholars propose that provision of pubertal suppression and/or gender-affirming hormones meets the principle of *beneficence*, as eligible adolescents have shown persistence of gender incongruence or dysphoria [32] and as longitudinal studies have shown improvement in mental health with endocrine treatment, as well as satisfaction with care [30,33,34]. However, other scholars argue that *non-maleficence* is not met as there may not be a permanence of current gender identity for youth into adulthood and as some hormonal treatments cause irreversible changes (eg, deepening of voice with testosterone) or do not have fully known long-term effects (eg, on fertility) [30,34]. Yet others argue that non-treatment in itself may cause harm, as transgender youth are at higher risk for homelessness, self-harm, depression and anxiety, and they may seek out non-regulated treatments, or may not address underlying mental health concerns such as suicidality, if unable to access medications through health care professionals [34–36].

WPATH guidelines stress the importance of *respect for autonomy* in care of transgender youth [30]. However, beyond the traditional health care mandates of obtaining informed consent/assent, pediatric endocrinology practitioners now need to be acutely aware of rapidly changing and diverse political and legal landscapes. For example, in the United States, numerous states have passed legislation either severely restricting, or outrightly banning, use of pubertal suppression and/or gender-affirming hormones for transgender adolescents [31]. Even in countries where care is not as legally or politically constrained, wait-lists for care in specialized clinics may be several years long [34]. Thus, external circumstances may affect the practitioner's ability to respect autonomy and may also play into considerations of *justice*. A youth's ability to access transgender care in a timely manner, or at all, is dependent on the region in which they happen to live. For example, it is estimated that a quarter of all transgender adolescents in the United States now live more than a day's drive away from a gender clinic [31]. Inequities are also inherently raised by this landscape, in terms of transportation, ability to miss school/work, and ability to pay (eg, if out-of-state clinics are not covered by insurance). As political and legal situations continue to evolve, it behooves practitioners to become aware of their local context in which they are applying ethical principles to the delivery of care to this vulnerable population.

DIABETES TECHNOLOGY

Management of diabetes was revolutionized with the discovery of insulin over 100 years ago by the surgeon Dr Frederick Banting and his medical student Charles Best [37]. Insulin was initially delivered subcutaneously via syringe and needles, and later by pen devices, requiring multiple daily injections [38]. Blood glucose was able to be measured intermittently by fingerstick.

Technology use, including continuous glucose monitors (CGMs) and insulin pumps, are now standard-of-care for treatment of pediatric patients with diabetes [39,40]. CGMs are wearable devices, which provide continuous measurements of interstitial glucose (approximations of blood glucose) and thus more information and dynamic trends than static fingerstick blood glucoses alone can provide. Insulin pumps are another wearable technology, which deliver small doses of subcutaneous insulin continuously with the ability to more precisely titrate dosing than with multiple daily injections. Over recent years, CGMs and insulin pumps have been integrated into hybrid closed loop systems or automated insulin delivery (AID) systems [37]. These AID systems have now received FDA approval for management of type 1 diabetes in pediatric patients, and AID systems have additional benefits for both glycemic management and safety in that the system algorithm can automatically increase or suspend insulin based on predictive glucose trends [41].

The ethical arguments for use of these devices are clear from the literature. *Beneficence* is met in that these devices have been shown to improve diabetes care by decreasing hemoglobin A1c and glucose variability [39,40,42]. These devices have also been shown to improve quality of life [43]. For example, parents of young children with type 1 diabetes have reported decreased fear of hypoglycemia and improvement of sleep when using these devices [44,45]. *Nonmaleficence* is met in that these devices in and of themselves do not cause harm. While there may be risks of bleeding and infection at insertion sites, most would consider these risks minimal especially in the context of the aforementioned benefits.

While these devices are recommended as standard-of-care by many providers, as well as by international guidelines (eg, those by the International Society for Pediatric and Adolescent Diabetes), clinicians are ethically bound to respect patient *autonomy* [39,40]. Not all families and patients may opt for use of these devices, for varying reasons such as personal preferences, increased burden of device management, or cost [46]. For example, patients who have developmental delays or behavioral issues such as skin picking may have difficulties wearing these devices. Cost may also be a prohibitive factor in some countries. In fact, the distribution and availability of these devices have been shown repeatedly in the literature to be *unjust*. Studies from nations with differing health care systems have found significant socioeconomic disparities in uptake and use of diabetes technology. For example, a large population-based database study from the United States and Germany showed that those in the most deprived quintiles had lower use of these technologies [47]. Even in countries with universal health care such as Canada, disparities in uptake of pumps and use of CGM have been shown in terms of both material and social deprivation [48,49]. Thus, the drivers of these inequities must be more than monetary and may be related to other explicit or implicit prescribing biases [50]. For example, studies have shown disparities in technology use in terms of race/ethnicity, as well as education level [51,52]. Programs have been successful in increasing access to technology at new onset of type 1 diabetes in pediatrics [53], but more work needs to be done in maintaining this access and ensuring all groups benefit equitably from this technology.

GLUCAGON-LIKE PEPTIDE 1 RECEPTOR AGONISTS

Glucagon-like peptide 1 (GLP-1) is an incretin hormone produced by the intestine to help enhance insulin secretion, delay gastric emptying, reduce appetite, and improve satiety. A newer class of therapeutics, GLP-1 receptor agonists (GLP-1 RAs), has been developed to utilize these effects to improve glycemic management in diabetes in both adults and children [54]. The FDA has since approved use of injectable GLP-1 RAs for children aged 10 years and older with type 2 diabetes.

Similar to growth hormone therapy, the uses of GLP-1 RAs have rapidly expanded, moving from treatment of type 2 diabetes to weight management. While the prevalence of type 2 diabetes is growing with 1 multicenter study in the United States showing an increase from 0.34 per 1000 youth in 2001 to 0.67 per 1000 youth in 2017 [55], the prevalence of obesity is many, many fold higher with recent global estimates of 8.5% of all children and adolescents [56].

Thus, there is now a huge potential patient population for these medications. Currently, injectable GLP-1 RAs are now FDA-approved for obesity in children aged 12 years and older [57]. However, there are ongoing clinical studies, including 1 recently published [58], showing safety and efficacy of GLP-1 RAs in decreasing body mass index (BMI) in children as young as 6 years old. Notably, ages five to 7 years is the historical timing of the adiposity rebound (when BMI begins to increase from the physiologic nadir), but studies have shown that even earlier adiposity rebound is associated with adolescent obesity, controlling for confounders such as birth weight, puberty, and socioeconomic factors [59]. Thus, there could be future justification for testing or use of GLP-1 RAs in even younger populations. Fig. 2 shows the evolution GLP-RAs in the United States.

The FDA approval of GLP-1 RAs for adolescent obesity and the potential for approval of GLP-1 RAs in younger age groups in the near future bring up dilemmas for practitioners. It may be argued that the administration of GLP-1 RAs to children as young as 6 years for obesity adheres to *beneficence* as weight reduction may decrease risk of metabolic complications such as hypertension and type 2 diabetes, as well as may decrease joint pain, increase mobility, and promote physical activity. Not all children who have a BMI higher than the 95th percentile for age will develop these complications, yet obesity alone may be considered a chronic disease [60]. However, with limited long-term experience with this class of drugs in children, it is not clear that *non-maleficence* is met given the unknown effects of these drugs several decades later [57]. If GLP-1 RAs are stopped after starting, weight previously lost is often regained [57], thus necessitating continuation of these medications long-term for continued benefit. There is the added concern of pathologizing weight in a society, which already promotes thinness as the ideal

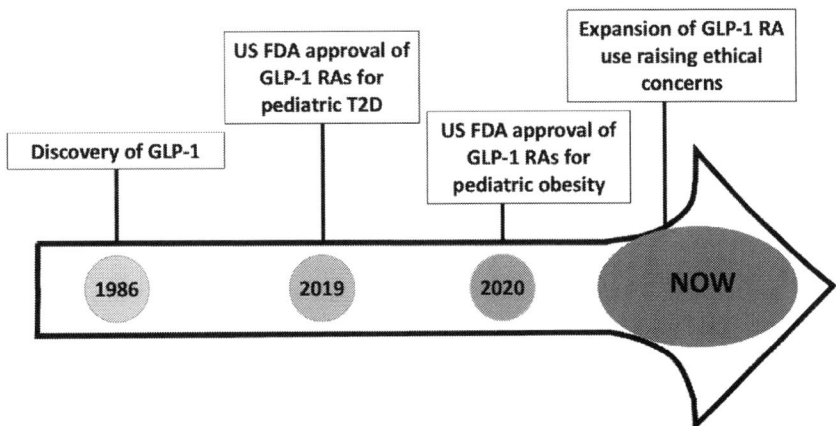

Fig. 2. Evolution of GLP-1 receptor agonist use. FDA, Food and Drug Administration; GLP-1, glucagon-like peptide 1; GLP-1 RAs, GLP-1 receptor agonists; US, United States.

through social media and other avenues; studies have even shown weight stigma is prevalent in children's movies [61]. Moreover, pediatric primary care providers and endocrinology practitioners may be approached by patients and families asking for medication without access to a comprehensive weight management program. Reliance on medication alone rather than simultaneous promotion of healthy active lifestyle habits and involvement of registered dieticians, physical therapists, and psychologists is contradictory to the 2023 American Academy of Pediatrics (AAP) expert guidelines. In fact, the guidelines are 100 pages, the majority of which are dedicated to comprehensive obesity treatment including healthy active lifestyle, with only a few pages on pharmacologic treatment including GLP-1 RAs [60]. Thus, a focus on development of healthy dietary habits (which are often at the root of obesity) should not be overlooked [62]. Regarding *respect for autonomy*, the 2023 AAP guidelines also highlight the need for shared decision-making amongst patients, their families, and their medical teams in terms of which treatment avenues to pursue [60].

In terms of *justice*, current access to GLP-1 RAs is inequitable given differing insurance coverage, high costs, and decreased availability. A fair allocation framework, including reduction of harm and maximizing benefit to those most disadvantaged, has been proposed in the literature to govern use of GLP-1 RAs in the setting of scarcity [63]. This framework could be used to argue for prioritization of GLP-1 RAs in adolescents with obesity (rather than in older adults) given the potential to reduce premature harm (eg, development of early cardiovascular morbidity), prevent premature mortality, and have more benefit over more potential years of life. Additionally, obesity disproportionately occurs in those adversely affected by social determinants of health such as poverty and lack of a safe built environment in which to exercise or access healthy foods [60]. Application of a fair allocation framework could promote justice by preferentially creating access to GLP-1 RAs in those least well-off. However, a recent simulated economic analysis showed that after taking into account both expense and effectiveness in the pediatric population, oral phentermine-topiramate was a more cost-effective option than were GLP-1 RAs in adolescents for weight management [64], and thus it may be prudent to consider other pharmacologic alternatives in pediatric obesity.

SUMMARY

The 5 areas of care broadly discussed herein raise ethical dilemmas for the pediatric endocrinology practitioner. The rapid expansion of technologies and treatments, and utilization of these in new populations, may raise concerns. By understanding the 4 pillars of Beauchamp and Childress, providers can recognize ethical issues in clinical situations seen in practice. Application of the principles of *beneficence, non-maleficence, respect for autonomy,* and *justice* can allow clinicians to make ethically sound treatment decisions in conjunction with patients and their families.

CLINICS CARE POINTS

- Based on the use of medications such as growth hormone and glucagon-like peptide 1 receptor agonists, beyond their original indications of treating growth hormone deficiency and type 2 diabetes, respectively, clinicians should be cognizant of the potential ethical dilemmas which may arise when delivering care.
- During the medical management involving the delivery of care to the neurologically devastated child, the caregivers desires should carefully weighed with the clinician's responsibility to protect this vulnerable patient population from harm.
- When applying ethical principles to the non-surgical management of the transgender patient, it is imperative that clinicians be aware of prevailing political and legal constraints which may affect the delivery of care.
- With technological advances being at the forefront in the delivery of care to pediatric patients with diabetes, clinicians should endeavor to ensure that patients from a variety of backgrounds have access to, and will benefit equitably from technology.

Disclosure

The authors have no disclosures.

References

[1] Lo B. Resolving ethical dilemmas A guide for clinicians. 6th edition. Philadelphia: Lippincott Williams and Wilkins; 2020.

[2] Zwitter M. Medical ethics in clinical practice, Springer nature; Switzerland. 2019. Available at: https://link.springer.com/book/10.1007/978-3-030-00719-5k (Accessed 7 June 2024).

[3] Raben MS. Treatment of a pituitary dwarf with human growth hormone. J Clin Endocrinol Metab 1958;18(8):901–3.

[4] Frasier SD. The not-so-good old days: working with pituitary growth hormone in North America, 1956 to 1985. J Pediatr 1997;131(1 Pt 2):S1–4.

[5] Blizzard RM. History of growth hormone therapy. Indian J Pediatr 2012;79(1):87–91.

[6] Degenerative neurologic disease in patients formerly treated with human growth hormone. Report of the committee on growth hormone use of the Lawson Wilkins pediatric endocrine society, may 1985. J Pediatr 1985;107(1):10–2.

[7] Dean HJ, Friesen HG. Growth hormone therapy in Canada: end of one era and beginning of another. CMAJ (Can Med Assoc J) 1986;135(4):297–301.

[8] Meideros A. Heightened expectations: the rise of the human growth hormone industry in America. 2nd edition. Tuscaloosa: University of Alabama Press; 2016.

[9] Buchanan A. Growth hormone: a paradigm of expansive biotechnologies. Endocrinololgist 2001;11(4):78s–+.

[10] Sandberg DE, Voss LD. The psychosocial consequences of short stature: a review of the evidence. Best Pract Res Clin Endocrinol Metab 2002;16(3):449–63.

[11] Backeljauw P, Cappa M, Kiess W, et al. Impact of short stature on quality of life: a systematic literature review. Growth Horm IGF Res 2021;57-58:101392.

[12] Vance ML, Mauras N. Growth hormone therapy in adults and children. N Engl J Med 1999;341(16):1206–16.

[13] Grimberg A, Feemster KA, Pati S, et al. Medically underserved girls receive less evaluation for short stature. Pediatrics 2011;127(4):696–702.

[14] Grimberg A, Kutikov JK, Cucchiara AJ. Sex differences in patients referred for evaluation of poor growth. J Pediatr 2005;146(2):212–6.

[15] Tanaka T, Soneda S, Sato N, et al. The boy:Girl ratio of children diagnosed with growth hormone deficiency-induced short stature is associated with the boy:Girl ratio of children visiting short stature clinics. Horm Res Paediatr 2021;94(5–6):211–8.

[16] Miller BS. What do we do now that the long-acting growth hormone is here? Front Endocrinol 2022;13:980979.

[17] Bell J, Parker KL, Swinford RD, et al. Long-term safety of recombinant human growth hormone in children. J Clin Endocrinol Metab 2010;95(1):167–77.

[18] Stochholm K, Kiess W. Long-term safety of growth hormone-A combined registry analysis. Clin Endocrinol 2018;88(4):515–28.

[19] Allen DB. Growth hormone post-marketing surveillance: safety, sales, and the unfinished task ahead. J Clin Endocrinol Metab 2010;95(1):52–5.

[20] Daniels N. Normal functioning and the treatment-enhancement distinction. Camb Q Healthc Ethics 2000;9(3):309–22.

[21] Allen DB. Growth promotion ethics and the challenge to resist cosmetic endocrinology. Horm Res Paediatr 2017;87(3):145–52.

[22] Daniels N. Justice, health, and healthcare. Am J Bioeth 2001;1(2):2–16.

[23] Allen DB, Fost N. hGH for short stature: ethical issues raised by expanded access. J Pediatr 2004;144(5):648–52.

[24] Gunther DF, Diekema DS. Attenuating growth in children with profound developmental disability: a new approach to an old dilemma. Arch Pediatr Adolesc Med 2006;160(10): 1013–7.

[25] Tan N, Brassington I. Agency, duties and the "Ashley treatment". J Med Ethics 2009;35(11): 658–61.

[26] Ashley GG. Two born as one, and the best interests of a child. Camb Q Healthc Ethics 2016;25(1):22–37.

[27] EB S. Making someone child-sized forever? Ethical considerations in inhibiting the growth of a developmentally disabled child. Clin Ethics 2007;2(1):46–9.

[28] Diekema DS, Fost N. Ashley revisited: a response to the critics. Am J Bioeth 2010;10(1): 30–44.

[29] Edwards SD. The Ashley treatment: a step too far, or not far enough? J Med Ethics 2008;34(5):341–3.

[30] Coleman E, Radix AE, Bouman WP, et al. Standards of care for the health of transgender and gender diverse people, version 8. Int J Transgend Health 2022;23(Suppl 1):S1–259.

[31] McNamara M, Gentry KR, Sequeira GM, et al. State-level bans on the care of transgender and gender diverse youth in the United States: implications for ethics and advocacy. J Pediatr 2024;274:114182.

[32] Hembree WC, Cohen-Kettenis PT, Gooren L, et al. Endocrine treatment of gender-dysphoric/gender-incongruent persons: an endocrine society clinical practice guideline. J Clin Endocrinol Metab 2017;102(11):3869–903.

[33] Achille C, Taggart T, Eaton NR, et al. Longitudinal impact of gender-affirming endocrine intervention on the mental health and well-being of transgender youths: preliminary results. Int J Pediatr Endocrinol 2020;2020:8.

[34] Maung HH. Gender affirming hormone treatment for trans adolescents: a four principles analysis. J bioeth Inq 2024;21(2):345–63.

[35] Kimberly LL, Folkers KM, Friesen P, et al. Ethical issues in gender-affirming care for youth. Pediatrics 2018;142(6):e20181537.

[36] Tordoff DM, Wanta JW, Collin A, et al. Mental health outcomes in transgender and nonbinary youths receiving gender-affirming care. JAMA Netw Open 2022;5(2):e220978.

[37] Sims EK, Carr AlJ, Oram RA, et al. 100 years of insulin: celebrating the past, present and future of diabetes therapy. Nat Med 2021;27(7):1154–64.

[38] Home P. The evolution of insulin therapy. Diabetes Res Clin Pract 2021;175:108816.

[39] Sherr JL, Schoelwer M, Dos Santos TJ, et al. ISPAD clinical practice consensus guidelines 2022: diabetes technologies: insulin delivery. Pediatr Diabetes 2022;23(8):1406–31.

[40] Tauschmann M, Forlenza G, Hood K, et al. ISPAD clinical practice consensus guidelines 2022: diabetes technologies: glucose monitoring. Pediatr Diabetes 2022;23(8):1390–405.

[41] Phillip M, Nimri R, Bergenstal RM, et al. Consensus recommendations for the use of automated insulin delivery technologies in clinical practice. Endocr Rev 2023;44(2):254–80.

[42] Laffel LM, Kanapka LG, Beck RW, et al. Effect of continuous glucose monitoring on glycemic control in adolescents and young adults with type 1 diabetes: a randomized clinical trial. JAMA 2020;323(23):2388–96.

[43] Speight J, Choudhary P, Wilmot EG, et al. Impact of glycaemic technologies on quality of life and related outcomes in adults with type 1 diabetes: a narrative review. Diabet Med 2023;40(1):e14944.

[44] Hilliard ME, Levy W, Anderson BJ, et al. Benefits and barriers of continuous glucose monitoring in young children with type 1 diabetes. Diabetes Technol Ther 2019;21(9):493–8.

[45] Verbeeten KC, Perez Trejo ME, Tang K, et al. Fear of hypoglycemia in children with type 1 diabetes and their parents: effect of pump therapy and continuous glucose monitoring with option of low glucose suspend in the CGM TIME trial. Pediatr Diabetes 2021;22(2):288–93.

[46] Messer LH, Johnson R, Driscoll KA, et al. Best friend or spy: a qualitative meta-synthesis on the impact of continuous glucose monitoring on life with Type 1 diabetes. Diabet Med 2018;35(4):409–18.

[47] Addala A, Auzanneau M, Miller K, et al. A decade of disparities in diabetes technology use and HbA(1c) in pediatric type 1 diabetes: a transatlantic comparison. Diabetes Care 2021;44(1):133–40.

[48] Ladd JM, Sharma A, Rahme E, et al. Comparison of socioeconomic disparities in pump uptake among children with type 1 diabetes in 2 Canadian provinces with different payment models. JAMA Netw Open 2022;5(5):e2210464.

[49] Stanley JR, Clarke ABM, Shulman R, et al. Mediating effects of technology-based therapy on the relationship between socioeconomic status and glycemic management in pediatric type 1 diabetes. Diabetes Technol Ther 2023;25(3):186–93.

[50] Odugbesan O, Addala A, Nelson G, et al. Implicit racial-ethnic and insurance-mediated bias to recommending diabetes technology: insights from T1D exchange multicenter pediatric and adult diabetes provider cohort. Diabetes Technol Ther 2022;24(9):619–27.

[51] Lai CW, Lipman TH, Willi SM, et al. Racial and ethnic disparities in rates of continuous glucose monitor initiation and continued use in children with type 1 diabetes. Diabetes Care 2021;44(1):255–7.

[52] Mönkemöller K, Müller-Godeffroy E, Lilienthal E, et al. The association between socioeconomic status and diabetes care and outcome in children with diabetes type 1 in Germany: the DIAS study (diabetes and social disparities). Pediatr Diabetes 2019;20(5):637–44.

[53] Prahalad P, Ding VY, Zaharieva DP, et al. Teamwork, targets, technology, and tight control in newly diagnosed type 1 diabetes: the pilot 4T study. J Clin Endocrinol Metab 2022;107(4):998–1008.

[54] Holst JJ. From the incretin concept and the discovery of GLP-1 to today's diabetes therapy. Front Endocrinol 2019;10:260.

[55] Lawrence JM, Divers J, Isom S, et al. Trends in prevalence of type 1 and type 2 diabetes in children and adolescents in the US, 2001-2017. JAMA 2021;326(8):717–27.

[56] Zhang X, Liu J, Ni Y, et al. Global prevalence of overweight and obesity in children and adolescents: a systematic review and meta-analysis. JAMA Pediatr 2024;178(8):800–13.

[57] Torbahn G, Lischka J, Brown T, et al. Anti-obesity medication in the management of children and adolescents with obesity: recent developments and research Gaps. Clin Endocrinol 2024;102(1):51–61.

[58] Fox CK, Barrientos-Pérez M, Bomberg EM, et al. Liraglutide for children 6 to <12 Years of age with obesity - a randomized trial. N Engl J Med 2024; https://doi.org/10.1056/NEJMoa2407379.

[59] Hughes AR, Sherriff A, Ness AR, et al. Timing of adiposity rebound and adiposity in adolescence. Pediatrics 2014;134(5):e1354–61.
[60] Hampl SE, Hassink SG, Skinner AC, et al. Clinical practice guideline for the evaluation and treatment of children and adolescents with obesity. Pediatrics 2023;151(2):e2022060640.
[61] Howard JB, Skinner AC, Ravanbakht SN, et al. Obesogenic behavior and weight-based stigma in popular children's movies, 2012 to 2015. Pediatrics 2017;140(6):e20172126.
[62] Ludwig DS, Holst JJ. Childhood obesity at the crossroads of science and social justice. JAMA 2023;329(22):1909–10.
[63] Emanuel EJ, Dellgren JL, McCoy MS, et al. Fair allocation of GLP-1 and dual GLP-1-GIP receptor agonists. N Engl J Med 2024;390(20):1839–42.
[64] Mital S, Nguyen HV. Cost-effectiveness of antiobesity drugs for adolescents with severe obesity. JAMA Netw Open 2023;6(10):e2336400.

Advances in Pediatrics 72 (2025) 185–195

ADVANCES IN PEDIATRICS

ELSEVIER
MOSBY

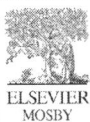

Artificial Intelligence in Pediatric Endocrinology

Sabitha Sasidharan Pillai, MD[a,b,*],
Ambika P. Ashraf, MD, FNLA[c]

[a]Department of Pediatrics, Keck School of Medicine, University of Southern California, Los Angeles, CA, USA; [b]Center for Endocrinology, Diabetes and Metabolism, Children's Hospital, 4650 W Sunset Boulevard, Los Angeles, CA 90027, USA; [c]Department of Pediatrics, University of Alabama, Lowder Building 1600 7th Avenue South, Birmingham, AL 35233-1771, USA

Keywords
- Artificial intelligence • Machine learning • Diabetes • Bone age

Key points
- Artificial intelligence (AI) models using deep learning can enhance diagnostic performance, particularly when paired with human expertise, for example, accuracy in bone age assessments.
- AI-driven hybrid closed-loop insulin delivery systems significantly improve glycemic control in diabetic patients.
- Facial recognition AI demonstrates potential for diagnosing Turner syndrome, Cushing syndrome, acromegaly, and congenital adrenal hyperplasia (CAH) with high accuracy.
- AI algorithms can identify endocrine tumors and assess thyroid nodule malignancy, improving sensitivity in pediatric cases.
- AI chatbots outperform physicians in empathetic and high-quality responses in simulated patient interactions.

INTRODUCTION

The rapid technological progress over the last couple of decades has paved the way for innovative methods capable of solving scientific questions at a rate far exceeding human capabilities. One prime example is the field of artificial intelligence (AI) [1]. The term AI was coined by John McCarthy, an American computer and cognitive scientist, in 1955, and defined it as "the science and engineering of making machines that are smart." AI systems use data to learn

*Corresponding author. Center for Endocrinology, Diabetes and Metabolism, Children's Hospital Los Angeles, Los Angeles, CA. E-mail address: ssasidharanpillai@chla.usc.edu

https://doi.org/10.1016/j.yapd.2024.12.003

and improve, identifying patterns and relationships that humans might miss and perform tasks that are usually associated with human intelligence [2]. AI comprises several technologies, such as machine learning (ML), deep learning (DL), natural language processing, robotics, speech processing, and other automation technologies [3]. AI, with its significant potential, has found its place in both medical care and clinical research. AI and ML are valuable tools in advancing the field for pediatric endocrinology.

Physical and virtual components are the 2 forms of AI application. Examples of physical applications of AI include robot-assisted surgery of adrenal cancers while examples of virtual applications of AI include electronic medical records (EMRs), where specific algorithms are used to identify subjects, and mobilize health-related data [1]. ML encompasses a group of technologies that learn from a set of examples on how to perform a task, creating a model which capsulizes the knowledge to execute the task. Then, when new data are assigned, the model is able to correctly perform the learned task within an acceptable accuracy [4]. DL is a form of representation learning which is made of multiple layers of representations. When raw data are imputed, a machine creates its own representations needed for pattern recognition. As data pass through the layers of the system, the input space becomes repetitively distorted until data points become distinguishable. In this way, highly complex functions can be learned [5]. AI technology can have marked influence at the level of physicians, by enhancing the diagnostic accuracy and facilitating therapeutic and surgical interventions, at the level of health systems, by promoting better workflow and reducing errors and at the patient level, through personalized diagnostic and treatment approaches based on the unique phenotypic and genetic features of individual patients [1]. In this article, we focus on the use of AI applications in the field of pediatric endocrinology and limitations or concerns associated with its use.

ARTIFICIAL INTELLIGENCE IN DIAGNOSIS

AI technology has attained physician-level accuracy at a broad variety of diagnostic tasks. AI technology has been applied across a broad variety of medical scans, including bone films for fractures and bone age (BA) estimation [6].

Bone age assessment

BA radiography of the nondominant hand is used to assess the skeletal maturity in children with endocrine disorders. The patient's BA is determined by comparing his left hand and wrist X ray image with a reference standard image from the Greulich-Pyle atlas and reported as advanced, normal, and delayed skeletal maturity [7]. However, manual estimation of BA is subject to inter-rater and intra-rater variability and may be affected by ethnicity, region, economic status, and nutrition [4]. Recently, several innovative approaches, based on DL, have been utilized for BA assessment. A systematic review and meta-analysis that analyzed the research related to BA assessment studies which utilized ML techniques was reported in 26 studies. Many of these studies suggested automated systems for BA assessment and examined methods for BA estimation based on hand and wrist radiographs. The data of origin in these studies were mostly from the United States and West Europe. Few studies investigated ethnic differences and socioeconomic but other aspects that could influence BA were not addressed [4,8]. Thodberg and colleagues proposed a BA assessment system in 2009 that is in commercial use–the BoneXpert, which studied BA assessment using samples from Japanese, Dutch, and American subjects of 4 ethnicities (African American, Asian, Caucasian, and Hispanic) [9,10].

A study comparing the BA assessment performance of 6 pediatric radiologists with and without an AI model that was developed based on ML and deep neural networks demonstrated that use of AI model by radiologists improved performance by increasing accuracy and decreasing variability compared with AI alone, a radiologist alone, or a pooled cohort of experts [8,11]. Another study observed significant disagreement between AI and human clinical determinations of BA. This study from China evaluated the effects of data site differences, interpretation bias, and interobserver variability on BA assessment of 3 AI models developed using DL methods: the USA model, the China model, and a joint model combining the USA and China data set in assessing BA. The authors evaluated the AI models' and radiologists' clinical determinations of BA and studied the results of internal and external validation to analyze AI performance: the internal validation being the training and test datasets from the same institution and external validation being the training and test datasets from the 2 separate institutions. This study observed that performance of AI was better with internal validation than with external validation. Heatmaps of the hand generated using the gradient weighted class activation mapping (Grad-CAM) method demonstrated that AI heatmaps were not fully consistent with human focusing areas based on the Greulich-Pyle atlas. The authors proposed that variable performance in BA estimation by different AI models and the disagreement between AI and radiologists' clinical determinations of BA may be due to data biases, including patients' sex and age, institutions, and radiologists [7].

Diabetes retinopathy screening

Enhanced image classification systems through AI technology have eased diabetes retinopathy detection. A meta-analysis of 60 studies suggested high diagnostic accuracy of ML algorithms in diabetes retinopathy screening. US Food and Drug Administration (FDA) approved the first AI device in 2018 that provides screening decisions for diabetic retinopathy without the clinician's assisted interpretation [12]. This was the first system in any field of medicine to receive FDA approval for an autonomous AI. Another AI diagnostic system received FDA clearance for autonomous diagnosis of diabetic retinopathy in 2020 [13]. The SEE study from the United States that involved 310 youth with diabetes aged 5 to 21 years observed that the implementation of a non-mydriatic fundus camera with an autonomous AI system for the detection of diabetic retinopathy in a multidisciplinary pediatric diabetes center was safe and effective for diabetic eye screening and improved the adherence to screening recommendations [14]. However, recent data suggest poorer performance of these algorithms in real-world settings. Researchers have also raised concerns due to lack of detail in grading as well as explanation of how the algorithm determined the grading [13].

Prediction of diabetic foot ulcers
Recently, AI algorithm has been developed to predict the risk for diabetic foot ulcers. It used 6 risk factors that incorporated both physical and demographic parameters: cellulitis, Charcot joint, peripheral arterial disease, uncontrolled diabetes mellitus, peripheral vascular disease, and male gender to predict the likelihood of developing diabetic foot ulcers with 80% accuracy [15].

Predicting obesity-associated disorders
ML algorithms can build models to make correct disease predictions. Researchers from China observed that logistic regression model developed using ML could be used as a screening tool to predict metabolic dysfunction associated steatotic liver disease (MASLD) among school children with overweight and obesity [16]. Researches from India developed an ML model, XGB model to screen for prediabetes among youth aged 5 to 19 years in the community setting. The clinical and anthropometric measurements such as triceps skin fold thickness, mid upper arm circumference, waist circumference, age, and height determined the model accuracy. The authors reported about 90% 10-fold cross-validation accuracy without considering any biomarkers for the XGB model in the initial screening of prediabetes [17].

Predicting adult height
Another study that assessed ML algorithms to predict adult height based on growth parameters until age 6 years observed that the model random forest with 51 regression trees generated the most precise predictions. Observed and predicted adult height were 173.9 ± 8.9 cm and 173.9 ± 7.7 cm, respectively, with prediction average error of −0.4 ± 4.0 cm that resulted in over or underestimation of adult height for short and tall subjects, respectively [18].

Diagnosis of diabetes insipidus
A study from Switzerland observed that ML-based algorithm eased the differentiation between arginine vasopressin deficiency and primary polydipsia with

high accuracy even when only clinical information and laboratory data were available avoiding the need for hypertonic saline infusion test [19].

Diagnosis of genetic conditions

AI technology has been used to identify genetic conditions using automated facial recognition technology based on deep learning. The facial diagnostic system for Turner syndrome developed using deep convolutional neural networks demonstrated high accuracy in real clinical setting suggesting its potential role in the screening of Turner syndrome [20]. Similarly another study reported a multiple facial feature extraction and processing method for computer-aided diagnosis of Turner syndrome that could facilitate large-scale screening in underdeveloped areas enabling early detection and treatment [21].

Diagnosis of endocrine conditions

Automated facial recognition technology has also been utilized to detect certain endocrine conditions. A model developed using pretrained deep-learning network to identify Cushing syndrome and acromegaly based on distinguishing facial changes demonstrated an accuracy of 0.96 and 0.95 and recalls of 0.8 each respectively and outperformed endocrine experts [22]. Another study observed that facial morphologic features in patients with congenital adrenal hyperplasia (CAH) are distinct and that DL can identify subtle facial features to predict CAH [23].

ARTIFICIAL INTELLIGENCE IN TREATMENT PLANNING AND DECISION MAKING

In the field of clinical decision making, AI has exhibited marked capabilities for predicting and classifying diagnoses, as well as providing recommendations and insights. Current literature proposes that knowledge-based computerized decision support, and knowledge-based clinical decision support systems have the capability to augment doctor performance. By assisting health care professionals in diagnosing diseases, deciding most appropriate treatment, and predicting outcomes, AI improves the quality and efficiency of health care decision making, as well as the contentment and involvement of users [3]. Advances in AI-based decision support systems are gaining more attention as technological tools to support personalized health care in many fields of medicine. An exciting field is exploration of AI's potential in early-stage disease prediction through wearable devices.

Insulin delivery systems

AI is a rapidly advancing field for endocrinology and has already been made use of in the treatment of diabetes [24]. The introduction of closed loop systems (artificial pancreas or automated insulin delivery systems) revolutionized the care of patients with diabetes with marked improvement in time in range [25]. Hybrid closed-loop automated insulin delivery systems, pairing continuous blood glucose monitoring with an insulin infusion device, illustrate one of the most noteworthy AI developments in the field of endocrinology. Initial trials of fully automated closed loop control system with automatic prandial dosing that did not require meal announcements have been reported to be very safe and feasible among adolescents [26]. AI algorithms have also been utilized in the management of diabetic foot ulcers. Advanced ML algorithms can detect, localize, and segment diabetic foot ulcers in images [13].

Precision medicine

AI algorithms have been widely utilized to evaluate pediatric obesity, both for recognizing different intervention goals and for speculating future weight outcomes. AI may help detect patients at risk for obesity and obesity-associated comorbidities using predictor variables such as sex, age, height, weight, body mass index (BMI), exclusive breast feeding, parental education, parental BMI, maternal smoking, home environment, diet variables, physical activity. AI algorithms considering parameters such as genetic profile, family history, medical history, environmental and behavioral background, and laboratory evaluation may help predict the best treatment plan for patients with obesity, thereby helping health care providers to provide personalized care and improve outcome [27–30]. AI models can also predict success of antiobesity therapies among youth. A study from Switzerland used different ML methods to predict success of 6 month weight loss therapy defined as BMI after therapy less than 0.4 BMI units than before among a small cohort of 20 children aged 11 to 16 years with overweight or obesity. The predictors used were heart rate at several intervals during a run test and a cooldown period, weight, age, BMI, and height. The researchers reported that the best model had an accuracy of 85%, and the ML models outperformed the prediction of 2 domain experts [31].

Evaluation and management of childhood thyroid nodules

The risk of being malignant is higher in childhood thyroid nodules compared with adult onset disease (22%–26% vs 5%–10% in adults) and fine needle aspiration is warranted in those with size greater than 1 cm or abnormal ultrasound features (hypoechogenicity, irregular margins, microcalcification, increased vascularity, and lymph node involvement) and clinical characteristics (history of radiation therapy, familial differentiated thyroid cancer (DTC) or hereditary tumor syndromes associated with DTC such as adenomatous polyposis coli (APC)-associated polyposis, DICER1 syndrome, Carney complex) irrespective of the nodule size [32]. The American College of Radiology - Thyroid Imaging Reporting and Data System (ACR TI-RADS) has been comprehensively studied in adults and is usually considered to be deficient in adequate sensitivity to be applied in children. Ultrasound findings of thyroid nodules in children are generally interpreted as per the radiologist's overall impression [33]. AI models have been utilized in the evaluation of thyroid nodules in adults [34]. A study from China reported higher sensitivity albeit lower specificity for both ACR TI-RADS and the DL algorithm in differentiating benign and malignant thyroid nodules on ultrasound in children and young adults compared with diagnostic performance of radiologists [33]. Through improvement in diagnostic performance, AI models may help reduce unnecessary fine needle aspiration for thyroid nodules.

Assistive tools in patient communication and care
A cross-sectional study that assessed the ability of an AI chatbot assistant (ChatGPT), to provide quality and empathetic responses to patient questions posed in an online forum compared with physician responses demonstrated that chatbot responses were of significantly higher quality and empathetic than physician responses and had higher prevalence of good or very good quality responses compared with physician responses. Future studies should analyze this technology in clinical settings and assess the use of AI assistant to improve responses, reduce provider burnout, and improve patient outcomes [35].

Research and data management
Finally, research in endocrinology may be immensely hastened by AI. Collection of clinical information can now be assisted by machines, thereby optimizing collection time and data structure. AI technology can help identify a cohort of patients with a particular condition from EMR. A pilot study from China that utilized semiautomated framework based on ML to liberalize filtering criteria to improve recall rate and minimize false positive rate for identifying patients with type 2 diabetes from EMR achieved higher identification performances compared with the state-of-the-art algorithm [36].

LIMITATIONS
AI promotes personalized health care by consolidating data from "omics" analysis, lifestyle tracking, medical records, laboratory and imaging, treatment response, and adherence from multiple sources. As data gathering and processing becomes basic, data privacy and protecting children's health data are important. AI intensifies existing cyber-security risks, undoubtedly threatening patient privacy and confidentiality. Susceptibility to adversarial attack or manipulation is a potential danger where planned hacking of an algorithm may harm people at a large scale, such as overdosing of insulin in those with diabetes [6,37]. Another concern is the increasing recognition of biases in AI algorithms. Even a hypothetical fair AI predictive model that is free of biases, implemented within the EMR, adaptive, nonautonomous, and operating in a decision support manner may have latent biases (biases that are waiting to happen) directly or indirectly. These latent biases need to be addressed urgently before the widespread application of AI algorithms in the health sector. The development of fair and unbiased AI algorithms address health care inequities, ensuring equitable access and accuracy across diverse populations. AI cannot generate the patient-doctor relationship or judge the determinants of care as a whole [37,38]. Other shortcoming of AI algorithms include unsuitability outside of the training domain, the challenge of generalization to diverse populations, brittleness with a tendency to be easily fooled, and lack of transparency and explainability. Another major drawback of these algorithms is that analytics are performed on previously generated data in silico, not prospectively in real-world clinical scenarios [6,39,40]. There

are also concerns over health equity due to underrepresentation of some populations in the ground truth data that are used to train the AI [13].

Recent evidence suggests that the use of AI as an assistive tool in health care may be less likely to have a negative effect on the doctor-patient relationship and may even advocate empathetic and trust-based doctor-patient relationships by providing enough time and space to the doctor to perform their role. They can also assist shared decision-making by allowing doctors and patients to take their own preferences into account [41]. In the future, use of federated learning to maintain data privacy could be considered while enabling collaborative AI model training.

FUTURE DIRECTIONS FOR ARTIFICIAL INTELLIGENCE IN ENDOCRINOLOGY

AI could be used to develop individualized nutrition and exercise plans for pediatric patients with obesity, metabolic syndrome, or prediabetes, enhancing the success of lifestyle interventions. AI-driven analysis of genetic and epigenetic data could identify predispositions to endocrine disorders like type 1 diabetes or thyroid cancer, enabling earlier interventions or preventive strategies. Beyond diabetes, AI could enable closed-loop systems for other hormone-related conditions, such as adrenal insufficiency, by automating hydrocortisone delivery during stress or illness. AI could optimize dosages for hormone replacement therapy (eg, thyroid hormones, growth hormones) based on real-time physiologic data and patient-specific factors, reducing side effects

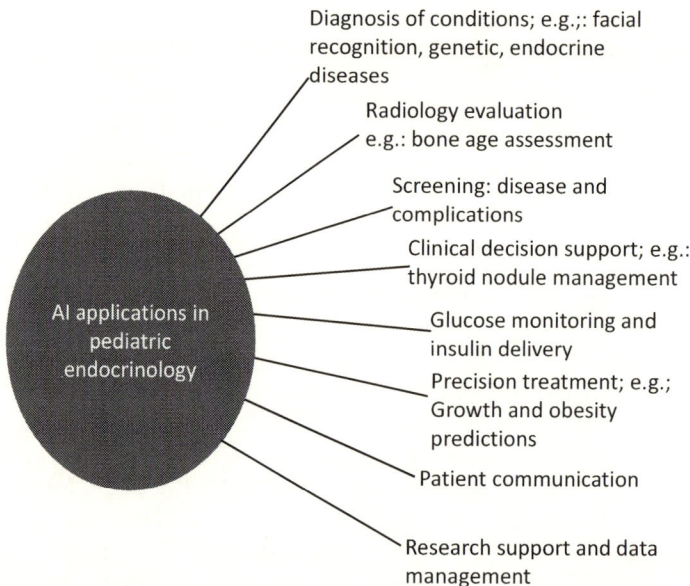

Fig. 1. AI applications in pediatric endocrinology.

and improving treatment outcomes. Advanced wearables equipped with AI could continuously monitor hormone levels (eg, cortisol, insulin) or vital parameters, providing early warnings for dysregulation in conditions such as diabetes, adrenal insufficiency, or hypoglycemia. AI could predict long-term outcomes for patients with chronic endocrine conditions, such as diabetes or Turner syndrome, helping clinicians tailor therapies to minimize complications. AI algorithms analyzing ovarian reserve, hormone fluctuations, and other fertility-related biomarkers could improve success rates for assisted reproductive technologies in pediatric and adolescent endocrinology contexts. Rare disorders like congenital adrenal hyperplasia or familial endocrine neoplasia could benefit from AI models trained on global datasets, improving diagnostic accuracy and management protocols. AI integrated with advanced imaging techniques could enhance the detection and monitoring of endocrine tumors, such as pituitary adenomas or adrenal masses, potentially improving early intervention and treatment success. AI-powered virtual assistants could support both clinicians and patients by providing decision support, medication adherence reminders, and lifestyle modification guidance, particularly for chronic endocrine conditions. AI could analyze large datasets to identify trends, risk factors, and disparities in endocrine disorders across populations, guiding public health initiatives, and resource allocation.

SUMMARY

AI complements, rather than replaces health care providers. The human–AI collaboration integrates the cognitive strengths of health care providers with the analytical capabilities of AI. A human-in-the-loop approach makes sure that the AI systems are guided, communicated, and supervised by human expertise while the AI technology complements and enhances the skills of clinicians resulting in improved safety and quality of health care services and patient outcomes (Fig. 1).

CLINICS CARE POINTS

- Artificial intelligence (AI) and machine learning are valuable tools in advancing the field for pediatric endocrinology.
- AI has exhibited marked capabilities for predicting and classifying diagnoses, as well as providing recommendations and insights.
- An exciting field is exploration of AI's potential in early-stage disease prediction through wearable devices.
- Shortcomings of AI technology include cyber-security risks, threatening patient privacy and confidentiality, latent biases in AI algorithms, unsuitability outside of the training domain, the challenge of generalization to diverse populations, brittleness with a tendency to be easily fooled, and lack of transparency and explainability.

Disclosure

The authors have nothing to disclose. No conflicts of interest.

References

[1] Gubbi S, Hamet P, Tremblay J, et al. Artificial intelligence and machine learning in endocrinology and metabolism: the dawn of a new era. Front Endocrinol (Lausanne) 2019;10: 185.

[2] Dimitri P, Savage MO. Artificial intelligence in paediatric endocrinology: conflict or cooperation. J Pediatr Endocrinol Metab 2024;37(3):209–21.

[3] Khosravi M, Zare Z, Mojtabaeian SM, et al. Artificial intelligence and decision-making in healthcare: a thematic analysis of a systematic review of reviews. Health Serv Res Manag Epidemiol 2024;11:23333928241234864.

[4] Dallora AL, Anderberg P, Kvist O, et al. Bone age assessment with various machine learning techniques: a systematic literature review and meta-analysis. PLoS One 2019;14(7): e0220242.

[5] Esteva A, Robicquet A, Ramsundar B, et al. A guide to deep learning in healthcare. Nat Med 2019;25(1):24–9.

[6] Topol EJ. High-performance medicine: the convergence of human and artificial intelligence. Nat Med 2019;25(1):44–56.

[7] Bai M, Gao L, Ji M, et al. The uncovered biases and errors in clinical determination of bone age by using deep learning models. Eur Radiol 2023;33(5):3544–56.

[8] Lee H, Tajmir S, Lee J, et al. Fully automated deep learning system for bone age assessment. J Digit Imaging 2017;30(4):427–41.

[9] Thodberg HH. An automated method for determination of bone age. J Clin Endocrinol Metab 2009;94(7):2239–44.

[10] Martin DD, Calder AD, Ranke MB, et al. Accuracy and self-validation of automated bone age determination. Sci Rep 2022;12(1):6388.

[11] Tajmir SH, Lee H, Shailam R, et al. Artificial intelligence-assisted interpretation of bone age radiographs improves accuracy and decreases variability. Skeletal Radiol 2019;48(2): 275–83.

[12] Bjerring JC, Busch J. Artificial intelligence and patient-centered decision-making. Philos Technol 2021;34(2):349–71.

[13] Huang J, Yeung AM, Armstrong DG, et al. Artificial intelligence for predicting and diagnosing complications of diabetes. J Diabetes Sci Technol 2023;17(1):224–38.

[14] Wolf RM, Liu TYA, Thomas C, et al. The SEE study: safety, efficacy, and equity of implementing autonomous artificial intelligence for diagnosing diabetic retinopathy in youth. Diabetes Care 2021;44(3):781–7.

[15] Stefanopoulos S, Ayoub S, Qiu Q, et al. Machine learning prediction of diabetic foot ulcers in the inpatient population. Vascular 2022;30(6):1115–23.

[16] Xing Y, Zhang PP, Li X, et al. New predictive models and indices for screening MAFLD in school-aged overweight/obese children. Eur J Pediatr 2023;182(11):5025–36.

[17] Kushwaha S, Srivastava R, Jain R, et al. Harnessing machine learning models for non-invasive pre-diabetes screening in children and adolescents. Comput Methods Programs Biomed 2022;226:107180.

[18] Shmoish M, German A, Devir N, et al. Prediction of adult height by machine learning technique. J Clin Endocrinol Metab 2021;106(7):e2700–10.

[19] Nahum U, Refardt J, Chifu I, et al. Machine learning-based algorithm as an innovative approach for the differentiation between diabetes insipidus and primary polydipsia in clinical practice. Eur J Endocrinol 2022;187(6):777–86.

[20] Pan Z, Shen Z, Zhu H, et al. Clinical application of an automatic facial recognition system based on deep learning for diagnosis of Turner syndrome. Endocrine 2021;72(3):865–73.

[21] Song W, Lei Y, Chen S, et al. Multiple facial image features-based recognition for the automatic diagnosis of turner syndrome. Comput Ind 2018;100:85–95.

[22] Wei R, Jiang C, Gao J, et al. Deep-learning approach to automatic identification of facial anomalies in endocrine disorders _ neuroendocrinology _ karger publishers. Neuroendocrinology 2020;110(5):328–37.

[23] Abdalmageed W, Mirzaalian H, Guo X, et al. Assessment of facial morphologic features in patients with congenital adrenal hyperplasia using deep learning. JAMA Netw Open 2020;3(11):e2022199.

[24] Webb-Robertson BJM. Explainable artificial intelligence in endocrinological medical research. J Clin Endocrinol Metab 2021;106(7):e2809–10.

[25] Nimri R, Phillip M, Kovatchev B. Closed-loop and artificial intelligence-based decision support systems. Diabetes Technol Ther 2023;25(S1):S70–89.

[26] Garcia-Tirado J, Diaz JL, Esquivel-Zuniga R, et al. Advanced closed-loop control system improves postprandial glycemic control compared with a hybrid closed-loop system following unannounced meal. Diabetes Care 2021;44(10):2379–87.

[27] Colmenarejo G. Machine learning models to predict childhood and adolescent obesity: a review. Nutrients 2020;12(8):2466.

[28] Alghalyini B. Applications of artificial intelligence in the management of childhood obesity. J Fam Med Prim Care 2023;12(11):2558–64.

[29] Bays HE, Fitch A, Cuda S, et al. Artificial intelligence and obesity management: an obesity medicine association (OMA) clinical practice statement (CPS) 2023. Obes Pillars 2023;6: 100065.

[30] Dugan TM, Mukhopadhyay S, Carroll A, et al. Machine learning techniques for prediction of early childhood obesity. Appl Clin Inform 2015;6(3):506–20.

[31] Öksüz N, Shcherbatyi I, Kowatsch T, et al. A data-analytical system to predict therapy success for obese children. In: ICIS 2018 - international conference on information systems international conference on information systems (ICIS-2018), December 13–16, San Francisco, CA, Springer, 2018.

[32] Francis GL, Waguespack SG, Bauer AJ, et al. Management guidelines for children with thyroid nodules and differentiated thyroid cancer. Thyroid 2015;25(7):716–59.

[33] Yang J, Page LC, Wagner L, et al. Thyroid nodules on ultrasound in children and young adults: comparison of diagnostic performance of radiologists' impressions, ACR TI-RADS, and a deep learning algorithm. Am J Roentgenol 2023;220(3):408–17.

[34] Peng S, Liu Y, Lv W, et al. Deep learning-based artificial intelligence model to assist thyroid nodule diagnosis and management: a multicentre diagnostic study. Lancet Digit Health 2021;3(4):e250–9 [published correction appears in Lancet Digit Health 202;3(7):e413.

[35] Ayers JW, Poliak A, Dredze M, et al. Comparing physician and artificial intelligence chatbot responses to patient questions posted to a public social media forum. JAMA Intern Med 2023;183(6):589–96.

[36] Zheng T, Xie W, Xu L, et al. A machine learning-based framework to identify type 2 diabetes through electronic health records. Int J Med Inform 2017;97:120–7.

[37] Quinn TP, Senadeera M, Jacobs S, et al. Trust and medical AI: the challenges we face and the expertise needed to overcome them. J Am Med Inform Assoc 2021;28(4):890–4.

[38] DeCamp M, Lindvall C. Latent bias and the implementation of artificial intelligence in medicine. J Am Med Inform Assoc 2020;27(12):2020–3.

[39] Kelly CJ, Karthikesalingam A, Suleyman M, et al. Key challenges for delivering clinical impact with artificial intelligence. BMC Med 2019;17(1):195.

[40] khan B, Fatima H, Qureshi A, et al. Drawbacks of artificial intelligence and their potential solutions in the healthcare sector. Biomed Mater Devices 2023;1(2):731–8.

[41] Sauerbrei A, Kerasidou A, Lucivero F, et al. The impact of artificial intelligence on the person-centred, doctor-patient relationship: some problems and solutions. BMC Med Inform Decis Mak 2023;23(1):73.

Advances in Pediatrics 72 (2025) 197–217

ADVANCES IN PEDIATRICS

ELSEVIER
MOSBY

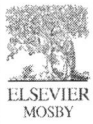

Pharmacology in Pediatric Renal Solid Organ Transplantation

Check for updates

Christine Tabulov, PharmD[a],*, Kelly McGee, MD[b],
Beatriz Fabiola Marin Ruiz, MD[c]

[a]Department of Pharmacotherapeutics and Clinical Research, University of South Florida Taneja College of Pharmacy, 12901 Bruce B. Downs Boulevard, MDC 30, Tampa, FL 33612, USA; [b]Department of Pediatrics, University of South Florida, 17 Davis Boulevard, Suite 200, Tampa, FL 33606, USA; [c]Division of Pediatric Nephrology, Department of Pediatrics, University of South Florida, 2 Tampa General Circle, 5026, Tampa, FL 33606, USA

Keywords
- Immunosuppression • Pediatric • Renal transplantation • Pharmacokinetics
- Pharmacology

Key points
- Maintenance regimens for pediatric renal transplantation frequently comprise a combination of a calcineurin inhibitor, antiproliferative agent, and corticosteroid.
- Alterations in pharmacokinetics within the pediatric population may significantly affect drug absorption, distribution, metabolism, and elimination.
- Therapeutic drug monitoring for immunosuppressant medications is essential to prevent toxicity and reduce the risk of renal transplant rejection.
- Immunosuppressive therapy elevates the risk of infections and malignancies; therefore, regular screenings are necessary to address these risks proactively.

INTRODUCTION

Pediatric end-stage renal disease is associated with high morbidity and mortality, with mortality rates 30 times greater than those of healthy children [1,2]. Transplantation has been reported to improve these children's quality of life and life expectancy [3,4]. The first pediatric kidney transplant (PKT) in the United States was performed in 1959 at the University of Oregon [5]. As of 2022, the Scientific Registry of Transplant Recipients (SRTR) reported that 34 programs perform PKTs with various demographics (Box 1) [6]. Immunosuppression (IS) medications are critical for preventing rejection of the

*Corresponding author. E-mail address: ctabulov@usf.edu

https://doi.org/10.1016/j.yapd.2024.12.001

Abbreviations

AR	acute rejection
ATG	antithymocyte globulin
CNI	calcineurin inhibitors
CS	corticosteroid
DDKT	deceased donor kidney transplant
EBV	Epstein-Barr virus
HLA	human leukocyte antigen
IL	interleukin
IS	immunosuppression
LDKT	living donor pediatric kidney transplant
MPA	mycophenolic acid
mTOR	mammalian target of rapamycin
OPTN	Organ Procurement and Transplantation Network
PKT	pediatric kidney transplant
rATG	rabbit-based antithymocyte globulin
SRTR	Scientific Registry of Transplant Recipients

transplanted kidney and maintaining adequate kidney function for as long as possible [7]. However, IS comes with adverse effects, infection, and malignancy risks [4,8]. IS in PKT encompasses 3 stages: induction, maintenance, and rejection. This article discusses the pharmacology of IS used in PKT induction and maintenance, with its implications in clinical practice.

INDUCTION AGENTS

Induction is the first phase of PKT. Induction aims to prevent rejection by decreasing the number of T cells before, during, and after transplantation

---

Box 1: 2022 Scientific Registry of Transplant Recipients report of characteristics of children who received a kidney transplant

- 705 PKTs performed
  - 71.2% deceased donor (DDKT) (n = 502) versus 28.8% living donor (LDKT) (n = 203).
- 59.6% of DDKT and 44.8% LDKT between ages 12 and 17 years.
- Racial demographics:
  - DDKT: White (39.6%); Hispanic (30.9%); Black (21.3%); Asian (5.2%); Multiracial (2.8%); Native American (0.2%)
  - LDKT: White (63.5%), Hispanic (16.7%), Black (11.8%), Asian (4.9%), Multiracial (2.5%), Native American (0.5%)

Data from [Organ Procurement and Transplantation Network (OPTN) and Scientific Registry of Transplant Recipients (SRTR). OPTN/SRTR 2022 Annual Data Report. U.S. Department of Health and Human Services, Health Resources and Services Administration; 2024. Accessed September 20, 2024. http://srtr.transplant.hrsa.gov/annual_reports/Default.aspx].

[4,7]. Rejection risk is highest at the time of transplant and in the first 3 to 6 months post transplant. Induction agents utilized in PKT include basiliximab, antithymocyte globulin (ATG), and alemtuzumab [9–11]. Two ATG products are approved by the United States Food and Drug Administration, both rabbit and equine-based, but the rabbit-based ATG (rATG) is utilized more often in clinical practice. A randomized, double-blind clinical trial of adults found acute rejection (AR) incidence to be 4% with rATG versus 25% with equine-based ATG ($P = .014$), with AR rates lower with rATG compared with equine-based ATG (relative risk $= 0.09$; $P = .009$) [12]. Similar results were seen in a single center, with the incidence of AR being lower in PKT patients who received rATG versus equine-based ATG (33% vs 50%, $P = .02$) [13]. The selection of an induction agent is determined by evaluating the patient's immunologic risk and comorbidities and considering the donor type, human leukocyte antigen (HLA) matching, institutional protocols, and physician preference. An assessment of SRTR data from 2000 to 2018 found no significant difference in 6-month (alemtuzumab 8.6% vs rATG 7.8% vs basiliximab 9.2%, $P = .30$) and 12-month rejection rates (alemtuzumab 17.2% vs rATG 15.7% vs basiliximab 16.5%, $P = .70$) [14]. The 2009 Kidney Disease: Improving Global Outcomes Clinical Practice Guideline for the Care of Kidney Transplant Recipients recommends first-line use of an interleukin-2 receptor antagonist (eg, basiliximab) unless the patient has high immunologic risk (Box 2). A lymphocyte-depleting agent (ATG, alemtuzumab) is indicated [4]. A summary of the various induction agents and their clinical implications is found in Table 1.

Box 2: Factors contributing to high immunologic risk in pediatric renal transplantation [4,15]

- Human leukocyte antigen (HLA) Mismatch
  - The methodology(ies) of detecting anti-HLA antibodies in transplant patient candidates may be used to determine different levels of immunologic risk.
  - Methodologies include complement-dependent cytotoxic cross-match, flow cytometric cross-match, and pretransplant donor-specific antibodies.
  - Patients with positive results from all 3 methodologies represent the group of highest immunologic risk, followed by the group of patients with a negative complement-dependent cytotoxic cross-match but positive flow cytometric cross-match and pretransplant donor-specific antibodies.
- Young recipient age
- Mature donor age
- African American
- Delayed graft function
- Panel reactive antibody presence
- Donor-specific antibody existence
- Cold ischemic time beyond 24 hours

Table 1
Induction agents in pediatric kidney transplant

Agent	Mechanism of action	Adverse effects	Clinical pearls
Basiliximab	A chimeric (human/murine) monoclonal antibody binds to interleukin (IL)-2 receptor on T-lymphocytes, decreases IL-2 and IL-15-related proliferation of T-lymphocytes [7].	Gastrointestinal most common (based on adult data): constipation, nausea, vomiting, diarrhea, dyspepsia, and abdominal pain [16,17]. In pediatric patients, hypertension (49%), hypertrichosis (49%), rhinitis (49%), urinary tract infections (46%), and fever (39%) were reported when given in combination with cyclosporine (modified), corticosteroids, azathioprine, or mycophenolate mofetil [17].	Generally well tolerated, thus premedication not required; hypersensitivity reactions are rare [7,16]. If hypersensitivity reaction occurs, discontinue basiliximab and treat reaction. Contraindicated in patients with a known hypersensitivity to the drug or its components [16,17]. Clearance is not dose dependent. Slower clearance seen in infants and children but not dependent on age, body surface area, or weight [16]. Associated with lower incidence of post-transplant lymphoproliferative disorder (PTLD) and infections [16].

	Description	Adverse effects	Notes
Antithymocyte globulin	Polyclonal antibody that targets T-cell surface antigens, B-cell surface antigens, natural killer cell antigens, adhesion molecules, and chemokine receptors. Through means are not completely understood, complement-dependent lysis and antibody-dependent cellular toxicity are likely means by which lymphocyte depletion is achieved [7].	Cytokine release syndrome, hemolytic anemia, thrombocytopenia, neutropenia, and serum sickness [16]. There is inconclusive evidence regarding possible increased risk of malignancies (eg, post transplant lymphoproliferative disorder) [7].	Premedications are recommended: corticosteroid, diphenhydramine, and acetaminophen [16]. Preferably administered through central venous access with 0.22 μm filter given risk of phlebitis or thrombosis [18,19]. Some centers report using peripheral administration when heparin and hydrocortisone are added [19]. Dose adjustments necessary for low white blood cell or platelet counts [7,18]. Half-life of 2–3 d; however, lymphocyte-depleting effects may be present for 9–12 mo [18,19].
Alemtuzumab	Humanized recombinant monoclonal antibody that binds to the cluster of differentiation 52) antigen on lymphocytes causing antibody-dependent lysis [7].	Cytopenias, cytokine release syndrome, infections, hemolytic anemia, thyroid disease, and malignancy [7].	Premedications are recommended: corticosteroids, diphenhydramine, and acetaminophen [7]. Only available through a restricted distribution program [20]. Half-life reported to be 11 h to 6 d [19]. Found to have rapid B cell depletion with effects lasting for several months to a year or more [7].

Recent studies have investigated the efficacy and safety of lower doses of rATG. A retrospective multicenter study by the Pediatric Nephrology Research Consortium found the AR rates were similar between low-dose rATG ($\leq$4.5 mg/kg) and standard-dose rATG (>4.5 mg/kg) (17% vs 19%, P = .13) [21]. In addition, a single-center retrospective study found that patients who received standard-dose basiliximab had higher incidences of biopsy-proven AR than those who received rATG 3 mg/kg single dose (21% vs 10%, P = .015). In the same study, survival free from the composite endpoint (treated AR, graft loss, or death) was 78% in the rATG group compared to 61% in the basiliximab group (P = .0025) [22].

MAINTENANCE IMMUNOSUPPRESSIVE AGENTS

An immunosuppressive regimen for PKT typically includes a calcineurin inhibitor and an antiproliferative agent, with or without a corticosteroid (CS) [7]. These regimens are often standardized through center-specific protocols but can also be customized to meet the specific needs of individual patients. According to the 2022 Scientific Registry of Transplant Recipients Data, the most commonly used regimens in PKT recipients were tacrolimus, mycophenolate mofetil, and CS [6].

Calcineurin inhibitors (cyclosporine, tacrolimus)

Calcineurin inhibitors (CNI) are a cornerstone of therapy in PKT. Cyclosporine was widely used; however, most centers have transitioned to tacrolimus. This shift is supported by evidence indicating a lower incidence of AR with tacrolimus (8.3%) compared to cyclosporine (16.6%), as demonstrated in a nonrandomized clinical trial involving 12 recipients on tacrolimus, azathioprine, and prednisone versus 12 recipients on cyclosporine, mycophenolate mofetil (MMF), and CS (both groups received basiliximab induction) [23]. CNI exert their mechanism of action by binding to FK506 binding protein to inhibit calcineurin phosphatase to decrease cytokine transcription (eg, interleukin (IL)-2, IL-4, tumor necrosis factor-a, and interferon-Y), which prevents T-lymphocyte activation and proliferation [24,25]. CNI can be impacted by various pharmacokinetic parameters, with unique pediatric considerations highlighted (Table 2). Therapeutic drug monitoring with trough levels is standard of care and should be performed, although there is no consensus on target trough levels among PKT centers.

Antiproliferative agents

Mycophenolate and azathioprine are antiproliferative agents used in PKT recipients. Mycophenolate use is more common in most PKT centers [6].

Mycophenolate

Currently, 2 forms of mycophenolate are available: mycophenolate mofetil and mycophenolic acid (MPA). Mycophenolate mofetil is a prodrug converted in the liver through hydrolysis to MPA, its active metabolite [47]. MPA is also available as an enteric-coated tablet that can bypass the stomach and enter

Table 2
Clinical considerations for calcineurin inhibitors pharmacokinetics

Pharmacokinetic parameter	Tacrolimus	Cyclosporine
Absorption	• Take with or without food consistently at the same times [26–28].	• Modified formulation provides more consistent absorption (not dependent on bile emulsification) [27,28].
	• Absorption may be erratic with administration via feeding tube [29–31].	
	• Reduced absorption associated with compounded suspension compared to immediate-release capsule in pediatric liver transplant patients [19,32].	
	• Immediate release capsule may be administered sublingually; however, associated with doubled tacrolimus exposure [19].	
	• Available as granules, utilize equivalent dosing to immediate-release capsule [19].	
	• Extended-release tablet [lifecycle pharma [LCP]-tacrolimus] associated with enhanced bioavailability and lower maximum concentrations than immediate release tacrolimus. Therefore, daily dose is not equivalent.	
	○ Based on adult data (not approved in pediatric population but may be utilized off-label in adolescent population), decrease dose (by 30% in non-African American, 20% in African American) when converting from immediate release tacrolimus to LCP-tacrolimus [19,33,34]	

(continued on next page)

Table 2
(continued)

Pharmacokinetic parameter	Tacrolimus	Cyclosporine
Distribution	• Trough levels may need to be interpreted differently in the case of low hematocrit as hematocrit levels <33% are associated with elevated clearance rates [35,36]. • Hypoalbuminemia is often seen in pediatric patients, which may increase metabolism and elimination [36].	
Metabolism	• Adjust dose for drug-drug interactions with cytochrome P450 3A4 (CYP3A4) and CYP3A5 inducers and inhibitors [26–28]. • Increased CYP3A4 activity may be seen in younger pediatric kidney transplant (PKT) patients after 1 year of age resulting in larger dosages [36]. • Avoid grapefruit and pomegranate [27,28,37]. • African Americans may require higher dosages due to CYP3A5 variants (*3, *6, *7) [38,39]. • Diarrhea reduces CYP3A4 and p-glycoprotein activity which increases tacrolimus trough levels [40,41].	• Diarrhea may not impact cyclosporine trough levels [42].
Elimination	Younger children may require 3 times daily dosing [43,44] • Half-life of immediate-release tacrolimus reported to average 12.4 h (8–16.8 h) in pediatric patients [19,45] • Half-life of extended-release capsule reported to be 35–41 h in adults [19]	• Half-life of nonmodified cyclosporine is 7.3 h (6.1–16.6 h) in PKT patients with its clearance being 11.8 mL/min/kg (9.8–15.5 mL/min/kg) [46]

the small intestine to release MPA [48]. Both mycophenolate formulations work as noncompetitive, reversible inhibitors of inosine monophosphate dehydrogenase to inhibit the de novo purine guanosine synthesis pathway, affecting T and B lymphocyte development [49]. The pharmacokinetic properties of MPA in pediatric populations are comparable to those observed in adults; however, it is noteworthy that the area under the curve exposure is approximately 25% greater, which can be attributed to the body surface area dosing method commonly employed in pediatric practice [50].

Common side effects of mycophenolate include nausea, vomiting, diarrhea, leukopenia, and anemia [51]. (Box 3) Patients younger than 6 years of age may have higher incidences of diarrhea, leukopenia, and anemia [52]. MPA may help decrease gastrointestinal adverse effects; however, usage is limited to patients who can swallow tablets since the enteric-coated pills cannot be crushed. For patients unable to swallow pills, taking mycophenolate mofetil with food or splitting the total daily dose into 3 or 4 doses may be helpful. It is important to note that switching from mycophenolate mofetil to MPA is not a 1:1 dose conversion [19], with 500 mg of mycophenolate mofetil being equivalent to 360 mg of MPA. Diarrhea is often dose-dependent, and fluid replacement must be utilized to mitigate the increased risk of dehydration in pediatric patients [53,54]. Antidiarrheal medications and probiotics may also be helpful once a gastrointestinal infection is ruled out, and their use depends on each center's guidelines. Mycophenolate is a part of a risk evaluation and mitigation strategy program in the United States due to its risk for congenital malformations and first-trimester pregnancy loss. Data for individuals of reproductive potential are limited to females at this time, with the recommendations that females of reproductive age use 2 forms of birth control unless an intrauterine device, tubal sterilization, or vasectomy is utilized [55]. Therapeutic drug monitoring of mycophenolate has been described in the literature; however, not all centers currently use it. If therapeutic drug monitoring is used, a trough concentration of 1 to 4.5 mg/L is targeted to prevent rejection. It has also been used to confirm nonadherence and to make significant adjustments to CNI therapy (reduced dosage, switch, withdrawal), high immunologic risk, altered gastrointestinal, hepatic, or kidney function, and drug interactions [56].

Box 3: Clinical considerations for mycophenolate

- Common adverse effects of mycophenolate mofetil/mycophenolic acid (MPA) include diarrhea, leukopenia, and anemia.
- MPA can help decrease the incidence of diarrhea; however, its utilization in PKTs may be limited since these enteric-coated tablets cannot be crushed.
- Double-check conversion to avoid dosing errors when converting a patient from mycophenolate mofetil to MPA.
- A pregnancy test is recommended before initiation of mycophenolate mofetil/ MPA and during therapy in female patients who have started menarche.

Azathioprine

Azathioprine is a prodrug that gets converted to 6-mercaptopurine in the liver and erythrocytes; its active metabolite 6-thiouric acid blocks active T and B lymphocytes from proliferating and inhibiting de novo purine synthesis [57]. Pharmacogenomic testing has been implemented in practice for thiopurine S-methyltransferase (TPMT) and nucleoside diphosphate-linked moiety X-type motif 15 (NUDT15), enzymes responsible for converting 6-mercaptopurine to inactive metabolites [58]. Individuals deficient in these enzymes are at increased risk for adverse effects and require dose adjustment if the deficiency is identified. The most common side effects are dose-related myelosuppression (leukopenia, thrombocytopenia, anemia) and gastrointestinal (nausea, vomiting) [57]. Gastrointestinal side effects may be relieved by giving food or splitting the dose further. Patients with hepatic or renal dysfunction require dose adjustments [57]. A critical drug-drug interaction for azathioprine is allopurinol, which can result in increased mercaptopurine exposure; therefore, it is recommended that the dose of azathioprine be reduced by 75% [19]. Currently, azathioprine is not used as first-line therapy as it is used mainly in female patients considering pregnancy or who are pregnant [59].

CORTICOSTEROIDS

Corticosteroids(CS) (eg, prednisone, prednisolone) can be a part of maintenance therapy for PKTs. CS affect many parts of the T and B cell lines to decrease T and B cell proliferation. CS also decrease prostaglandin and cytokine synthesis, histamine and bradykinin release, and capillary permeability. Methylprednisolone is often administered in a high dose intravenously preoperatively and immediately post transplant. For post-transplant maintenance therapy, CS are typically switched to either prednisone or prednisolone and tapered to a lower dose. There is no standard CS taper, as the transplant program often determines tapers [19]. This drug class is associated with dermatologic (eg, Cushingoid appearance), skeletal, muscular, gastric, metabolic, cardiovascular, and psychiatric adverse effects (Box 4). In addition, a retrospective cohort review found greater CS exposure may be associated with lower morning cortisol levels and adrenal insufficiency diagnoses [60]. As a result, some centers participate in CS a minimization protocol, which specifies CS administration during the induction period with rATG [61]. The withdrawal of CS has been reported at various time points, including the first week post transplant (rapid discontinuation) and within the first year post transplant (late withdrawal) [62]. Rapid discontinuation and late withdrawal of CS have similar patient and graft outcomes compared to steroid-based regimens [62], thus avoiding long-term CS use and minimizing side effects.

Prednisolone is the active metabolite of prednisone in the liver. It is rapidly absorbed, with peak plasma levels often occurring 1 to 3 hours after oral dose [63]. The time to peak levels is prolonged with food [64]. CS may be taken with food to prevent stomach upset and ulcerations. In addition, it is recommended that drug-drug interactions be monitored since CS acts on CYP3A4/CYP3A5 [63].

Box 4: Corticosteroid side effects [65,66]

- General Side Effects
  - ○ Increased risk of glaucoma and cataracts in a dose-dependent and duration-dependent manner.
  - ○ Some studies have shown that with regular corticosteroid (CS), risk of heart failure, ischemic heart disease, and other cardiovascular conditions increases.
  - ○ May increase risk of hypertension, although the exact mechanism behind this effect is not fully known.
  - ○ CS-induced myopathy is possible, higher doses of steroids for longer periods of time increase this risk.
  - ○ CS also associated with side effects of mood disorders, behavioral symptoms, and cognitive deficits.
- Specific Concerns for Pediatric Populations
  - ○ There is significant overlap in the side effects/complications seen in adult and pediatric populations.
  - ○ Children who take glucocorticoids may be more at risk for cataract development compared to adults.
  - ○ CS have, in several studies, been shown to frequently result in growth suppression in pediatric patients.
  - ○ Medication-induced diabetes is also a risk in pediatric patients taking CS.
  - ○ CS may also lead to adrenal suppression in pediatric patients, the risk correlating with both the dose and duration of the therapy.
  - ○ CS side effects in the pediatric population may also include cushingoid features, hypertension, behavioral disturbances, weight gain, and growth impairment.

MAMMALIAN TARGET OF RAPAMYCIN INHIBITORS

There are 2 mammalian target of rapamycin (mTOR) inhibitors currently on the market: sirolimus and everolimus. This drug class is utilized as a later-line agent in PKT. mTOR inhibitors bind to the cytosolic FK-binding protein 12 to form a complex inhibiting mammalian target of rapamycin complex 1 (mTORC1) to block T cell proliferation [67]. Sirolimus may be combined with CNI (cyclosporine) and CS for adolescent kidney transplant patients. Likewise, everolimus is combined with CNI (cyclosporine) and CS. Exclusion criteria include a prior history of AR, proteinuria, and low CNI toxicity scores. There are few studies on the use of mTOR inhibitors in pediatric patients. In addition, best practices regarding when to convert to mTOR inhibitors remain under discussion. When utilizing everolimus, it is imperative to use the Zortress brand as Afinitor is not approved for solid organ transplantation; however, Zortress is not approved in pediatrics. A multicenter, open-label study with 106 children (ages 1–18 years of age receiving their first or second kidney transplant) found there was no difference in the incidence of biopsy-proven acute

AR, graft loss, or death from randomization to 1-year post transplant between patients who received everolimus and reduced dosages of tacrolimus (10.3%) compared to those who received standard dosing of tacrolimus and mycophenolate mofetil 5.8% (4.4% difference; $P = .417$). In addition, there was no difference in glomerular filtration rate between the 2 groups (76.2 mL/min/1.73m^2 and 72.5 mL/min/1.73m^2 [difference of 3.8 mL/min/1.73m^2] $P = .49$) [68]. The pharmacokinetic variations observed within the pediatric population are prominently illustrated in Table 3.

BELATACEPT

Some transplant centers have utilized belatacept for maintenance immunosuppression (IS) for Epstein-Barr virus (EBV) seropositive kidney transplant patients, particularly in adolescent patients. A fusion protein binds to CD80 and CD86 to prevent binding to the costimulatory receptor CD28 and decrease T cell proliferation [73]. Adverse effects from CNI and reports that belatacept is less toxic have led to its increased usage; however, belatacept is associated with higher rejection rates [74]. Blew and colleagues, reported a

Table 3
Clinical considerations for pharmacokinetics of mammalian target of rapamycin inhibitors

Pharmacokinetic parameter	Sirolimus	Everolimus
Half-life	Approximately 62 h in children—may require twice daily dosing [69]	Approximately 35 h in children [70]
Metabolism	• Mammalian target of rapamycin (mTOR) inhibitors are metabolized in the gut and liver by CYP3A4 and p-glyco-protein; therefore, monitoring of drug-drug interactions is crucial. • Therapeutic drug monitoring is recommended to be utilized to guide dosing • Avoid grapefruit	
Adverse Effects	Hyperlipidemia, hypertension, leukopenia, thrombocytopenia, anemia, proteinuria, oral ulcers, poor wound healing (mTOR inhibitors are typically avoided immediately post transplant)	
Administration Considerations	Available as a tablet and oral solution • Not recommended to crush the tablet [71] • Solution must be mixed into at least 60 mL of water or orange juice in a cup to drink immediately. Cup is to be refilled with another 120 mL of water or orange juice to be ingested immediately [71].	Available as a tablet • Data from studies of pediatric heart transplant patients indicate the tablet can be crushed and dissolved in an oral syringe and mixed with 5 mL of water within the same syringe [72]

case series with 3 patients adherent to belatacept maintenance therapy after alemtuzumab and methylprednisolone induction, with 1 CS-responsive acute cellular rejection in adolescent patients [75]. Lerch and colleagues, found conversion to belatacept-based IS can be an option for EBV-seropositive adolescents who are nonadherent before deterioration of graft function [76]. The dosing of belatacept is extrapolated from adult data. Post-transplant lymphoproliferative disorder is a potential adverse effect of belatacept. Thus, there is a black box warning for its use in EBV-seronegative patients [77]. Also, belatacept increases the risk of cytomegalovirus infection, and prophylaxis with valganciclovir is recommended for at least 3 months [77]. When administering antithymocyte globulin for induction or rejection therapy, a 12-h interval between the medications is needed to avoid venous thrombosis of the renal allograft [77].

SPECIAL CONSIDERATIONS FOR PEDIATRIC IMMUNOSUPPRESSION

Challenges of therapeutic drug monitoring in pediatric kidney transplant patients during illness

As described previously, various immunosuppressant medications require therapeutic drug monitoring, including CNIs (tacrolimus, cyclosporine) and mTOR inhibitors (sirolimus, everolimus). Therapeutic drug monitoring may also be used for azathioprine and mycophenolate. These medications have narrow therapeutic windows to ensure appropriate safety and efficacy, especially during times of illness when there may be pharmacokinetic changes that cause delayed or erratic absorption and/or nonadherence to medication regimens. For example, persistent diarrhea can increase tacrolimus levels through inhibition of p-glycoprotein; therefore, closer monitoring and potential dosage reduction or switching immunosuppression medications may be required during illness to avoid risk of rejection or toxicity [54,78]. Changing immunosuppressant medications from oral/enteral to intravenous routes is also performed to minimize the need for first-pass metabolism. In addition, mycophenolate mofetil is associated with nausea, vomiting, and diarrhea. If pediatric patients can swallow solid dosage forms, a conversion from mycophenolate mofetil to enteric-coated mycophenolic acid may be utilized; however, it is important to keep in mind that this dosage form is not ideal for younger pediatric patients who cannot swallow solid dosage forms as described previously. Therapeutic drug monitoring of mycophenolate may be performed in cases of hypoalbuminemia and/or loss of renal function [78]. In general, during times of diarrhea and vomiting, hydration is critical in pediatric patients, given their higher total body water composition. Oral rehydration solution may be used for mild to moderate dehydration until vomiting and diarrhea resolve. Intravenous bolus and fluids (normal saline, Lactated Ringer's) are used for severe dehydration or hypovolemic shock cases. Additionally, for diarrhea cases, gastrointestinal infection must be ruled out [54]. Younger pediatric patients are often colonized with *Clostridioides difficile*, with the highest risk age group being between 1 and

4 years of age; however, only 2.3% of PKT recipients were reported to be infected with *C difficile* (less than other transplanted organs) [79]. Further treatment of infection and symptoms (diarrhea, vomiting) is often determined by the transplant center.

Growth and development

Because CS can cause growth suppression in pediatric patients, CS minimization protocols have been developed to decrease this risk, which is highest in prepubertal patients [62,80]. The TWIST study determined that the minimization of corticosteroids (CS) was correlated with a greater mean change in height standard deviation scores in comparison to the standard utilization of CS (0.16 with tacrolimus/mycophenolate mofetil/daclizumab/steroids until day 4 vs 0.03 with tacrolimus/mycophenolate mofetil/standard-dose steroids). This effect was particularly pronounced in prepubertal children, exhibiting a mean treatment group difference of 0.21 (P=.009 [95% confidence interval 0.05–0.36]). In contrast, pubertal children displayed a mean difference of 0.05 (p = not significant), all without a corresponding increase in graft rejection rates [81]. The advantages of steroid minimization must be carefully weighed against the potential risk of allograft rejection. The following patient characteristics have been documented as less likely to benefit from corticosteroid minimization: African American ethnicity, preemptive transplantation, deceased donor transplants, pretransplant dialysis requirements, panel reactive antibodies exceeding 80%, underlying primary glomerular diseases, and delayed graft function. Furthermore, living donor transplantation has been correlated with an increased utilization of corticosteroid minimization strategies [62]. If prepubertal patients need to be on CS, it should be tapered to the lowest dosage as soon as possible, following institutional protocols [19].

Adherence to therapy

Nonadherence to the immunosuppression regimen has been linked to a shorter duration of graft survival; thus, adherence is essential. Nonadherence in PKT ranges from 30% to 70%; reportedly, each 10% decrease in nonadherence is associated with an 8% higher risk of graft failure and mortality [82–84]. Younger pediatric patients are at decreased risk due to increased caregiver involvement with medication regimens. Adolescents are at the highest risk for nonadherence, given increased independence with managing their medication regimen and cosmetic side effects from the therapy (mostly with CNI and CS) [85]. Different strategies have been proposed for ways to assist adolescents with the complex transplant medication regimen [86]. When managing care for adolescents, it is important to simplify medication routines, offer continuous education, utilize technology (such as smartphones, alarms, and text messaging), encourage shared decision-making between adolescents and their parents, and evaluate psychological barriers to adherence. Furthermore, regularly assessing trough levels (for example, CNIs, mTOR inhibitors, and mycophenolate) can aid in supporting adherence [87].

Transition to adult care

The American Society of Transplantation and the American Academy of Pediatrics recommend assisting adolescents with the pediatric-to-adult transition [87,88]. The focus is on medications, and the goal is for adolescents to know their medications (their names, indications, typical side effects, and how to mitigate them). Adolescents should also be taught how to request refills from the pharmacy. Overall, it is recommended that multidisciplinary teams develop individualized transition plans throughout adolescence to prepare patients for adulthood [89].

Increased malignancy risk

Immunosuppression medications have been linked to malignancies. Although the incidences of malignancies other than lymphoproliferative diseases (eg, post-transplant lymphoproliferative disorder) are rare in PKT patients, they are at 5 to 10 times higher risk of developing cancer compared to the general population [90]. PKT patients who are seronegative for Epstein Barr virus should be monitored closely for symptoms and signs such as fever, lymphadenopathy, diarrhea, and renal transplant dysfunction. Those receiving a seropositive Epstein Barr virus donor kidney may require weekly to biweekly monitoring of the Epstein Barr virus viral load (in plasma or whole blood) during the first year after transplantation. Beyond the first year, monitoring of viral load is typically advised for PKT patients experiencing fluctuating immunosuppression, episodes of rejection, or lacking a defined viral "set point." [91] Skin cancers are the most common. Thus, pediatricians must screen for skin cancers during routine visits. Other types of malignancies reported include sarcoma, renal cell carcinoma, and neuroblastoma [90,92].

Metabolic and cardiovascular health

Post-transplant diabetes is associated with CNI (tacrolimus >cyclosporine) and CS, as is hypertension. Hypertension has been reported in 60% to 90% of PKT patients, which is significantly influenced by tacrolimus and CS usage [93]. Approximately 50% of PKT patients have developed dyslipidemia in adulthood, with cyclosporine and mTOR inhibitors contributing [94].

SUMMARY

Immunosuppression for pediatric renal transplant involves a backbone of CNI (most commonly tacrolimus) and mycophenolate, with or without a CS. More data on the pediatric population are needed, and ongoing research and collaboration are required.

CLINICS CARE POINTS

- Collaborate closely with the transplant team to ensure accurate immunosuppressive medication dosing. This reduces the risk of rejection while minimizing side effects such as nephrotoxicity, infections, and malignancies.

- Assess growth parameters regularly, including height, weight, and pubertal progression. Monitor vital signs such as blood pressure and laboratory markers, including renal function, electrolytes, and complete blood counts, to evaluate the impact of immunosuppressive therapy.
- Reinforce the importance of strict adherence to immunosuppressive medications, particularly in adolescents. Proactively address potential barriers, such as socioeconomic challenges, side effects, and gaps in knowledge.
- Vigilantly monitor for drug-drug and drug-food interactions, especially with antibiotics, antifungals, and over-the-counter medications commonly prescribed in pediatric care.
- Recognize and manage calcineurin inhibitor-related side effects such as nephrotoxicity, tremors, and hyperglycemia. Ensure therapeutic drug monitoring is performed consistently.
- Be alert to gastrointestinal symptoms, such as diarrhea, and bone marrow suppression associated with mycophenolate use. To reduce infection and bleeding risks, monitor and promptly address cytopenias, including leukopenia, anemia, and thrombocytopenia.
- When corticosteroids are prescribed, regularly monitor for side effects, including weight gain, mood changes, growth suppression, and bone health. Tailor dosing and taper regimens according to patient needs.
- Confirm that patients are up to date on vaccinations. Live vaccines, such as MMR and varicella, are contraindicated post-transplant. Coordinate with the transplant team for guidance on immunization schedules.
- Stay vigilant for early signs of opportunistic infections, such as fever, respiratory symptoms, or gastrointestinal complaints. Communicate promptly with the transplant team to ensure timely evaluation and treatment.
- Foster multidisciplinary collaboration to optimize patient outcomes and ensure long-term graft survival. Address both medical and psychosocial aspects of care to provide comprehensive support for the patient and family.

Disclosure

The authors have nothing to disclose.

References

[1] McDonald SP, Craig JC. Australian and New Zealand Paediatric Nephrology Association. Long-term survival of children with end-stage renal disease. N Engl J Med 2004;350(26): 2654–62.
[2] Tjaden L, Tong A, Henning P, et al. Children's experiences of dialysis: a systematic review of qualitative studies. Arch Dis Child 2012;97(5):395–402.
[3] Czyżewski L, Sańko-Resmer J, Wyzgał J, et al. Assessment of health-related quality of life of patients after kidney transplantation in comparison with hemodialysis and peritoneal dialysis. Ann Transplant 2014;19:576–85, Published 2014 Nov 9.
[4] Kidney Disease: Improving Global Outcomes (KDIGO) Transplant Work Group. KDIGO clinical practice guideline for the care of kidney transplant recipients. Am J Transplant 2009;9(Suppl 3):S1–155.
[5] Papalois VE, Najarian JS. Pediatric kidney transplantation: historic hallmarks and a personal perspective. Pediatr Transplant 2001;5(4):239–45.

[6] Organ Procurement and Transplantation Network (OPTN) and Scientific Registry of Transplant Recipients (SRTR). OPTN/SRTR 2022 annual data report. U.S. Department of Health and Human Services, Health Resources and Services Administration; 2024. Available at: https://srtr.transplant.hrsa.gov/. Accessed November 20, 2024.

[7] Balani SS, Jensen CJ, Kouri AM, et al. Induction and maintenance immunosuppression in pediatric kidney transplantation-Advances and controversies. Pediatr Transplant 2021;25(7):e14077.

[8] Hussain Y, Khan H. Immunosuppressive drugs. Encyclopedia of Infection and Immunity 2022;726–40.

[9] Offner G, Toenshoff B, Höcker B, et al. Efficacy and safety of basiliximab in pediatric renal transplant patients receiving cyclosporine, mycophenolate mofetil, and steroids. Transplantation 2008;86(9):1241–8.

[10] Velez C, Zuluaga G, Ocampo C, et al. Clinical description and evolution of renal transplant pediatric patients treated with alemtuzumab. Transplant Proc 2011;43(9):3350–4.

[11] Moudgil A, Puliyanda D. Induction therapy in pediatric renal transplant recipients: an overview. Paediatr Drugs 2007;9(5):323–41.

[12] Brennan DC, Flavin K, Lowell JA, et al. A randomized, double-blinded comparison of Thymoglobulin versus Atgam for induction immunosuppressive therapy in adult renal transplant recipients [published correction appears in Transplantation 1999 May 27;67(10):1386]. Transplantation 1999;67(7):1011–8.

[13] Khositseth S, Matas A, Cook ME, et al. Thymoglobulin versus ATGAM induction therapy in pediatric kidney transplant recipients: a single-center report. Transplantation 2005;79(8): 958–63.

[14] Riad S, Jackson S, Chinnakotla S, et al. Primary pediatric deceased-donor kidney transplant recipients outcomes by immunosuppression induction received in the United States. Pediatr Transplant 2021;25(5):e13928.

[15] Sharma A, Durkan AM. Desensitisation strategies in high-risk children before kidney transplantation. Pediatr Nephrol 2018;33(12):2239–51.

[16] Chapman TM, Keating GM. Basiliximab: a review of its use as induction therapy in renal transplantation. Drugs 2003;63(24):2803–35.

[17] Simulect® (basiliximab) [package insert]. Bridgewater, NJ: Novartis Pharmaceutical Corp; 2003.

[18] THYMOGLOBULIN® (anti-thymocyte globulin [rabbit]) [package insert]. Cambridge, MA: Genzyme Corporation; 2024.

[19] Crowther B. Solid organ transplantation. In: Bernhardt MB, Blackmer AB, Cho HJ, et al, editors. Updates in Therapeutics®: Pediatric Pharmacy Preparatory Review and e.L. and Recertification Course, KS: American College of Clinical Pharmacy, 2022, p. 643-685.

[20] CAMPATH® (alemtuzumab) injection [package insert]. Cambridge, MA: Genzyme Corporation; 2020.

[21] Ashoor IF, Beyl RA, Gupta C, et al. Low-dose antithymocyte globulin has No disadvantages to standard higher dose in pediatric kidney transplant recipients: report from the pediatric Nephrology research Consortium. Kidney Int Rep 2021;6(4):995–1002, Published 2021 Jan 17.

[22] Custodio LFP, Martins SBS, Viana LA, et al. Efficacy and safety of single-dose anti-thymocyte globulin versus basiliximab induction therapy in pediatric kidney transplant recipients: a retrospective comparative cohort study. Pediatr Transplant 2024;28(3):e14713.

[23] Garcia CD, Schneider L, Barros VR, et al. Pediatric renal transplantation under tacrolimus or cyclosporine immunosuppression and basiliximab induction. Transplant Proc 2002;34(7): 2533–4.

[24] Hamawy MM. Molecular actions of calcineurin inhibitors. Drug News Perspect 2003;16(5):277–82.

[25] Thomson AW, Bonham CA, Zeevi A. Mode of action of tacrolimus (FK506): molecular and cellular mechanisms. Ther Drug Monit 1995;17(6):584–91.

[26] Prograf (tacrolimus) capsules/injection [package insert]. Deerfield, IL: Astellas Pharma US, Inc; 2012.

[27] Sandimmune (cyclosporine capsules, USP) [package insert]. East Hanover, NJ: Novartis pharmaceuticals corporation; 2006.

[28] Neoral (cyclosporine capsules, USP) Modified. East Hanover, NJ: Novartis Pharmaceuticals Corporation; 2009.

[29] Aldieri A, Bae E, Chandran MM. Effect of jejunal administration on tacrolimus trough concentrations in a pediatric liver transplant recipient. J Pediatr Pharmacol Ther 2022;27(4): 390–5.

[30] McIntyre CM, Monk HM. Medication absorption considerations in patients with postpyloric enteral feeding tubes. Am J Health Syst Pharm 2014;71(7):549–56.

[31] Goorhuis JF, Scheenstra R, Peeters PM, et al. Buccal vs. nasogastric tube administration of tacrolimus after pediatric liver transplantation. Pediatr Transplant 2006;10(1):74–7.

[32] Reding R, Sokal E, Paul K, et al. Efficacy and pharmacokinetics of tacrolimus oral suspension in pediatric liver transplant recipients. Pediatr Transplant 2002;6(2):124–6.

[33] Tremblay S, Nigro V, Weinberg J, et al. A steady-state head-to-head pharmacokinetic comparison of all FK-506 (tacrolimus) formulations (ASTCOFF): an open-label, prospective, randomized, two-arm, three-period crossover study. Am J Transplant 2017;17(2):432–42.

[34] Trofe-Clark J, Brennan DC, West-Thielke P, et al. Results of ASERTAA, a randomized prospective crossover pharmacogenetic study of immediate-release versus extended-release tacrolimus in african American kidney transplant recipients. Am J Kidney Dis 2018;71(3):315–26.

[35] Schijvens AM, van Hesteren FHS, Cornelissen EAM, et al. The potential impact of hematocrit correction on evaluation of tacrolimus target exposure in pediatric kidney transplant patients. Pediatr Nephrol 2019;34(3):507–15.

[36] Marfo K, Altshuler J, Lu A. Tacrolimus pharmacokinetic and pharmacogenomic differences between adults and pediatric solid organ transplant recipients. Pharmaceutics 2010;2(3): 291–9, Published 2010 Sep 9.

[37] Miedziaszczyk M, Bajon A, Jakielska E, et al. Controversial interactions of tacrolimus with dietary supplements, herbs and food. Pharmaceutics 2022;14(10):2154, Published 2022 Oct 10.

[38] Sanghavi K, Brundage RC, Miller MB, et al. Genotype-guided tacrolimus dosing in African-American kidney transplant recipients. Pharmacogenomics J 2017;17(1):61–8.

[39] Mohamed ME, Schladt DP, Guan W, et al. Tacrolimus troughs and genetic determinants of metabolism in kidney transplant recipients: a comparison of four ancestry groups. Am J Transplant 2019;19(10):2795–804.

[40] Asano T, Nishimoto K, Hayakawa M. Increased tacrolimus trough levels in association with severe diarrhea, a case report. Transplant Proc 2004;36(7):2096–7.

[41] Lemahieu W, Maes B, Verbeke K, et al. Cytochrome P450 3A4 and P-glycoprotein activity and assimilation of tacrolimus in transplant patients with persistent diarrhea. Am J Transplant 2005;5(6):1383–91.

[42] Maes BD, Lemahieu W, Kuypers D, et al. Differential effect of diarrhea on FK506 versus cyclosporine A trough levels and resultant prevention of allograft rejection in renal transplant recipients. Am J Transplant 2002;2(10):989–92.

[43] Alabdulkarim Z, Al-Jedai A, Alkortas D, et al. Efficacy and safety of three times daily dosing of tacrolimus in pediatric kidney transplantation patients: a single-center comparative study. Pediatr Transplant 2020;24(6):e13733.

[44] Cooney GF, Habucky K, Hoppu K. Cyclosporin pharmacokinetics in paediatric transplant recipients. Clin Pharmacokinet 1997;32(6):481–95.

[45] Wallemacq PE, Verbeeck RK. Comparative clinical pharmacokinetics of tacrolimus in paediatric and adult patients. Clin Pharmacokinet 2001;40(4):283–95.

[46] Burckart GJ, Venkataramanan R, Ptachcinski RJ, et al. Cyclosporine pharmacokinetic profiles in liver, heart, and kidney transplant patients as determined by high-performance liquid chromatography. Transplant Proc 1986;18(6 Suppl 5):129–36.

[47] Cellcept (mycophenolate mofetil) [package insert]. Nutley, NJ: Roche Laboratories Inc; 1998.

[48] Myfortic (mycophenolic acid) [package insert]. East hanover, NJ: Novartis Pharmaceuticals Corporation; 2009.

[49] Allison AC. Mechanisms of action of mycophenolate mofetil in preventing chronic rejection. Transplant Proc 2002;34(7):2863–6.

[50] Ettenger R, Bartosh S, Choi L, et al. Pharmacokinetics of enteric-coated mycophenolate sodium in stable pediatric renal transplant recipients. Pediatr Transplant 2005;9(6):780–7.

[51] Arns W. Noninfectious gastrointestinal (GI) complications of mycophenolic acid therapy: a consequence of local GI toxicity? Transplant Proc 2007;39(1):88–93.

[52] Bunchman T, Navarro M, Broyer M, et al. The use of mycophenolate mofetil suspension in pediatric renal allograft recipients. Pediatr Nephrol 2001;16(12):978–84.

[53] Hartling L, Bellemare S, Wiebe N, et al. Oral versus intravenous rehydration for treating dehydration due to gastroenteritis in children. Cochrane Database Syst Rev 2006;2006-(3):CD004390:Published 2006 Jul 19.

[54] Angarone M, Snydman DR, AST ID Community of Practice. Diagnosis and management of diarrhea in solid-organ transplant recipients: guidelines from the American society of transplantation infectious diseases community of practice. Clin Transplant 2019;33(9):e13550.

[55] What you need to know about mycophenolate use, first trimester pregnancy loss, and congenital malformations. Healthcare Provider Brochure. Mycophenolate REMS. Available at: https://www.mycophenolaterems.com/Resources/Docs/PrescriberProgramBrochur-e.pdf. Accessed September 26, 2024.

[56] Tönshoff B, David-Neto E, Ettenger R, et al. Pediatric aspects of therapeutic drug monitoring of mycophenolic acid in renal transplantation. Transplant Rev 2011;25(2):78–89.

[57] Imuran (azathioprine) [package insert]. Roswell, GA: Sebela Pharmaceuticals Inc; 2018.

[58] Relling MV, Schwab M, Whirl-Carrillo M, et al. Clinical pharmacogenetics implementation Consortium guideline for thiopurine dosing based on TPMT and NUDT15 genotypes: 2018 update. Clin Pharmacol Ther 2019;105(5):1095–105.

[59] Chandra A, Midtvedt K, Åsberg A, et al. Immunosuppression and reproductive health after kidney transplantation. Transplantation 2019;103(11):e325–33.

[60] Chae HH, Ahmed A, Bone JN, et al. Adrenal insufficiency in pediatric kidney transplantation recipients. Pediatr Transplant 2024;28(4):e14768.

[61] Oberholzer J, John E, Lumpaopong A, et al. Early discontinuation of steroids is safe and effective in pediatric kidney transplant recipients. Pediatr Transplant 2005;9(4):456–63.

[62] Kizilbash SJ, Jensen CJ, Kouri AM, et al. Steroid avoidance/withdrawal and maintenance immunosuppression in pediatric kidney transplantation. Pediatr Transplant 2022;26(2):e14189.

[63] Skauby RH, Bjerre A, Sæves I, et al. Prednisolone and prednisone pharmacokinetics in pediatric renal transplant recipients-A prospective study. Ther Drug Monit 2017;39(5):472–82.

[64] Al-Habet SM, Rogers HJ. Effect of food on the absorption and pharmacokinetics of prednisolone from enteric-coated tablets. Eur J Clin Pharmacol 1989;37(4):423–6.

[65] Caplan A, Fett N, Rosenbach M, et al. Prevention and management of glucocorticoid-induced side effects: a comprehensive review: ocular, cardiovascular, muscular, and psychiatric side effects and issues unique to pediatric patients. J Am Acad Dermatol 2017;76(2):201–7.

[66] Croitoru A, Balgradean M. Treatment-associated side effects in patients with steroid-dependent nephrotic syndrome. Maedica (Bucur) 2022;17(2):285–90.

[67] Pape L, Ahlenstiel T. mTOR inhibitors in pediatric kidney transplantation. Pediatr Nephrol 2014;29(7):1119–29.

[68] Tönshoff B, Ettenger R, Dello Strologo L, et al. Early conversion of pediatric kidney transplant patients to everolimus with reduced tacrolimus and steroid elimination: results of a randomized trial. Am J Transplant 2019;19(3):811–22.

[69] Stenton SB, Partovi N, Ensom MH. Sirolimus: the evidence for clinical pharmacokinetic monitoring. Clin Pharmacokinet 2005;44(8):769–86.

[70] Van Damme-Lombaerts R, Webb NA, Hoyer PF, et al. Single-dose pharmacokinetics and tolerability of everolimus in stable pediatric renal transplant patients. Pediatr Transplant 2002;6(2):147–52.

[71] RAPAMUNE (sirolimus) [package insert]. Philadelphia, PA: Pfizer, Inc; 2015.

[72] Almond CS, Sleeper LA, Rossano JW, et al. The teammate trial: study design and rationale tacrolimus and everolimus against tacrolimus and MMF in pediatric heart transplantation using the major adverse transplant event (MATE) score. Am Heart J 2023;260:100–12.

[73] Vincenti F, Rostaing L, Grinyo J, et al. Belatacept and long-term outcomes in kidney transplantation. N Engl J Med 2016;374(4):333–43 [published correction appears in N Engl J Med. 2016 Feb 18;374(7):698. doi: 10.1056/NEJMx160003].

[74] Kirk AD, Guasch A, Xu H, et al. Renal transplantation using belatacept without maintenance steroids or calcineurin inhibitors. Am J Transplant 2014;14(5):1142–51.

[75] Blew KH, Chua A, Foreman J, et al. Tailored use of belatacept in adolescent kidney transplantation. Am J Transplant 2020;20(3):884–8.

[76] Lerch C, Kanzelmeyer NK, Ahlenstiel-Grunow T, et al. Belatacept after kidney transplantation in adolescents: a retrospective study. Transpl Int 2017;30(5):494–501.

[77] NULOJIX (belatacept) for injection, for intravenous use [package insert]. Princeton, NJ: Bristol-Myers Squibb Company; 2011.

[78] Weber LT. Therapeutic drug monitoring in pediatric renal transplantation. Pediatr Nephrol 2015;30(2):253–65.

[79] Pant C, Deshpande A, Desai M, et al. Outcomes of Clostridium difficile infection in pediatric solid organ transplant recipients. Transpl Infect Dis 2016;18(1):31–6.

[80] Tsampalieros A, Knoll GA, Molnar AO, et al. Corticosteroid use and growth after pediatric solid organ transplantation: a systematic review and meta-analysis. Transplantation 2017;101(4):694–703.

[81] Grenda R, Watson A, Trompeter R, et al. A randomized trial to assess the impact of early steroid withdrawal on growth in pediatric renal transplantation: the TWIST study. Am J Transplant 2010;10(4):828–36.

[82] Steinberg EA, Moss M, Buchanan CL, et al. Adherence in pediatric kidney transplant recipients: solutions for the system. Pediatr Nephrol 2018;33(3):361–72.

[83] Chisholm-Burns MA, Spivey CA, Rehfeld R, et al. Immunosuppressant therapy adherence and graft failure among pediatric renal transplant recipients. Am J Transplant 2009;9(11):2497–504.

[84] Simons LE, Gilleland J, Blount RL, et al. Multidimensional Adherence Classification System: initial development with adolescent transplant recipients. Pediatr Transplant 2009;13(5):590–8.

[85] Kindem IA, Bjerre A, Hammarstrøm C, et al. Kidney-transplanted adolescents-nonadherence and graft outcomes during the transition phase: a nationwide analysis, 2000-2020. Transplantation 2023;107(5):1206–12.

[86] Richards VL, Johnson CK, Blosser CD, et al. Strategies to improve patient engagement in Young kidney transplant recipients: a review. Ann Transplant 2018;23:654–8.

[87] Katz DT, Torres NS, Chatani B, et al. Care of pediatric solid organ transplant recipients: an overview for primary care providers. Pediatrics 2020;146(6):e20200696.

[88] Pediatric transition portal. American society of transplantation. 2024. Available at: https://www.myast.org/pediatric-transition-portal. Accessed October 16, 2024.

[89] Molitor SJ, Aguilera V, Lerret S. Educational needs of the adolescent transplant recipient: a developmental approach to understanding transplant. Pediatr Transplant 2024;28(5):e14812.

[90] Aoki Y, Satoh H, Hamasaki Y, et al. Incidence of malignancy after pediatric kidney transplantation: a single-center experience over the past three decades in Japan. Clin Exp Nephrol 2022;26(3):294–302.

[91] Allen UD, Preiksaitis JK, AST Infectious Diseases Community of Practice. Post-transplant lymphoproliferative disorders, epstein-barr virus infection, and disease in solid organ transplantation: guidelines from the American society of transplantation infectious diseases community of practice. Clin Transplant 2019;33(9):e13652.

[92] Order KE, Rodig NM. Pediatric kidney transplantation: cancer and cancer risk. Semin Nephrol 2024;44(1):151501.

[93] Bae SR, Bicki A, Coufal S, et al. Cardiovascular disease risk factors and lifestyle modification strategies after pediatric kidney transplantation: what are we dealing with, and what can we target? Pediatr Nephrol 2023;38(3):663–71.

[94] Silverstein DM. Risk factors for cardiovascular disease in pediatric renal transplant recipients. Pediatr Transplant 2004;8(4):386–93.

Advances in Pediatrics 72 (2025) 219–234

ADVANCES IN PEDIATRICS

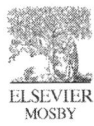

A Practical Approach to Functional Abdominal Pain and Irritable Bowel Syndrome in Children and Adolescents

Biren J. Desai, DO[a,b], Hannibal Person, MD[a,b,*]

[a]Department of Pediatrics, University of Washington, Seattle, WA, USA; [b]Division of Gastroenterology, Hepatology, and Nutrition, Seattle Children's Hospital, Seattle, WA, USA

Keywords

- Disorders of gut brain interaction (DGBI) • Functional disorders • Rome criteria
- Abdominal pain • Irritable bowel syndrome • Functional abdominal pain
- Pediatric • Adolescent

Key points

- Disorders of gut-brain interaction (DGBI), formally called functional gastrointestinal disorders, are common in children and adolescents, and not diagnoses of exclusion, requiring only the application of appropriate diagnostic criteria.
- DGBI should be conceptualized and relayed to the patient and family within the biopsychosocial model, taking into consideration the often-multifaceted nature of the genesis and maintenance of these disorders.
- There are a variety of treatment strategies for DGBI, ranging from lifestyle and dietary changes to neuromodulation, and care should be taken to personalize treatment to the needs and goals of the patient.

INTRODUCTION AND BACKGROUND

Disorders of gut-brain interaction (DGBI) are common in children and adolescents and describe a variety of conditions with gastrointestinal (GI) symptoms that lead to a substantial impact on health care utilization, psychosocial distress, and school absenteeism [1]. Previously called functional gastrointestinal disorders, this nomenclature has been changed to better represent the pathophysiology, increase patient acceptance of a DGBI diagnosis, and reduce stigma.

---

*Corresponding author. Division of Gastroenterology and Hepatology, Seattle Children's Hospital, 4800 Sand Point Way NE, MS OB.9.620.1, PO Box 5371, Seattle, WA 98145-5005. E-mail address: Hannibal.Person@seattlechildrens.org

https://doi.org/10.1016/j.yapd.2025.03.002

Abbreviations

ARFID	avoided restrictive food intake disorder
CBT	cognitive behavioral therapy
DGBI	disorders of gut brain interaction
FAP	functional abdominal pain
GI	gastroenterology
IBS	irritable bowel syndrome
PCP	primary care provider
PENFS	percutaneous electrical nerve field stimulation

General practice and pediatric gastroenterology clinics should expect to see patients with DGBI frequently. Additionally, there are comorbid chronic pain disorders including headaches, chronic musculoskeletal pain, and chronic pelvic pain as well as anxiety and depression [2]. The classification of these conditions has relied on the Rome criteria, which define the necessary symptom duration and symptom qualities in the diagnosis of all DGBI [3]. Over time, there has been refinement of the Rome criteria with the publication of Rome IV in 2016 as well as Rome V set to be released in 2026. As our understanding of these conditions has increased, there has been more precision in the diagnostic criteria, and these same criteria have supported ongoing scientific investigation into DGBI by more clearly defining disease states for inquiry.

The exact pathophysiology of DGBI remains unclear, and their genesis are multifactorial, including internal and external factors. Internal factors might include personal genetic susceptibility, postinfection, other gut inflammation, microbiome abnormalities, other physiologic disturbances, adverse childhood experiences, and a child's experience and response to pain [4]. Meanwhile, external stressors, cultural factors, and the caregiver's response to symptoms may be important external factors. For example, a child might develop irritable bowel syndrome with constipation (see definitions later in discussion) after an enteric infection, marked by inflammation and transient disruption of healthy gut mucosa, and changes in gut permeability and motility. The disease experience might be further heightened by the child psychologically interpreting symptoms, such as abdominal pain, as highly threatening to their wellbeing, possibly in the setting of a past adverse childhood experience. If that child then has a caregiver with health anxiety who continues to ask the child about their symptoms, seeks excessive medical evaluation and intervention, and models distress about the symptom process, the child may experience more persistent and significant symptoms as well as impaired functioning and development.

Definitions and diagnostic criteria

- *Disorders of Gut–Brain Interaction (DGBI)* - a group of disorders classified by GI symptoms related to any combination of motility disturbances, visceral hypersensitivity, altered mucosal and immune function, gut microbiota, and/or central nervous system [2–4].

- *Irritable Bowel Syndrome (IBS)* - Recurrent abdominal pain on average at least 1 day/week in the last 3 months, associated with 2 additional criteria (pain related to defecation, the associated change in frequency of stool, the associated change in appearance of stool as defined by the Bristol Stool Chart).
  - *IBS-Predominant Constipation subtype (IBS-C)* – greater than 25% of bowel movements as Bristol type 1 or 2 stools (consistent with constipation) and less than 25% of bowel movements as Bristol type 6 or 7 (consistent with diarrhea).
  - *IBS-Predominant Diarrhea subtype (IBS-D)* – greater than 25% of bowel movements as Bristol type 6 or 7 stools and less than 25% of bowel movements as Bristol type 1 or 2.
- *Functional Abdominal Pain* – At least 2 months of episodic or continuous abdominal pain that does not occur solely during physiologic events (eg, eating, stooling, menses) and cannot be explained by another medical condition but with insufficient criteria for irritable bowel syndrome, functional dyspepsia, or abdominal migraine.
- *Functional Dyspepsia* – At least one symptom for 2 months, which includes postprandial fullness, early satiation, epigastric pain, or burning not associated with defectaion.
- *Abdominal Migraine* – Must include all of the following and must occur at least twice:
  - Paroxysmal episodes of intense, acute periumbilical, midline, or diffuse abdominal pain lasting 1 hour or more (the most distressing symptom).
  - Episodes are separated by weeks to months.
  - Pain is incapacitating and interferes with normal activities.
  - Sterotypical pattern and symptoms in the individual patient.
  - The pain is associated with 2 or more of the following: anorexia, nausea, vomiting, headache, photophobia, pallor.
  - Symptoms cannot be explained by another medical condition.

Epidemiologic data for pediatric DGBI varies and is limited by most pediatric studies being survey-based, limited to select groups, and relying on nonrepresentative sampling. The worldwide pooled prevalence of functional abdominal pain was 13.5% and irritable bowel syndrome was 8.8% [1]. The prevalence was higher in South America (16.8%) and Asia (16.5%) compared with Europe (10.5%). Functional abdominal pain also occurs more frequently in females at 15.9% vs 11.5% in males [1]. When a child is experiencing a DGBI, quality of life scores (QoL) are significantly lower compared with healthy peers. Additionally, DGBI conditions were ranked as the second most common reason for school absence emphasizing not only the high prevalence of these disorders but their negative impact on both quality of life and functioning [5].

The purpose of this review article is to assist health care providers as they navigate the changing landscape of the diagnosis and treatment of DGBI [6]. This review article will focus on 2 specific diagnoses in the DGBI umbrella: irritable bowel syndrome (IBS) and functional abdominal pain (FAP). It is important to acknowledge that while literature to guide the evaluation and management of pediatric DGBI is growing, no one pathway in caring for pediatric patients with DGBI exists, and both potential medical testing and treatment decisions must be based on a comprehensive history and physical with a plan personalized to the patient and their caregiver/family. To help solidify these discussion points, we invite readers to review the later in discussion case presentation, which we will continue to reference as we discuss the evaluation and management of pediatric DGBI.

CASE PRESENTATION

Jeanie is a 16-year-old cisgender young woman who is seen by her primary care provider (PCP) for evaluation after experiencing symptoms of central abdominal pain and constipation for the past 2 months. She reports that after a camping trip with her family, she developed acute symptoms of low-grade fever, diffuse abdominal cramping, and nonbloody diarrhea for 5 days. While the abdominal pain gradually improved in severity and the diarrhea resolved, she then developed constipation, with Bristol 1 to 2 stools once to twice weekly. Her abdominal pain is central, nonradiating, and has been more manageable, though she has missed 4 days of school in the past 2 months due to pain. The pain is not associated with eating but is often associated with an urge to have a bowel movement. A warming pad and acetaminophen have been helpful. She started polyethylene glycol for constipation which has been successful in her achieving a Bristol 3 to 4 bowel movement daily, which is ideal, but she still complains of abdominal pain that is unchanged. She continues to eat and maintain her weight. There are no other concerning symptoms including hematochezia, vomiting, fevers, arthralgias, dysphagia, or odynophagia. Her physical examination is significant for a soft abdomen with mild tenderness to deep palpation throughout, no localization of pain, no organomegaly, and no mass.

DIAGNOSTIC EVALUATION

The diagnosis of pediatric DGBI relies on taking a comprehensive history and a complete physical examination, specifically assessing for symptoms or examination findings called "alarm symptoms" (Fig. 1) [4]. Alarm symptoms are more suggestive of the presence of an organic disorder and should prompt additional evaluation as indicated, though not every child with alarm symptoms will have a non-DGBI diagnosis. For example, a patient with IBS-C might report intermittent hematochezia, an alarm symptom, related to traumatic stooling in the setting of ongoing constipation despite having a DGBI. Diagnostic options for gastrointestinal disorders are broad, ranging from less-invasive serum, stool, breath, and radiographic evaluations, to more invasive endoscopic, manometry, and pH impedance testing. If diagnostics are pursued, it may be beneficial to perform a tiered and staggered approach based on how concerning the patient's symptoms are and the level of clinical suspicion. Discussion should occur with the patient and caregiver prior to ordering these studies that testing may be normal or nondiagnostically important, as some families may benefit from this expectation setting and early conversations about the possibility of DGBI. For example, a child with abdominal pain

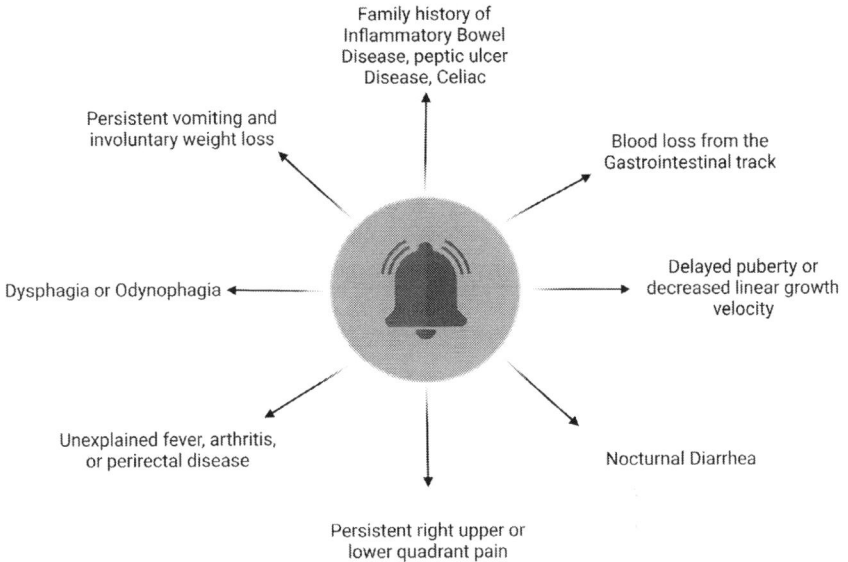

Fig. 1. Alarm symptoms requiring further investigation.

and chronic diarrhea may benefit from stool testing to assess for enteric infection or inflammation, but if this testing is reassuring and there are no alarm symptoms, endoscopic evaluation of the digestive system may not be needed. A child with unintentional weight loss and chronic abdominal pain may benefit from serum testing for nutritional deficiencies and screening for conditions such as celiac disease; however, in a child with isolated pain, no alarm symptoms, including weight loss, and a normal physical examination this testing might be best reserved if conservative intervention for DGBI is not successful in ameliorating their symptoms.

Decisions about the diagnostic evaluation of a child with DGBI can be challenging, as patients, and parents may be concerned about an organic condition and present to care expecting medical testing to be performed. Health care providers may feel reassured by negative results, yet the diagnosis of these conditions is largely based on a comprehensive history and physical examination and application of Rome IV diagnostic criteria. There is a difficult balance between wanting to rule out non-DGBI conditions and "not miss anything," and not wanting to contribute to overmedicalizing and potential iatrogenic harm. Currently, it is recommended to use laboratory testing, stool studies, imaging, and endoscopy sparingly [7]. In fact, it has been estimated that the diagnostic yield is just 3% when pursuing serum testing and abdominal ultrasound in pediatric patients with chronic abdominal pain without alarm symptoms [8].

Celiac serologies in the form of a total IgA level and tissue transglutaminase IgA (TTG-IgA) are appropriate if there is evidence of delayed puberty, decreased linear growth velocity, or weight loss. They can also be considered when a child has chronic abdominal pain and changes to their bowel habits, particularly chronic diarrhea [4]. Additionally, if there are bloody stools, a fecal calprotectin can help inform the decision to move forward with a referral to gastroenterology for the consideration of an esophagogastroduodenoscopy (EGD) and colonoscopy. Of note, it is important to appropriately counsel families on how to collect and submit a fecal specimen for calprotectin testing, as literature has showed the molecule assessed in the assay can degrade at room temperature [9]. Advising families to submit a fresh stool sample to the laboratory for this testing or refrigerating the specimen prior to submission if there will be a delay is important in ensuring a false negative result from an inappropriately stored specimen does not occur. It should be noted that excessive diagnostic evaluation with multiple repeated studies that have been normal can cause iatrogenic harm to a patient and lead to delays in proper diagnosis and treatment [10].

The biopsychosocial model

The biopsychosocial model is a valuable tool in conceptualizing and managing DGBI, as it examines and integrates the biological, social, and psychological aspects of illness. The model gained popularity in the 1970s after George Engel described its utility to address the social and psychological components of illness that are sometimes neglected [11]. Over time, the biopsychosocial model has gained traction, and it has been used more readily in the health care realm. The model relies on patient and provider participation with the goal of pinpointing other contributing factors to an individual's disease state [12]. The model's primary goal is to understand the genesis of a disease process by looking at biological factors, psychological factors (thoughts, feelings, emotions), and social factors (relationships, support systems, stress). It relies on providers taking a comprehensive history during their evaluations. When a provider can pinpoint concerns in any of the 3 spheres, it offers the opportunity for intervention on modifiable factors, which in turn will help improve the disease state. Additionally, patient education and understanding of nonmodifiable factors can still be helpful in building their insight into the condition and supporting their personal agency in disease management.

Once a diagnosis of a DGBI is established, it is crucial that the diagnostic conversation focus on validating symptoms and patient experiences, clearly and positively communicating the diagnosis, and providing education [13]. Further, patients will often benefit from regular provider follow-up to continue to build a therapeutic treatment relationship and re-evaluate response to treatment. The Rome Foundation has many provider resources that can lead to successful conversations when discussing a DGBI diagnosis, which in turn are thought to improve patient health outcomes [14].

Revisiting our case presentation

Jeanie's PCP recognizes she meets the criteria for postinfection irritable bowel syndrome with constipation (IBS-C). This is supported by her lack of alarm symptoms, reassuring examination, and predisposing history of enteric infection. It is also supported by the fact that even with polyethylene glycol and regular Bristol 3 to 4 bowel movements, she is still having pain, speaking against a diagnosis of functional constipation whereby pain would be alleviated by the resolution of the constipation. Jeanie's PCP provides reassurance as part of a diagnostic conversation, validating the pain Jeanie has been experiencing and relaying she meets the criteria for a DGBI called IBS-C. In a shared discussion, Jeanie, her parents, and her PCP decide to defer laboratories, stool studies, and referral to gastroenterology. By implementing the biopsychosocial model in their discussion, Jeanie's PCP was able to learn that Jeanie's mother was prone to abdominal pain as a child as well and ultimately diagnosed with IBS-C after an exhaustive diagnostic evaluation that led to worsening anxiety. Jeanie has also been thinking about career opportunities and has had lower self-esteem when comparing herself to her peers who she feels are smarter. If Jeanie pursues higher education, she will be the first member of her family to attend college, which Jeanie privately notes to her PCP as a source of added stress, creating even more tension when she misses school because of her abdominal pain.

TREATMENT OPTIONS

After a diagnosis has been made, it is important to partner with patients and their families to find the treatment regimen that is most likely to be beneficial, with the understanding that no 2 individuals are the same. Some providers and families struggle to navigate the landscape of treatment options (Fig. 2). Providers should initially focus on understanding symptom severity, which symptoms are the most bothersome, minimize polypharmacy, and set expectations

Therapies					
Lifestyle	**Diet**	**Psychological Therapies**	**Microbiome**	**Medications**	**Other**
Sleep Hygiene	Consult with Dietician	Cognitive Behavioral Therapy	*Lactobacillus rhamnosus* and *Lactobacillus reuteri*	Cyproheptadine	Percutaneous electrical nerve field stimulation
Stress Management	Evaluate for disordered eating (ARFID)	Hypnotherapy		Tricyclic antidepressants	
Diaphragmatic breathing		Biofeedback	Rifaximin	Enteric Peppermint	
Physical Therapy	Soluble fiber		Fecal microbiota transplant	Antipsychotics	
Acupuncture and Massage	Gluten free/ dietary restriction			SNRIs	
			Prebiotics and post biotics	SSRIs	
Exercise	Low FODMAPs			Gabapentin	
Yoga				Hyoscyamine and Dicyclomine	
Dance					

Fig. 2. Therapies for DGBI conditions.

as DGBI symptoms often vacillate, which may be confusing as to whether the patient is experiencing a therapeutic response. It is helpful to maximize non-pharmacologic treatments in attempts to minimize polypharmacy. The non-pharmacologic strategies can continue on an ongoing basis for the patient's self-management of DGBI beyond their possible need for pharmacologic or other therapies. Additionally, typical nonpharmacologic approaches to DGBI, including stress reduction exercises, exercise, and dietary modification may offer more global benefits to the patient beyond gut-specific therapies.

Over the course of the last 30 years, there have been an increasing number of therapies for the various DGBI. Unfortunately, given the nature of these conditions and lack of objective physiologic markers, drug studies are sometimes confounded by the robust placebo effects seen in DGBI, difficulties generalizing outcomes to the heterogeneous pediatric DGBI population, and reliance on patient and caregiver symptom reporting [15].

Therapies are commonly grouped into several categories including changes to lifestyle, diet, psychological therapies, interventions that impact the microbiome, and medications. Additionally, there are other therapies becoming available, such as percutaneous electrical nerve field stimulation (PENFS), which involves the transmission of electrical impulses to cranial nerve bundles in multiple pain disorders [16]. The most common therapies used for the management of pediatric FAP and IBS are listed in Fig. 2. The multiple treatment options available for DGBI conditions allow for the creation of a tailored therapeutic plan based on each individual patient, focusing on their most bothersome symptoms and the family's treatment goals and preferences. It is important to note these therapies are used in other chronic pain conditions, and consideration should be taken to maximize the benefits of any treatment modality in not only managing GI symptoms but also other pain conditions. For example, many patients with DGBI will also experience a headache disorder, and some DGBI medications also are used as headache prophylaxis.

Lifestyle modifications

It is often considered best practice to maximize lifestyle changes to avoid polypharmacy and adverse drug reactions from medications. Lifestyle modifications that promote behavior activation can be helpful as they promote the restoration of functionality and protect against descending into disability and maladaptive responses [17]. Put simply, behavioral activation involves an individual increasing participation in positive activities and decreasing participation in negative activities and has been well-studied in both pediatric and adult mood disorders. In both primary care and subspecialty settings, a health care professional can coach a patient and encourage more participation in positive activities to build feelings of accomplishment and mastery to support their functionality and work to reduce disability [18].

Sleep hygiene has not only been shown to improve all DGBI conditions but there are overall health benefits [19]. Patients also report improved symptoms with stress management techniques, diaphragmatic breathing, exercise, and physical therapy [20]. Diaphragmatic breathing is easy to teach in an ambulatory setting and provides the patient with an easily accessible tool to manage symptoms of abdominal pain, bloating, and nausea [20]. Select patients have improved when pursuing acupuncture and massage, though the evidence is limited. There is also less evidence for the use of yoga and dance, but it is important to encourage patients to trial these modifications as they may have benefits [21,22].

Dietary modifications

In general, there are no specific dietary changes that have been documented to be universally helpful, but patients often find clinical benefit in having a discussion with a dietitian. Patients should be encouraged to chew their food well and avoid irritating foods (caffeine, carbonated beverages, spicy, fatty foods). There is conflicting data about the utility of a low FODMAP diet (Fermentable Oligo-, Di- and Mono-saccharides and Polyols, which refers to choosing foods that have a lower content of fermentable sugars), but can be useful if the main symptom is bloating [23]. Soluble fiber, such as Benefiber or Metamuscil, is particularly helpful for IBS-C and functional constipation [24]. Many patients may also benefit from a discussion clarifying the difference between food sensitivities (difficulty digesting) and allergies (immune system activation via IgE mechanisms), as this may lead to unnecessary restricted eating. When counseling on dietary therapies, it is important to avoid the over-restriction of foods as it can encourage disordered eating, such as Avoided Restrictive Food Intake Disorder (ARFID, whereby individuals are extremely selective eaters and often with little interest in eating) which has been a bourgeoning problem in the post-COVID era for unclear reasons [25–27]. For this reason, consultation with a dietitian can be helpful in establishing the patient's current nutritional intake versus their needs and avoiding overly restrictive diets that can lead to nutritional deficiencies. In certain situations, when disordered eating such as ARFID, anorexia nervosa, and bulimia is suspected, referral should be made to appropriate care for the condition prior to any consideration of dietary modification to address GI symptoms.

Psychological therapies

Psychological therapies, such as cognitive behavioral therapy (CBT) and hypnotherapy are helpful to many patients and have the strongest evidence base for the management of pediatric FAP and IBS [28]. CBT was originally developed to help treat depression, but its applications have since been diversified. Through CBT, patients can better recognize associations of situations, thoughts, emotions, behaviors, sensations, and maladaptive behaviors. As patients are better able to pinpoint these triggers, they can begin challenging these disordered thoughts [28]. The core of CBT involves psychoeducation, and this education empowers the patient through demystifying their symptom process and encouraging them to consistently engage in concrete strategies to feel better. The exact mechanism for the utility of hypnotherapy is unknown. This treatment modality first requires patients to learn how to achieve and deepen a hypnotic state, thus promoting relaxation. Subsequent sessions involve gut-focused imagery and hypnotic suggestions emphasizing a cooperative and appropriate relationship between the brain and the digestive system. Hypnosis also provides relaxation and other self-hypnosis skills to practice at home [28]. Currently, there are no set protocols for the number of sessions needed to promote recovery, and are limited by the relationship a patient develops with their psychologist, time, cost, and patient acceptance of this therapeutic modality. Psychological therapies are particularly helpful in patients with co-morbid anxiety and depression [28]. It should be noted that there is currently a lack of access to GI psychologists, who are trained and have an interest in treating DGBI-related conditions, at the national level. Community mental health providers may not always be well-versed in these specific treatments and can cause iatrogenic harm by reinforcing maladaptive behaviors, such as hypervigilance of bodily symptoms or seeking medical evaluation for ongoing DGBI symptoms.

Microbiome

There has been an increased interest in the role of the microbiome in DGBI conditions; there appears to be bidirectional signaling between the GI tract and brain via the vagus nerve, the hypothalamic-pituitary-adrenal axis, immune, and metabolic pathways which all interconnect to the microbiome. It has been hypothesized that dysbiosis, or imbalance of microbial populations in the intestinal tract, is part of the pathogenesis of DGBI diagnoses [29]. There is mixed evidence for probiotics such as *Lactobacillus rhammosus* GG and *Lactobacillus reuteri* in IBS [30]. There is no current evidence for prebiotics (non-digestible food ingredients that promote the growth of beneficial bacteria), postbiotics (bioactive compounds produced by beneficial bacteria ex-vivo), synbiotics (combination of prebiotics and probiotics), or fecal microbiota transplants.

Medications

Medications for DGBI include agents acting on the peripheral, central, and the enteric nervous systems [31]. Antispasmodics available in the United States of America include hyoscyamine and dicyclomine. It is postulated that they exhibit their effect by relaxing the smooth muscle surrounding the digestive system via anticholinergic mechanisms to reduce pain. There is no evidence to support their use for pediatric FAP or IBS, though they are still commonly used for short-term pain relief. It should be noted that their anticholinergic properties can cause side effects including worsening constipation.

Cyproheptadine is thought to be helpful via several pathways including acting as an antihistamine, anticholinergic, and an anti-serotonergic. Cyproheptadine notably stimulates appetite and helps reduce pain in functional abdominal pain disorder [32]. Use is sometimes limited by its sedating properties and constipation. It can also be helpful in chronic nausea, functional dyspepsia and prophylaxis against headaches [33].

Peppermint promotes the relaxation of intestinal smooth muscle via blockade of calcium channels and helps reduce abdominal pain and improves quality of life [34] in patients with functional abdominal pain. It comes in different formulations including an enteric peppermint preparation, which is preferred because it facilitates effective delivery to the intestines. Enteric peppermint should be avoided in those patients with gastrointestinal reflux disorder (GERD) as it will lower the tone of the lower esophageal sphincter and may worsen reflux symptoms [6].

There has been increased attention paid to the use of neuromodulators, which are medications that have both central and peripheral nervous system effects, and which have been found to reduce pain and other gastrointestinal symptoms. Many of these medications were formerly called psychotropics (anti-depressants, anti-psychotics); however, their name was changed in the management of DGBI and other chronic pain disorders to better represent their mechanism of action and reduce stigma toward medications identified for psychiatric indications. Tricyclic antidepressants (TCAs) have been found to be helpful in patients with refractory GI symptoms, however, use is often limited by anticholinergic side effects. Their use also requires monitoring for QTc prolongation [31,35–37]. Of selective serotonin reuptake inhibitors (SSRI), citalopram is the most studied and seems to be most helpful in patients with comorbid depression, anxiety, or obsessive-compulsive disorder [38]. SNRIs, such as Venlafaxine and Duloxetine, on the other hand, have been helpful for pain control and mood disorders and are approved by the Food and Drug Administration for children ages 7 and above with generalized anxiety disorder, and ages 13 and above with chronic musculoskeletal pain [39–42]. There is no pediatric evidence for their use in FAP and IBS, though it is believed their shared noradrenergic properties with amitriptyline explain their pain reduction benefit in other chronic pain conditions.

Other agents such as mirtazapine, buspirone, atypical antipsychotics, such as olanzapine and quetiapine, and delta ligand agents, such as gabapentin and pregabalin, have also been explored in pediatric DGBI. There is limited literature both in pediatrics and adults for their use, and they are often used off-label in patients with more severe and refractory DGBI symptoms. Anecdotally, mirtazapine, an atypical anti-depressant with serotonergic properties, is helpful for chronic nausea and aids in sleep initiation and promoting appetite. Buspirone, an azapirone serotonin agonist, can be helpful for esophageal sensitivity and dyspepsia, though is widely used as a treatment for anxiety. Atypical antipsychotics may aid sleep and be helpful for digestive symptoms via serotonergic mechanisms. Delta ligand agents, such as gabapentin and pregabalin, may impact both the central nervous system and peripheral nerves of the enteric nervous system to reduce gastrointestinal sensation and are often best used for chronic abdominal wall pain. The use of these agents is often challenging given the need for clinical monitoring while on these therapies and their side-effect profiles. Additionally, it is often difficult to pinpoint a specific practitioner who would be responsible for prescribing and monitoring the response to these agents. Consultation with a neurogastroenterologist, pain specialist, or behavioral health care practitioner may be helpful in guiding therapy decision-making and monitoring [25,26,43].

Other neuromodulation therapies

PENFS has also been used to treat DGBI [16]. It involves the nonsurgical placement of a device (worn for several sequential weeks) that sends electrical impulses to cranial nerves [44]. This therapy is currently FDA approved for children as young as 11 years of age with IBS, whereby there is the best evidence for this therapeutic modality [44]. The mechanism of action is unclear, but the effect seems to be mediated by the central nervous system, including the modification of cranial nerve output to the gut [16].

Bowel medications

Management with bowel medications is common in patients suffering from IBS who are experiencing either constipation, diarrhea, or both. Medications are typically classified as laxatives or antidiarrheal, though caution should be exercised in patients with mixed bowel symptoms as these therapies may precipitate worsening diarrhea or constipation. Common laxatives used include polyethylene glycol, lactulose, milk of magnesia, bisacodyl, and senna. All these therapies are over the counter and can be titrated to effect for each individual patient. For antidiarrheal, the most common treatments are loperamide and bismuth subsalicylate [45]. Care should be taken in any patient with new diarrhea, as anti-diarrheal are contraindicated in the setting of enteric infection or inflammatory bowel disease. Newer therapies for IBS-C and functional constipation include linaclotide (aguanylate cyclase-C agonists) [46]. For IBS-D, newer options include bile acid sequestrants (Cholestyramine and Colestipol), serum-derived bovine immunoglobulin/protein isolate (a medical food product), and glutamine [47].

Revisiting our case presentation

Jeanie opts to trial lifestyle modifications and dietary changes. She was initially successful with a combination of exercise, hydration, and increased dietary or soluble fiber. She was referred to outpatient psychological services and did not find a meaningful therapeutic relationship with her first psychologist. At the encouragement of her PCP, Jeanie sought treatment with a second psychologist and underwent a productive 8 sessions of CBT. She felt like she learned coping and relaxation skills to address her feelings of inadequacy when comparing herself to her friends and dealing with the pressure of trying to be the first person in her family to attend college. Two years later, Jeanie matriculated into her first-choice undergraduate institution and initially had challenges maintaining her previous dietary/lifestyle changes living on campus, with her prime symptom being constipation. After additional shared decision-making discussions, Jeanie agreed to try medications and had an excellent therapeutic response to linaclotide, which works by activating guanylate cyclase-C receptors.

FUTURE CONSIDERATIONS

There are ongoing efforts to improve the care for children and adolescents with DGBI who often face a lack of recognition of these conditions, unnecessary medical testing, and inadequate treatment opportunities. Future work in pediatric DGBI should include professional society-sponsored guidelines to better support health care professionals in providing evidence-based assessment and management. There is also a need to have multi-institutional research that leads to increased therapeutic options and better personalization of therapies as well as expand options for the preventive management of DGBI. It is also important to note the dearth of information to help inform patients and their caregivers about navigating school and other social obligations as well as the lack of clear systems for the transfer of medical care from pediatric to adult settings. Further, there are growing concerns about workforce shortages in both the primary care and specialty care settings [48], with many institutions facing shortages of dedicated pediatric psychology providers as well as pediatric gastroenterology physicians [49,50]. Given these shortages, it is important we provide prompt the recognition and effective management of these conditions to prevent further patient disability and health care utilization while engaging the public to better understand these conditions with the goal of increasing patient acceptance of DGBI diagnosis and reducing stigma.

SUMMARY

DGBI conditions are commonly encountered in clinical practice, which requires providers to be familiar with diagnostic criteria and common treatments. The diagnosis relies heavily on history gathering, physical examination, and using the biopsychosocial model, and less on diagnostic tests. It is important to exclude red flag/alarm symptoms in the history, which, if present, would compel further diagnostic workup. When a diagnosis is made, the patient's symptoms should be validated to help build a collaborative and productive relationship between patients, families, and practitioners. When considering treatment options, it is desirable to maximize lifestyle and dietary therapies and consider medical therapies as appropriate while monitoring for adverse drug reactions and polypharmacy.

CLINICS CARE POINTS

- When making a diagnosis within the DGBI umbrella, it is important to review diagnostic criteria and obtain a detailed history using the biopsychosocial model. Once a diagnosis is made, it should be delivered confidently with patients and their families.

- Treatment for functional abdominal pain must be individualized for each patient and can involve a combination of lifestyle changes, medication, and psychotherapy.

- Red flag gastrointestinal symptoms should typically prompt appropriate evaluation for a non-DGBI disorder.

- It is important to be remain aware of the possibility of iatrogenic harm through unecessary medical testing or pharmacotherapy in this population.

Disclosures

The authors have no disclosures. The authors have no pertinent sources of funding related to this article

References

[1] Korterink JJ, Diederen K, Benninga MA, et al. Epidemiology of pediatric functional abdominal pain disorders: a meta-analysis. PLoS One 2015;10(5):e0126982.

[2] Sperber AD, Bangdiwala SI, Drossman DA, et al. Worldwide prevalence and burden of functional gastrointestinal disorders, results of Rome foundation global study. Gastroenterology 2021;160(1):99–114.e3.

[3] Schmulson MJ, Drossman DA. What is new in Rome IV. J Neurogastroenterol Motil 2017;23(2):151–63.

[4] Hyams JS, Di Lorenzo C, Saps M, et al. Functional disorders: children and adolescents. Gastroenterology 2016;S0016-5085(16):00181-5.

[5] Youssef NN, Atienza K, Langseder AL, et al. Chronic abdominal pain and depressive symptoms: analysis of the national longitudinal study of adolescent health. Clin Gastroenterol Hepatol 2008;6(3):329–32.

[6] Rexwinkel R, de Bruijn CMA, Gordon M, et al. Pharmacologic treatment in functional abdominal pain disorders in children: a systematic review. Pediatrics 2021;147(6):e2020042101.

[7] Lacy BE, Parikh M, Taylor DC, et al. S512 prevalence and impact of abdominal symptoms in patients with IBS-C. Am J Gastroenterol 2021;116(1):S229–30.

[8] Llanos-Chea A, Saps M. Utility of diagnostic tests in children with functional abdominal pain disorders. Gastroenterol Hepatol 2019;15(8):414–22.

[9] Haisma SM, van Rheenen PF, Wagenmakers L, et al. Calprotectin instability may lead to undertreatment in children with IBD. Arch Dis Child 2020;105(10):996–8.

[10] Reedy RA, Filipp SL, Gurka MJ, et al. Utility of esophagogastroduodenoscopy in the evaluation of uncomplicated abdominal pain in children. Glob Pediatr Health 2019;6:2333794X19898345.

[11] Wade DT, Halligan PW. The biopsychosocial model of illness: a model whose time has come. Clin Rehabil 2017;31(8):995–1004.

[12] Madani S, Parikh S, Madani RS, et al. Long-term study of children with ROME III functional gastrointestinal disorders managed symptomatically in a biopsychosocial model. Gastroenterol Res 2017;10(2):84–91.

[13] Luo Y, Shah BJ, Keefer LA. Special considerations for the management of disorders of gut-brain interaction in older adults. Curr Treat Options Gastroenterol 2022;20(4):582–93.

[14] Drossman DA, Chang L, Deutsch JK, et al. A review of the evidence and recommendations on communication skills and the patient-provider relationship: A Rome foundation working team report. Gastroenterology 2021;161(5):1670–88.e7.

[15] Nurko S, Saps M, Kossowsky J, et al. Effect of open-label placebo on children and adolescents with functional abdominal pain or irritable bowel syndrome: a randomized clinical trial. JAMA Pediatr 2022;176(4):349.

[16] Kovacic K, Hainsworth K, Sood M, et al. Neurostimulation for abdominal pain-related functional gastrointestinal disorders in adolescents: a randomised, double-blind, sham-controlled trial. Lancet Gastroenterol Hepatol 2017;2(10):727–37.

[17] Ciharova M, Furukawa TA, Efthimiou O, et al. Cognitive restructuring, behavioral activation and cognitive-behavioral therapy in the treatment of adult depression: a network meta-analysis. J Consult Clin Psychol 2021;89(6):563–74.

[18] Malik K, Ibrahim M, Bernstein A, et al. Behavioral Activation as an "active ingredient" of interventions addressing depression and anxiety among young people: a systematic review and evidence synthesis. BMC Psychol 2021;9(1):150.

[19] Robbertz AS, Shneider C, Cohen LL, et al. Sleep problems in pediatric disorders of gut-brain interaction: a systematic review. J Pediatr Psychol 2023;48(9):778–86.

[20] Burgell RE, Hoey L, Norton K, et al. Treating disorders of brain-gut interaction with multidisciplinary integrated care. Moving towards a new standard of care. JGH Open Open Access J Gastroenterol Hepatol 2024;8(5):e13072.

[21] Högström S, Philipson A, Ekstav L, et al. Dance and yoga reduced functional abdominal pain in young girls: a randomized controlled trial. Eur J Pain Lond Engl 2022;26(2): 336–48.

[22] Okawa Y. A discussion of whether various lifestyle changes can alleviate the symptoms of irritable bowel syndrome. Healthc Basel Switz 2022;10(10):2011.

[23] Altobelli E, Del Negro V, Angeletti PM, et al. Low-FODMAP diet improves irritable bowel syndrome symptoms: a meta-analysis. Nutrients 2017;9(9):940.

[24] Menon J, Thapa BR, Kumari R, et al. Efficacy of oral psyllium in pediatric irritable bowel syndrome: a double-blind randomized control trial. J Pediatr Gastroenterol Nutr 2023;76(1): 14–9.

[25] Chumpitazi BP, Cope JL, Hollister EB, et al. Randomised clinical trial: gut microbiome biomarkers are associated with clinical response to a low FODMAP diet in children with the irritable bowel syndrome. Aliment Pharmacol Ther 2015;42(4):418–27.

[26] Thomassen RA, Luque V, Assa A, et al. An ESPGHAN position paper on the use of low-FODMAP diet in pediatric gastroenterology. J Pediatr Gastroenterol Nutr 2022;75(3): 356–68.

[27] Altomare A, Di Rosa C, Imperia E, et al. Diarrhea predominant-irritable bowel syndrome (IBS-D): effects of different nutritional patterns on intestinal dysbiosis and symptoms. Nutrients 2021;13(5):1506.

[28] Person H, Keefer L. Brain-gut therapies for pediatric functional gastrointestinal disorders and inflammatory bowel disease. Curr Gastroenterol Rep 2019;21(4):12.

[29] Sasso JM, Ammar RM, Tenchov R, et al. Gut microbiome-brain alliance: a landscape view into mental and gastrointestinal health and disorders. ACS Chem Neurosci 2023;14(10): 1717–63.

[30] Hillestad EMR, van der Meeren A, Nagaraja BH, et al. Gut bless you: the microbiota-gut-brain axis in irritable bowel syndrome. World J Gastroenterol 2022;28(4):412–31.

[31] Drossman DA, Tack J, Ford AC, et al. Neuromodulators for functional gastrointestinal disorders (disorders of gut-brain interaction): A Rome foundation working team report. Gastroenterology 2018;154(4):1140–71.e1.

[32] Madani S, Cortes O, Thomas R. Cyproheptadine use in children with functional gastrointestinal disorders. J Pediatr Gastroenterol Nutr 2016;62(3):409–13.

[33] Krasaelap A, Madani S. Cyproheptadine: a potentially effective treatment for functional gastrointestinal disorders in children. Pediatr Ann 2017;46(3):e120–5.

[34] Chumpitazi BP, Kearns GL, Shulman RJ. Review article: the physiological effects and safety of peppermint oil and its efficacy in irritable bowel syndrome and other functional disorders. Aliment Pharmacol Ther 2018;47(6):738–52.

[35] Bahar RJ, Collins BS, Steinmetz B, et al. Double-blind placebo-controlled trial of amitriptyline for the treatment of irritable bowel syndrome in adolescents. J Pediatr 2008;152(5):685–9.

[36] Saps M, Youssef N, Miranda A, et al. Multicenter, randomized, placebo-controlled trial of amitriptyline in children with functional gastrointestinal disorders. Gastroenterology 2009;137(4):1261–9.

[37] Seetharaman J, Poddar U, Yachha SK, et al. Efficacy of amitriptyline in pediatric functional abdominal pain disorders: a randomized placebo-controlled trial. J Gastroenterol Hepatol 2022;37(4):685–91.

[38] Roohafza H, Pourmoghaddas Z, Saneian H, et al. Citalopram for pediatric functional abdominal pain: a randomized, placebo-controlled trial. Neuro Gastroenterol Motil 2014;26(11):1642–50.

[39] Bonilla S, Nurko S. Focus on the use of antidepressants to treat pediatric functional abdominal pain: current perspectives. Clin Exp Gastroenterol 2018;11:365–72.

[40] Zar-Kessler CAM, Belkind-Gerson J, Bender S, et al. Treatment of functional abdominal pain with antidepressants: benefits, adverse effects, and the gastroenterologist's role. J Pediatr Gastroenterol Nutr 2017;65(1):16–21.

[41] Friedman G. Treatment of the irritable bowel syndrome. Gastroenterol Clin North Am 1991;20(2):325–33.

[42] Khalilian A, Ahmadimoghaddam D, Saki S, et al. A randomized, double-blind, placebo-controlled study to assess efficacy of mirtazapine for the treatment of diarrhea predominant irritable bowel syndrome. Biopsychosoc Med 2021;15(1):3.

[43] BouSaba J, Sannaa W, Camilleri M. Pain in irritable bowel syndrome: does anything really help? Neuro Gastroenterol Motil 2022;34(1):e14305.

[44] Karrento K, Zhang L, Conley W, et al. Percutaneous electrical nerve field stimulation improves comorbidities in children with cyclic vomiting syndrome. Front Pain Res Lausanne Switz 2023;4:1203541.

[45] Arnold MJ. Medications for irritable bowel syndrome: guidelines from the AGA. Am Fam Physician 2023;108(5):527–9.

[46] Baaleman DF, Gupta S, Benninga MA, et al. The use of linaclotide in children with functional constipation or irritable bowel syndrome: a retrospective Chart review. Paediatr Drugs 2021;23(3):307–14.

[47] Trinkley KE, Nahata MC. Medication management of irritable bowel syndrome. Digestion 2014;89(4):253–67.

[48] Ahmed H, Carmody JB. On the looming physician shortage and strategic expansion of graduate medical education. Cureus 2020;12(7):e9216.

[49] Sauer CG, Barnard JA, Vinci RJ, et al. Child health needs and the pediatric gastroenterology workforce: 2020-2040. Pediatrics 2024;153(Suppl 2):e2023063678K.

[50] Orr CJ, McCartha E, Vinci RJ, et al. Projecting the future pediatric subspecialty workforce: summary and recommendations. Pediatrics 2024;153(Suppl 2):e2023063678T.

Advances in Pediatrics 72 (2025) 235–244

ADVANCES IN PEDIATRICS

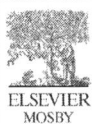

A Review of Wolff-Parkinson-White for the General Practitioner

Ismael Corral, MD, MBA[a,b,*],
Cherlyn Angela Perez-Corral, MD, MPP[c]

[a]Pediatric Cardiology, Department of Pediatrics, Los Angeles County Department of Health Services, Harbor-UCLA Medical Center, Torrance, CA, USA; [b]Pediatric Cardiology, Department of Pediatrics, Los Angeles County Department of Health Services, Olive View-UCLA Medical Center, Sylmar, CA, USA; [c]Department of Medicine, Los Angeles County Department of Health Services, Harbor-UCLA Medical Center, 1000 West Carson Street, Box #400, Torrance, CA 90509, USA

Keywords
- Wolff-Parkinson-White • Sudden cardiac death • Sudden cardiac arrest
- Arrhythmia • Tachyarrhythmia • Ventricular pre-excitation
- Ventricular preexcitation • WPW • VPE

Key points

- Review of Wolff-Parkinson-White (WPW) for the general practitioner.
- Understand how to identify and diagnose WPW on the surface electrocardiogram.
- Understand the importance of risk stratification of these patients.
- Develop a basic understanding of the treatment modalities.
- Have an overall understanding of the outcomes in these patients.

INTRODUCTION

The first description of Wolff-Parkinson-White (WPW) syndrome was published in the *American Heart Journal* in 1930 by Drs Wolff, Parkinson, and White. They described patients who had a short PR interval, widened QRS, and paroxysmal supraventricular tachycardia (PSVT) [1,2].

In the normal heart, the atrial and ventricles are insulated from one another. The conduction system, which consists of specialized cardiomyocytes, creates a

*Corresponding author. Harbor-UCLA Medical Center, Box #468 1000 West Carson Street, Torrance, CA 90502-2004. *E-mail address:* icorral@dhs.lacounty.gov

https://doi.org/10.1016/j.yapd.2025.03.007
0065-3101/25/

Abbreviations

AP	accessory pathway
AV	atrioventricular
AVRT	atrioventricular reentrant tachycardia
EPS	electrophysiology study
EST	exercise stress test
HRS	Heart Rhythm Society
PSVT	paroxysmal supraventricular tachycardia
RFA	radiofrequency ablation
SA	sinoatrial
SCD	sudden cardiac death
SPERRI	shortest preexcited R-R interval
TEEPS	transesophageal EP study
VPE	ventricular preexcitation
WPW	Wolff-Parkinson-White

method of communication that allows for cardiac synchronization of the upper and lower chambers, respectively [3]. This specialized tract includes the sinoatrial (SA) node, atrioventricular (AV) node, the bundle of His, and the ventricular network known as the Purkinje fibers. The SA node, also known as the cardiac pacemaker, initiates a wave of atrial depolarization which travels through the atria via internodal tracts to the AV node. The AV node is responsible for delay of the impulse propagation, followed by rapid distribution to the ventricles through the bundle of His and Purkinje fibers [4].

Patients with the aforementioned electrocardiogram (ECG) abnormality and no PSVT are classified as having asymptomatic ventricular preexcitation (VPE) or WPW pattern. In cases where there are episodes of PSVT, this is recognized as WPW syndrome [1].

The hallmark of VPE is anterograde conduction via an anomalous bypass or accessory pathway (AP) that is not part of the His-Purkinje pathway. This results in early ventricular depolarization that occurs before the normal His-Purkinje system leading to baseline ECG findings of a short PR interval, δ-wave (slurred QRS upstroke) resulting in a prolonged QRS duration (Fig. 1). Asymptomatic patients with these findings on a resting ECG are commonly defined as having asymptomatic WPW or VPE [5–8].

In rare cases, the presence of an AP in patients with WPW can result in sudden cardiac death (SCD) during atrial fibrillation (AFib). Antegrade conduction occurs through the AP leading to a high ventricular rate with the potential to deteriorate into ventricular fibrillation and death [9]. Although rare, the risk of SCD makes recognizing and understanding the need for further assessment in children and adolescents imperative for the general practitioner.

EPIDEMIOLOGY

The prevalence of WPW varies between asymptomatic WPW and WPW syndrome. With regards to asymptomatic WPW, the prevalence is estimated at 0.13% to 0.25% in the general population [5,10–13]. In patients with

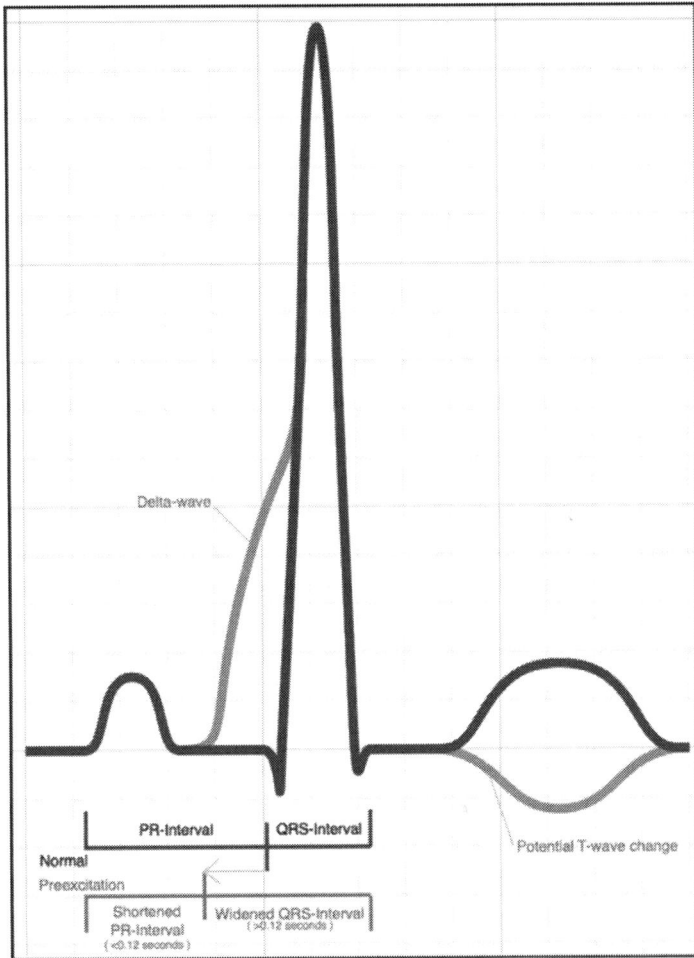

Fig. 1. ECG changes in WPW syndrome [5]. Walter Hoyt, Christopher S. Snyder, The asymptomatic Wolff–Parkinson–White syndrome, Progress in Pediatric Cardiology, 35 (1), 2013, 17-24, https://doi.org/10.1016/j.ppedcard.2012.11.003.

truly asymptomatic WPW, this may be an underestimate of the true prevalence.

The overall prevalence of WPW syndrome is lower, at an estimated 0.07% in patients 6 to 20 years of age [14]. Among patients with a first degree relative with WPW, the prevalence is up to 0.55%. This increased prevalence suggests a genetic component [15].

Within the asymptomatic population, the risk of sudden cardiac arrest has been found to range from 0.86 up to per 1000 person-years. This risk has been found to be much higher than in the adult population, 0.86 events per 1000 person-years [16,17].

It is worth noting that in some patients the diagnostic findings of WPW may be incomplete. In a landmark article by pediatric electrophysiologists Dr Perry and Dr Garson, they outlined the difficulty of diagnosing patients with subtle VPE using only a screening electrocardiogram [18]. In these cases, the classic VPE presentation of a δ-wave, short PR interval and prolonged QRS is incomplete with only partial features. Oftentimes elevated heart rates, AP location, and accessory tract refractory period can obscure clear preexcitation findings. This can manifest as subtle VPE findings demonstrating only a short PR interval or the presence of a δ-wave in certain leads on the ECG. Previous studies have described other, more subtle findings such as a left axis deviation and lack of Q-waves in the left chest leads in the setting of no obvious δ-wave [18].

CLINICAL PRESENTATION

The clinical manifestations in WPW can vary. Those with truly asymptomatic WPW or WPW pattern will present with a normal examination. Often, individuals will become aware of their diagnosis incidentally during routine ECG screening.

Individuals who develop a tachyarrhythmia as part of WPW syndrome, may present with symptoms of chest pain, palpitations, shortness of breath, dizziness, syncope, and/or sudden cardiac arrest/death [10]. The history of present illness (HPI) should focus on details surrounding a typical episode. This includes the initiation/onset of symptoms including common triggers, duration, associated symptoms (as detailed previously), and termination of the episode. The physical examination should focus the patient's neurologic status, cardiovascular, and pulmonary systems. In situations where a hemodynamically significant arrhythmia is present, the patient may be hypotensive, in cardiogenic shock and unresponsive. It should be noted that in the absence of tachyarrhythmia physical examination findings may be completely normal.

WPW has also been found to be associated with different forms of congenital heart disease, most notably Epstein's anomaly. There have also been cases of WPW in patients with cardiac tumors, like rhabdomyomas, and hypertrophic cardiomyopathy [10].

DISCUSSION

Diagnosis

The diagnosis of the WPW pattern typically occurs with the use of a surface ECG and has the findings first described by Drs Wolff, Parkinson, and White. Findings include a short PR interval, δ-wave, and a prolonged QRS duration (see Figs. 1 and 2) [1,5]. As mentioned previously, WPW syndrome will also have findings consistent with tachyarrhythmia.

Risk stratification

Asymptomatic patients with persistent ECG findings of preexcitation are at a higher overall risk for SCD relative to their counterparts that exhibit only intermittent findings. Further workup should be performed to risk stratify the AP.

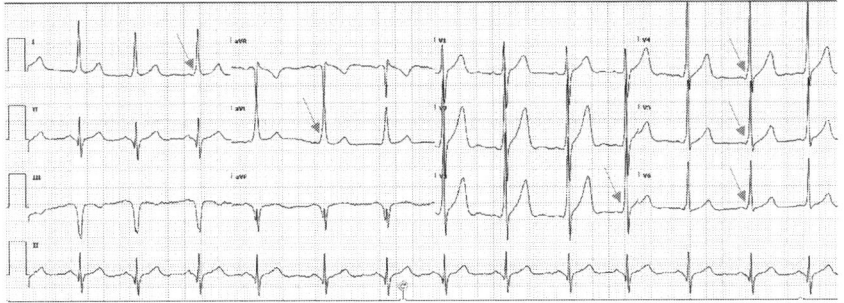

Fig. 2. A 12-lead ECG with WPW pattern.

These higher risk patients may have an AP capable of rapid anterograde conduction which opens the risk for SCD during rapid atrial conduction [5,9,10]. The rapid atrial conduction is able to bypass the protective decrement of the AV node via the AP leading to a high ventricular rate that can deteriorate to ventricular fibrillation and SCD [5,10]. Thus, making risk stratification of upmost importance in this patient population as those with WPW syndrome. Various methods such as wearable cardiac monitors, exercise stress test (EST), adenosine challenge, and electrophysiology studies have been used to further explore the conduction characteristics of the AP. As alluded to earlier, the lower risk subgroup with only intermittent preexcitation have been found to be at an overall lower risk for SCD and generally do not require more invasive diagnostic testing [10].

Holter monitor
Holter monitors are wearable devices that continuously record the cardiac ECG over extended periods of times, 24 to 48 hours or more. With regards to risk stratification in the asymptomatic WPW patient, monitoring for an intermittent delta wave can help identify patients with low-risk AP [19]. Those patients with persistent ECG findings require further workup to further risk stratify the AP.

Exercise stress test
In 1988, Daubert and colleagues found that abrupt and complete loss of preexcitation during exercise predicted a low-risk AP [20]. Thus, this has become a surrogate tool to aid in the risk stratification of patients with an AP. Patients who are old enough to engage in an EST, typically greater than 8 year of age and are able reasonably exert themselves can potentially avoid more invasive testing. For patients that have clear abrupt loss of preexcitation on the ECG tracing (Fig. 3), the AP properties pose a lower risk of SCD [10,20,21]. Those individuals with persistent WPW pattern or indeterminate findings should undergo further testing to help elucidate the AP properties and risk of SCD.

It is worth noting that an EST in patients with only subtle VPE findings on the baseline ECG may yield unclear results due to the incomplete findings at

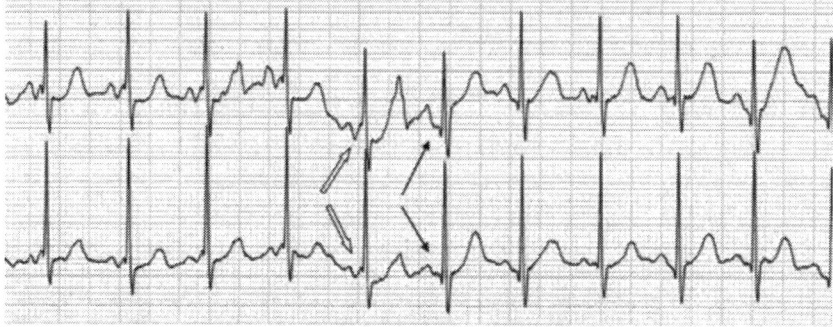

Fig. 3. Abrupt loss of preexcitation on EST [19]. Open arrows denote final preexcited beat. Closed arrows denote first beat after abrupt loss of preexcitation. Wackel, P. et al., (2012), Risk Stratification In Wolff-parkinson-white Syndrome: The Correlation Between Noninvasive And Invasive Testing In Pediatric Patients. Pacing And Clinical Electrophysiology, 35: 1451-1457. https://doi.org/10.1111/j.1540-8159. 2012.03518.x.

baseline. These individuals may also warrant further evaluation utilizing a different AP risk stratification modality.

Adenosine challenge

In patients with subtle findings of VPE on the ECG, adenosine challenge can be a useful tool to unmask an AP [22]. This medication has been traditionally used to rapidly terminate supraventricular tachyarrhythmias with a known side effect of inducing AFib. The mechanism by which this is accomplished is by binding A_1 receptors on cardiac nodal tissue resulting in decreased conduction velocity through the AV node and AV block [5]. During an adenosine challenge, patients with a surface ECG demonstrating a shortened PR interval and QRS widening are considered positive for an AP. Some institutions have elected to pursue more invasive electrophysiology study (EPS) in this patient population due to high correlation between positive AC and the presence of an AP [22].

Electrophysiology study

An EPS can stratify risk of SCD by evaluating the AP during periods of inducible AFib. Those pathways that exhibit characteristics that correlate with a high risk of SCD, shortest preexcited R-R interval (SPERRI) less than 250 ms, can then undergo ablation [5,10]. This form of risk stratification can either be performed via a transesophageal study or a transvenous study.

A transesophageal EP study (TEEPS) involves a specialized electrode catheter that is introduced into the esophagus via the oral or nasal passages. The catheter is advanced until the cardiac tracings are present and capture of the atrium achieved. The electrophysiologist is then able to induce AFib and analyze the AP characteristics. This minimally invasive procedure is appealing as it does not require central venous access, cost effectiveness, and quick recovery time [5,23].

A transvenous EPS, although more invasive, is considered the most effective manner to risk stratify WPW. Central venous access is acquired, and specialized electrode catheters are positioned within the heart. Afib is induced in a similar fashion to TEEPS, and the AP characteristics evaluated. If the AP is deemed high risk, then the electrophysiologist is able to convert the procedure to a curative study by ablating the AP [10]. Fig. 4 illustrates the management algorithm in the asymptomatic WPW patient [10].

Management. The first-line therapy for patients with a high-risk AP in asymptomatic WPW or WPW syndrome is radiofrequency ablation (RFA). Its

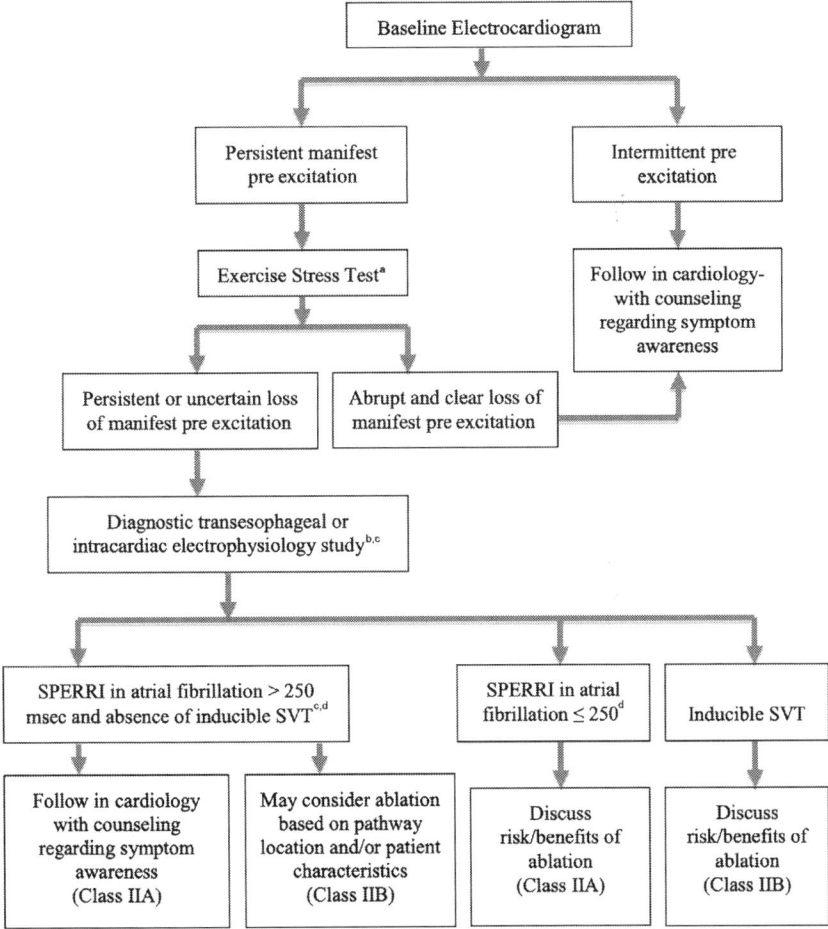

Fig. 4. Management algorithm in the asymptomatic WPW patient [10]. [a]Patients unable to perform an EST should undergo risk-stratification with an EP study. [b]Prior to invasive testing, patients and the parents/guardians should be counseled to discuss the risks and benefits of proceedings with invasive studies, risks of observation only, and risks of medication strategy. [c]Patients participating at moderate-high level competitive spots should be counseled with regards to risk-benefit of ablation (class IIA) and follow the 36th Bethesda Conference Guidelines [6]. [d]In the absence of inducible atrial fibrillation, the shortest preexcited R-R interval determined by rapid atrial pacing is a reasonable surrogate.

relatively low risk profile and high success rates [10]. Alternative forms of ablation include surgical and cryoablation, the latter is preferred when it is a septal AP or the AP is in close proximity to small coronary arteries [10].

In patients where ablation is not an option, medical therapy may be used. First-line pharmacologic therapy for orthodromic atrioventricular reentrant tachycardia (AVRT) includes class IC antiarrhythmics flecainide and propafenone [24–26]. Beta-blockers may be used as a second-line drug for chronic suppression of orthodromic AVRT in patients with a low-risk AP. While amiodarone can be used, the side effect profile of pulmonary, thyroid, and hepatic toxicity make it less appealing in the pediatric population. In cases where antidromic AVRT is a concern, class IC antiarrhythmics are again the agents of choice [26].

Generally speaking, in patients with antidromic AVRT, AV nodal blocking agents such as beta-blockers, calcium channel blockers, and digoxin should be avoided due to preferred conduction through the AP, potentially inducing ventricular fibrillation [27].

Overall outcomes of RFA are quite favorable with a success rate of approximately 90% and a recurrence rate of approximately 11% [28]. Cryoablation has similar success rates of 80%; however, the recurrence rate tends to be higher, around 30% [29].

Considerations in the athlete

The recent Heart Rhythm Society (HRS) expert consensus statement takes into account the increased risk of SCD within the pediatric population, relative to their adult counterparts, by lowering the threshold for intervention in those with a persistent WPW pattern on ECG. The statement put forth a class 1 recommendation for an EPS in these patients to identify a high-risk AP. Individuals with symptomatic WPW catheter ablation is recommended to reduce the risk of a life threatening event. Similarly, those with WPW pattern and evidence of left ventricular desynchrony ablation is also recommended regardless of the AP characteristics [16].

In the absence of symptoms, a documented arrhythmia or LV dysfunction on echocardiogram, athletes that are undergoing workup are able to return to play during their evaluation [16].

SUMMARY

In conclusion, WPW is a potential cause of SCD among the pediatric population, as such the ability to recognize and refer to a pediatric cardiologist for risk stratification and treatment is imperative.

CLINICS CARE POINTS

- Understanding the importance of a thorough HPI in patients that present with symptoms concerning for palpitations or a tachyarrhythmia.

- An ECG should be obtained in all patients where there is a concern for an arrhythmia.
- Patients that are diagnosed with a persistent Wolff-Parkinson-White (WPW) pattern, regardless of the presence of symptoms, should be referred to a cardiologist for further evaluation and workup.
- Utilizing noninvasive risk stratification may reduce the need for more invasive studies.
- Ablation can be curative in a vast majority of patients with low recurrence rates.
- Medications to avoid in patients with WPW are calcium channel blockers and Digoxin. Beta-blockers should be avoided in patients with antidromic atrioventricular tachycardia.
- Even though an ECG serves the primary mode of diagnosis in WPW, some forms are incomplete and need to be further evaluated for high-risk AP characteristics.

References

[1] Wolff L, Parkinson J, White PD. Bundle branch block with short pr interval in healthy young people prone to paroxysmal tachycardia. Am Heart J 1930;5:686–92.

[2] Scheinman MM. History of wolff-parkinson-white syndrome. Pacing Clin Electrophysiol 2005;28(2):152–6.

[3] Wessels A, Markman M, Vermeulen J, et al. The development of the atrioventricular junction in the human heart. Circ Res 1996;78(1):110–7.

[4] Shaddy RE, Penny DJ, Feltes TF, et al. Moss & Adams' Heart Disease in Infants, Children and Adolescents including the Fetus and Young Adult, 9e. Philadelphia (PA): Wolters kluwer health Adis (ESP); 2016.

[5] Hoyt W, Snyder CS. The asymptomatic Wolff Parkinson White syndrome. Prog Pediatr Cardiol 2013;35:17–24.

[6] Rosner MH, Brady WJ, Kefer MP, et al. Electrocardiography in the patient with the Wolff-Parkinson-White syndrome. AJEM (Am J Emerg Med) 1999;17(7):705–14.

[7] Scheinman M. History of wolff-parkinson-white syndrome. Pacing Clin Electrophysiol 2005;28(2):152–6.

[8] Chugh A, Morady F. Pre-excitation, atrioventricular reentry and variants. In: Zipes DP, Jalife J, Stevenson WG, editors. Cardiac Electrophysiology from cell to bedside. 7th Edition. Philadelphia, PA: Elsevier; 2018. p. 736.

[9] Klein GJ, Bashore TM, Sellers TD, et al. Ventricular fibrillation in the Wolff-Parkinson-white syndrome. N Engl J Med 1979;301(20):1080–5.

[10] Pediatric and Congenital Electrophysiology Society (PACES); Heart Rhythm Society (HRS); American College of Cardiology Foundation (ACCF); American Heart Association (AHA); American Academy of Pediatrics (AAP); Canadian Heart Rhythm Society (CHRS); Cohen MI, Triedman JK, Cannon BC, et al. PACES/HRS expert consensus statement on the management of the asymptomatic young patient with a wolff-parkinson-white (WPW, ventricular preexcitation) electrocardiographic pattern: developed in partnership between the pediatric and congenital electrophysiology society (PACES) and the heart Rhythm society (HRS). Endorsed by the governing bodies of PACES, HRS, the American college of cardiology foundation (ACCF), the American heart association (AHA), the American academy of pediatrics (AAP), and the Canadian heart Rhythm society (CHRS). Heart Rhythm 2012;9(6):1006–24.

[11] Liu S, Yuan S, Hertervig E, et al. Gender and atrioventricular conduction properties of patients with symptomatic atrioventricular nodal reentrant tachycardia and Wolff-Parkinson-White syndrome. J Electrocardiol 2001;34(4):295–301.

[12] Sorbo MD, Buja GF, Miorelli M, et al. The prevalence of the Wolff-Parkinson-White syndrome in a population of 116,542 young males. G Ital Cardiol 1995;25:681–7.

[13] De Bacquer D, De Backer G, Kornitzer M. Prevalences of ECG findings in large population-based samples of men and women. Heart 2000;84:625–33.

[14] Chiu SN, Wang JK, Wu MH, et al. Cardiac conduction disturbance detected in a pediatric population. J Pediatr 2008;152(1):85.

[15] Vidaillet HJ Jr, Pressley JC, Henke E, et al. Familial occurrence of accessory atrioventricular pathways (preexcitation syndrome). N Engl J Med 1987;317(2):65.

[16] Lampert R, Chung EH, Ackerman MJ, et al. 024 HRS expert consensus statement on arrhythmias in the athlete: evaluation, treatment, and return to play. Heart Rhythm 2024;21(10): e151–252.

[17] Rao AL, Salerno JC, Asif IM, et al. Evaluation and management of wolff-Parkinson-white in athletes. Sports Health 2014;6(4):326–32.

[18] Perry PC, Giuffre RM, Garson A. Clues to the electrocardiographic diagnosis of subtle Wolff- Parkinson-White syndrome in children. J Pediatr 1990;117(6):871–5.

[19] Wackel P, Irving C, Webber S, et al. Risk stratification in wolff Parkinson-white syndrome: the correlation between noninvasive and invasive testing in pediatric patients. Pacing Clin Electrophysiol 2012;35(12):1451–7.

[20] Daubert C, Ollitrault J, Descaves C, et al. Failure of the exercise test to predict the anterograde refractory period of the accessory pathway in Wolff-Parkinson- White syndrome. Pacing Clin Electrophysiol 1988;11:1130–8.

[21] Bricker JT, Porter CJ, Garson A Jr, et al. Exercise testing in children with Wolff-Parkinson-White syndrome. Am J Cardiol 1985;55(8):1001–4.

[22] Follansbee CW, Beerman LB, Wu L, et al. Utility and safety of adenosine challenge for subtle ventricular pre-excitation in the pediatric population. J Cardiovasc Electrophysiol 2019;30(7):1036–41.

[23] Hoyt WJ, Thomas PE, Snyder CS. Induction of atrial fibrillation with adenosine during a transesophageal electrophysiology study. Congenit Heart Dis 2013;8(4):E99–101.

[24] Ward DE, Jones S, Shinebourne EA. Use of flecainide acetate for refractory junctional tachycardias in children with Wolff-Parkinson-White syndrome. Am J Cardiol 1986;57(10):787.

[25] Musto B, D'Onofrio A, Cavallaro C, et al. Electrophysiological effects and clinical efficacy of propafenone in children with recurrent paroxysmal supraventricular tachycardia. Circulation 1988;78(4):863.

[26] Leoni L, Bronzetti G, Colonna D, et al. Diagnosis and treatment of fetal and pediatric age patients (0-12 years) with Wolff-Parkinson- White syndrome and atrioventricular accessory pathways. J Cardiovasc Med 2023;24(9):589–601.

[27] Khan IA, Nair CK, Singh N, et al. Acute ventricular rate control in atrial fibrillation and atrial flutter. Int J Cardiol 2004;97(1):7–13.

[28] Van Hare GR, Javitz H, Carmelli D, et al. Prospective assessment after pediatric cardiac ablation: recurrence at 1 year after initially successful ablation of supraventricular tachycardia. Heart Rhythm 2004;1:188–96.

[29] Collins KK, Rhee EK, Kirsh JA, et al. Cryoablation of accessory pathways in the coronary sinus in young patients: a multicenter study from the Pediatric and Congenital Electrophysiology Society's Working Group on Cryoablation. J Cardiovasc Electrophysiol 2007;18: 592–7.

Moving?

Make sure your subscription moves with you!

To notify us of your new address, find your **Clinics Account Number** (located on your mailing label above your name), and contact customer service at:

Email: journalscustomerservice-usa@elsevier.com

800-654-2452 (subscribers in the U.S. & Canada)
314-447-8871 (subscribers outside of the U.S. & Canada)

Fax number: 314-447-8029

Elsevier Health Sciences Division
Subscription Customer Service
3251 Riverport Lane
Maryland Heights, MO 63043

*To ensure uninterrupted delivery of your subscription, please notify us at least 4 weeks in advance of move.

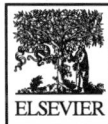

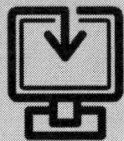

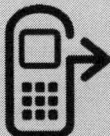

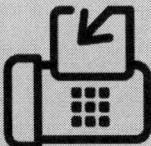

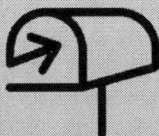

ELSEVIER

Made in the USA
Las Vegas, NV
06 December 2025

60fb969d-5aa3-4d02-bf76-d1d1817c1bb4R01